The Neuropsychiatry of Alzheimer's Disease and Related Dementias

The Neuropsychiatry of Alzheimer's Disease and Related Dementias

Edited by

Jeffrey L Cummings, MD

The Augustus S Rose Professor of Neurology
Professor of Psychiatry and Biobehavioral Sciences
Director of the UCLA Alzheimer's Disease Center
UCLA School of Medicine
Los Angeles, California, USA

Contributions by

Harry Vinters, MD

Professor of Neuropathology and Neurology
Chief, Section of Neuropathology
Department of Pathology and Laboratory Medicine
UCLA School of Medicine
Los Angeles, California, USA

and

Jenaro Felix, BS

Imaging Systems Analyst
Laboratory of Neuroimaging
Department of Neurology
UCLA School of Medicine
Los Angeles, California, USA

MARTIN DUNITZ

First published in the United Kingdom in 2003
by Martin Dunitz Ltd, Taylor and Francis Group plc, 11 New Fetter Lane,
London EC4P 4EE

Tel.: +44 (0) 20 7583 9855
Fax.: +44 (0) 20 7842 2298
E-mail: info@dunitz.co.uk
Website: http://www.dunitz.co.uk

A CIP record for this book is available from the British Library.

ISBN 1-84184-219-2

Distributed in the USA by
Fulfilment Center
Taylor & Francis
10650 Tobben Drive
Independence, KY 41051, USA
Toll Free Tel.: +1 800 634 7064
E-mail: taylorandfrancis@thomsonlearning.com

Distributed in Canada by
Taylor & Francis
74 Rolark Drive
Scarborough, Ontario M1R 4G2, Canada
Toll Free Tel.: +1 877 226 2237
E-mail: tal_fran@istar.ca

Distributed in the rest of the world by
Thomson Publishing Services
Cheriton House
North Way
Andover, Hampshire SP10 5BE, UK
Tel.:+44 (0)1264 332424
E-mail: salesorder.tandf@thomsonpublishingservices.co.uk

Composition by Wearset Ltd, Boldon, Tyne and Wear

Printed in Malta

This volume is dedicated to clinician–scientists around the world interested in improved understanding of the neurobiological basis and treatment of neuropsychiatric symptoms in patients with dementia, and to the patients and families affected by these disorders

Contents

Acknowledgments

I would like to acknowledge Cynthia Ishihara for her dedicated work in preparing this volume. Grant support from the National Institute on Aging and the State of California supported research presented in this volume. Enthusiastic support from Kate Johnson and the Deane F Johnson Foundation assisted the studies presented. The Sidell-Kagan Foundation has generously supported work described in this book. I have had the support of Robert C Collins, MD and John Mazziotta, MD, PhD, the Chairs of Neurology at UCLA, and thank them for their support of my work and of the Alzheimer's Disease Center. I am grateful to the many collaborators who have extended the use of the Neuropsychiatric Inventory into diverse domains of patient assessment. Many collaborators have helped advance the work and ideas presented here including Dag Aarsland, Judith Aharon-Peretz, David Ames, Clive Ballard, George Bartzokis, Frank Benson, Guiliano Binetti, Kyle Boone, Patricia Boyle, Tiffany Chow, Helen Chui, Helena Chui, Claudia Diaz-Olivarrieta, Steve Dekosky, Rochelle Doody, Teri Edwards-Lee, Lynn Fairbanks, J-L Fuh, Daniel Geschwind, Kevin Gray, Nobutusgu Hirono, Dilip Jeste, Dan Kaufer, David Knapman, Brian Lawlor, Morgan Levy, Irene Litvan, C-K Liu, Kostas Lyketsos, Ian McKeith, Susan McPherson, Donna Masterman, Michael Mega, Mario Mendez, Bruce Miller, John Morris, John O'Brien, Ron Peterson, Sara Petry, Peter Rabins, William Reichman, John Ringman, Philippe Robert, Lon Schneider, Gary Small, David Sultzer, Pierre Tariot, Sibel Tekin, Leon Thal, Arthur Toga, Michael

Trimble, Wilfred Van Gorp, Dianna VanLanker, Peter Whitehouse, Stacy Wood, Gorsev Yenner, and many others. I am particularly grateful to Vorapun Senanarong for her collaboration on projects in Thailand. I am eternally thankful to my wife, Inese, and my daughter, Juliana, for their tremendous support of my projects and who make life a joy.

Preface

Alzheimer's disease and related dementing disorders represent an increasing threat to public health as well as assaulting the lives of patients and their families. These disorders have cognitive, functional, and behavioral manifestations. Historically, the emphasis in studying Alzheimer's disease has been on cognitive decline. Investigation of the behavioral and neuropsychiatric disorders associated with dementing conditions has been of less concern. Increasingly, the marked importance of these symptoms for patients and caregivers is recognized. Progress has been made in developing and testing drugs relevant to treatment of neuropsychiatric symptoms in dementia. Management of neuropsychiatric manifestations of dementing disorders reduces patient and caregiver distress and improves quality of life. Excellence in management is fostered by comprehensive understanding of the complex pathophysiology of these behavioral changes, and the pathology, pathophysiology and molecular biology of the dementias is presented in this volume. Deciphering the neurobiology of behavioral symptoms provides insight into the mechanisms of psychiatric symptomatology and these insights may be applicable to other major mental illnesses including schizophrenia, bipolar illness, anxiety disorders, and obsessive-compulsive disorder. Studying these symptoms in patients with known neurobiological changes may facilitate understanding the pathophysiology of psychiatric disorders whose neurobiologic basis remains obscure. It is with the broad goal of synthesizing a comprehensive approach to neuropsychiatric syndromes and behavioral changes in dementing disorders, facilitating optimal management of these conditions in patients with dementia, reducing distress in patients manifesting symptoms, improving the lives of caregivers through improved management of patient behavioral changes, and providing insight into the pathophysiological basis of neuropsychiatric symptoms that development of this volume was undertaken.

Jeffrey L Cummings, MD
Los Angeles, CA, USA
March 30, 2002

The neuropsychiatry of dementing disorders

Dementia syndromes are defined as disorders with memory impairment and deficits in at least one other cognitive function that are acquired, produce occupational or social disability and are not present exclusively during a delirium.[1] Neuropsychiatric features are secondary descriptive characteristics in most definitions. As knowledge of the dementias has increased, the importance of the neuropsychiatric dimension of these disorders has become apparent.

Neuropsychiatric symptoms are distressing to patient and to caregiver and have dramatic effects on the quality of life of the patient and their family. Profiles of neuropsychiatric symptoms are sufficiently distinctive to provide important differential diagnostic information. In some cases dementia diagnosis depends on identifying characteristic neuropsychiatric features: both frontotemporal lobar degeneration and dementia with Lewy bodies have behavioral characteristics as part of their diagnostic clinical criteria (Chapters 4 and 5). A diagnosis of Alzheimer's disease requires exclusion of other potential causes of dementia and can be distinguished from frontotemporal lobar degeneration and dementia with Lewy bodies only after a neuropsychiatric assessment has been conducted. Increasingly, the neurobiology of the dementias can be linked to specific neuropsychiatric features of the diseases. Neuropsychiatric symptoms are often remediable and may benefit from treatment with disease-modifying agents, transmitter replacement therapy, or psychotropic agents. The growing importance of neuropsychiatric aspects of dementia syndromes and their characteristic features are described here.

Global aging

The demographic structure of the world's population is changing dramatically. There has been a rapid increase in the number of aged individuals in the population which is projected to continue through 2050.[2] Between 1997 and 2025 the number of individuals over the age of 65 in Africa will increase from 17.7 million to 37.9 million, in the Americas the increase will be from 62.7 million to 136.9 million, in the Eastern Mediterranean (including the Middle East) there will be an increase from 16.7 million to 44.1 million, in Europe the increase will be from 112.5 million to 169.8 million, in South East Asia (including India) the growth will be from 60.5 million to 166.7 million, and in the Western Pacific (including China) the increase will be from 110.7 million to 267.7 million (Figure 1.1). By 2025, most elderly individuals will live in South East Asia and the Western Pacific region. This increase in the elderly

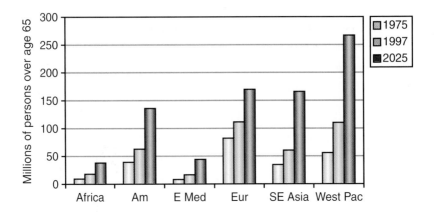

Figure 1.1 *Millions of persons over the age of 65 for the years 1975, 1997, and 2025 in Africa, the Americas (North and South America, Canada, and Mexico), the Eastern Mediterranean region (including all nations of the Middle East), Europe, South East Asia (including India), and the Western Pacific (including China).[2]*

population will have dramatic consequences for these nations, many of which are developing economies with limited health care budgets.

The increase in the number of aged individuals will inevitably be accompanied by an increase in age-related conditions including the dementia syndromes, stroke-related disorders, and Parkinson's disease.[3] Dementia doubles in frequency every 5 years after the age of 60 (Figure 1.2). Thus, approximately 1% of 60 year olds manifest a dementia syndrome, 2% of those aged 65–70, 4% of individuals aged 71–74, 8% of those 75–79 years of age, 16% of those aged 80–84, and 30–40% of those aged 85 and older.[4] This marked increase in dementias in the old-old becomes particularly relevant when the number of old-old individuals in the population is considered (Figure 1.3). Between 1997 and 2025, the number of old-old in Africa will increase from 2 million to 5.4 million, in the Americas from 13.8 million to 29.8 million, in the Eastern Mediterranean from 2 million to 6.6 million, in Europe from 23.2 million to 42.6 million, in South East Asia from 6.5 million to 24.3 million, and in the Western Pacific from 16.5 million to 51.8 million.[2] There will be a concomitant marked increase in the number of dementia patients.

The anticipated growth in the number of patients with dementia and the high frequency of neuropsychiatric symptoms in these individuals combine to make greater understanding and better treatment of the neuropsychiatric aspects of dementia urgent issues.

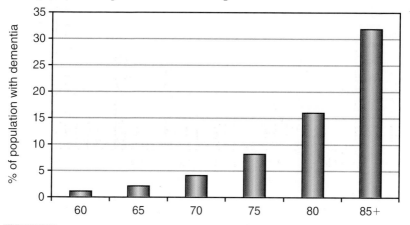

Figure 1.2 *Increasing percent of the population with dementia from age 60–85+.*[4]

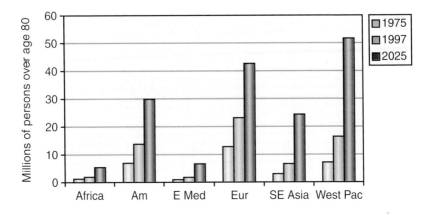

Figure 1.3 *Millions of persons over the age of 80 from 1997 to 2025 in Africa, the Americas (North and South America, Canada, and Mexico), the Eastern Mediterranean region (including all nations of the Middle East), Europe, South East Asia (including India), and the Western Pacific (including China).[2]*

Impact of neuropsychiatric symptoms in dementia syndromes

Neuropsychiatric symptoms have diverse impacts in patients with dementia (Figure 1.4). Neuropsychiatric symptoms produce an immediacy of distress for the patient that is often lacking with regard to neuropsychological symptoms. Patients often do not remember that they do not remember, may be unaware of cognitive abnormalities, and do not appear to be distressed by cognitive or memory decline. However, agitated patients are obviously upset or distressed by the causes of their agitated behavior; psychotic patients are fearful and filled with dread of thieves and pursuers; depressed patients are sad and experience feelings of worthlessness, hopelessness, and helplessness; anxious patients are uncomfortable, restless, and filled with feelings of foreboding. Neuropsychiatric symptoms produce disproportionate distress compared with other manifestations of dementia syndromes.

Neuropsychiatric symptoms also take a great toll on the caregivers, causing substantial distress and feelings of burden and role captivity.

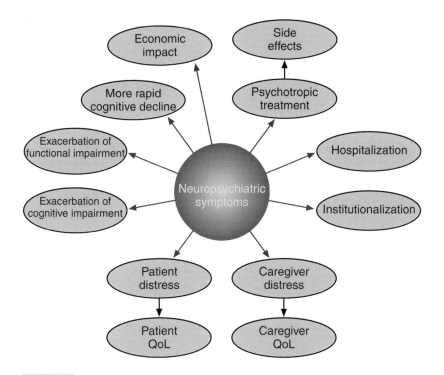

Figure 1.4 *Diverse consequences of neuropsychiatric symptoms in patients with dementia. QoL, Quality of life.*

Patients with behavioral symptoms are more likely to engage in physical altercations with their caregiver, to be the victims of physical abuse, and to strike those trying to provide assistance (Chapter 10).[5] Neuropsychiatric symptoms are among the most common causes of institutionalization of patients with dementia syndromes[6] and, when severe, may require at least temporary hospitalization for aggressive pharmacologic management.[7] Self-destructive behavior in patients residing in nursing homes is most common in patients with dementia.[8] Depression exaggerates functional disability and psychosis has been associated with more rapid cognitive decline and more severe cognitive impairment in patients with Alzheimer's disease (Chapter 3). Neuropsychiatric symptoms are commonly treated with psychotropic agents, leading to an increased risk of side effects including sedation, parkinsonism, falls, and postural hypotension.

Many of the aspects of dementia related to neuropsychiatric symptoms have financial consequences (Chapter 10). The increased caregiver stress associated with neuropsychiatric symptoms results in greater caregiver emotional and physical illness and the expense of treatment for these. Patient hospitalization and residential placement – precipitated by behavioral disturbances – are among the most expensive aspects of caring for dementia patients. Once institutionalized, patients with behavioral disturbances demand more staff time and require more expensive care. Psychotropic medications add to the direct costs of care and any side effects that require management (e.g. fractures from falls) further increase the expense of the disease. Neuropsychiatric symptoms are important drivers of the cost of care of dementia patients.

Principles of the neuropsychiatry of dementias

Some generalizations can be made regarding neuropsychiatric symptoms in patients with dementing disorders. More research has been devoted to investigation of neuropsychiatric phenomena of patients with Alzheimer's disease than to patients with other dementias, but the principles derived generalize to other dementing disorders.

Clinical features of neuropsychiatric symptoms in dementias

Neuropsychiatric symptoms are common in dementing disorders and affect most patients.[9-11] In epidemiologic examples,[11] the frequency of neuropsychiatric symptoms is lower than in clinical samples,[9] in part because care is sought when behavioral symptoms emerge.

Multiple symptoms are present simultaneously in patients with dementing disorders. Figure 1.5 shows the number of symptoms in Alzheimer's disease patients characterized with the Neuropsychiatric Inventory (NPI).[12] In all, 92% of patients had at least one symptom; 81% had two or more symptoms; and 51% had four or more symptoms. Thus, the majority of patients exhibited a multiplicity of neuropsychiatric symptoms simultaneously.

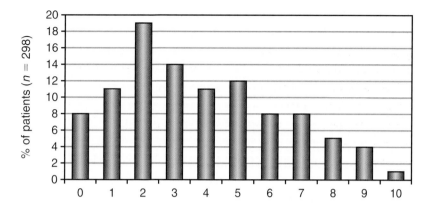

Figure 1.5 *The graph shows the percent of patients in an Alzheimer's disease clinical sample who exhibited 1, 2, 3, 4, etc. neuropsychiatric symptoms elicited through standard interview of the 10-item Neuropsychiatric Inventory. Note that 92% had at least one symptom; 81% had two or more symptoms; 51% had four or more symptoms.*

The presence of neuropsychiatric symptoms in dementia adversely affects prognosis. Decline in cognitive function is more rapid in Alzheimer's disease patients with psychosis,[13–17] and in Parkinson's disease when depression is evident.[18]

Analysis of clusters of symptoms in Alzheimer's disease[19] shows that approximately 40% of patients have few or only one neuropsychiatric symptom. A second group of patients exhibit primarily an affective disorder manifested by depression, anxiety, and irritability. Apathy is also common in conjunction with this symptom complex. A few patients exhibit agitation, delusions, or aberrant motor behavior. A third group of patients have primarily a psychotic disorder, suffering from delusions and hallucinations. A few of these patients exhibited apathy, agitation, depression, irritability, aberrant motor behavior, and anxiety. Similar findings emerged from a factor analysis of the NPI[20] where a mood factor (anxiety and depression), a psychosis factor (agitation, hallucinations, delusions, and irritability), and a frontal behavior factor (disinhibition and euphoria) were identified. Apathy and aberrant motor behavior did not load heavily on any of these factors. Similar analyses using other assessment approaches have identified three syndromes consisting of: 1) overactivity (walking, checking); 2) aggressive behavior; 3) psychosis.[21] Thus, the multiple symptoms occurring in patients with dementia syndromes can be grouped into syndromes or symptom complexes. The multiple simultaneous symptoms present in patients with dementia syndromes contrast with the relatively monosymptomatic presentation of patients with idiopathic psychiatric disorders.

Degenerative dementias have gradual onset and slow progression. Patients evolve from states with normal cognition through periods of limited cognitive impairment, eventually manifesting symptoms of sufficient severity to warrant a diagnosis of a dementia syndrome. Even vascular dementias often have prodromal periods of vascular cognitive impairment (VCI) that precede the onset of dementia (Chapter 6). In the case of Alzheimer's disease, the prodromal period is labeled mild cognitive impairment (MCI) (Chapter 3).[22] Neuropsychiatric symptoms commonly accompany other harbingers of the onset of dementia. Depression, anxiety, apathy, irritability and occasionally delusions or hallucinations may be present in the prodromal period, anticipating the occurrence of recognizable dementia (Chapter 3).[23-25]

Neuropsychiatric symptoms tend to become more frequent in populations of dementia patients as the underlying disease worsens, and the risk of emergent psychopathology is increased with disease progression. Figure 1.6 shows the relationship between the increasing prevalence of psychosis and stages of Alzheimer's disease as revealed by the Clinical Dementia Rating scale.[26] Figure 1.7 shows increasing agitation across Clinical Dementia Rating scale stages in an epidemiologically based sample.[11] Very advanced patients may be too severely disabled to exhibit behavioral changes or neuropsychiatric symptoms.

There is a relationship between increasing psychopathology and declining cognitive function across the course of the disease. However, correlations between individual neuropsychiatric symptoms and specific cognitive changes are limited and emerging neuropsychiatric symptoms are not readily attributable to cognitive disturbances.[27-31] Executive dysfunction indicative of prefrontal lobe involvement has the highest correlation with the occurrence of neuropsychiatric symptoms.[29,32] This is evident in the greater psychopathology of the frontal variant of

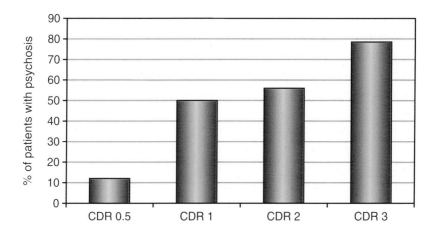

Figure 1.6 *Percent of patients exhibiting psychotic symptoms classified according to Clinical Dementia Rating (CDR) scale stage.[25]*

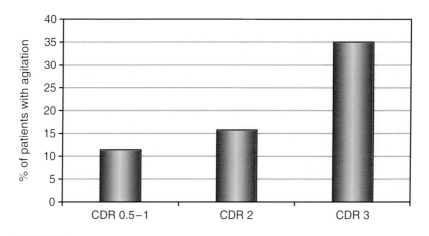

Figure 1.7 *Percent of patients with agitation by Clinical Dementia Rating scale stage.[11]*

Alzheimer's disease[33,34] (Chapter 3) and in the high rate of psychopathology in frontotemporal lobar degeneration (Chapter 7), where behavioral symptoms often precede the occurrence of cognitive abnormalities and predominate throughout the disease course.

Executive dysfunction and neuropsychiatric symptoms are strongly linked to functional ability[32,35] (Figure 1.8). Activities of daily living and functional integrity demand planning, programming, and implementing activities, functions that are compromised with prefrontal disturbances. Behavioral symptoms are more common in patients with frontal lobe dysfunction. Thus, there is a triad indicative of frontal involvement including neuropsychiatric symptoms, functional disability, and executive abnormalities.

Behavioral disturbances may exacerbate functional and cognitive deficits in patients with dementia. The presence of depression correlates with greater functional disability.[35-40]

Neuropsychiatric symptoms may fluctuate over time and are not present continuously but are highly recurrent once they emerge in the

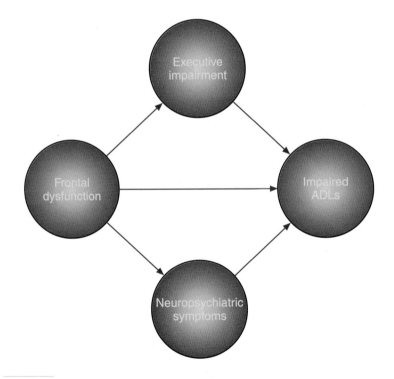

Figure 1.8 *Frontal dysfunction leads to a triad of related symptoms including executive deficits, impaired activities of daily living (ADLs), and neuropsychiatric symptoms.*

course of a dementing illness.[41,42] Psychosis and agitation, for example, may first occur in the early, middle, or late phases of the disease. Once present, they are likely to remain present during the course of the illness, although they may not be present on every examination if the patient is examined serially.

Emotional disorders in patients with dementing illnesses include both negative and positive phenomena (Table 1.1). Negative symptoms in patients with dementia include apathy, reduced motivation, poor emotional engagement, inability to recognize affective expression in other individuals, and reduced amplitude of emotional expression.[43,44] In addition, they exhibit positive symptoms of psychopathology including delusions, hallucinations, depression, anxiety, and agitation.[9]

Table 1.1 Positive and negative symptoms in dementia

Positive symptoms	Negative symptoms
Psychopathology	
• Psychosis	• Apathy
• Mania	• Impaired perception of
• Depression	emotional stimuli
• Agitation	• Reduced range of expression of normal
• Anxiety	emotions
• Irritability	• Reduced mood, affect and vocal
• Disinhibition	inflection
Cognitive abnormalities	
• Paraphasia	• Aphasia
• Confabulation	• Amnesia
	• Apraxia
	• Agnosia
	• Alexia, agraphia
	• Amusia
	• Anarithmetia
	• Anosognosia
	• Constructional disturbances
	• Attentional deficits

The profile of neuropsychiatric symptoms in different dementing disorders is sufficiently distinctive to provide differential diagnostic information. Patients with Alzheimer's disease have high rates of apathy, irritability, anxiety, and depression; patients with frontotemporal lobar degeneration have high rates of apathy and disinhibition; patients with progressive supranuclear palsy have marked apathy, modest disinhibition, and few other neuropsychiatric symptoms; patients with dementia with Lewy bodies have prominent visual hallucinations, delusions, and depression; patients with corticobasal degeneration have marked depression with relatively few other behavioral changes; patients with vascular dementia have apathy and depression.[9,11,45–47]

Neuropsychiatric symptoms cause substantial stress in caregivers. Symptoms such as apathy that reduce patient activity also reduce the patient's engagement in meaningful relationships and cause distress in couples. Symptoms such as agitation and delusions are disruptive to relationships and are related as highly distressing by caregivers[48] (Chapter 10).

Linking neurobiology to behavior

Neuroimaging studies suggest that dysfunction of frontal and anterior temporal regions are most closely linked to psychopathological symptoms in patients with dementia syndromes.[49–53] Among the most consistent imaging–behavior correlations is the reduction of medial frontal perfusion or metabolism in patients with apathy. This relationship is evident in patients with Alzheimer's disease, frontotemporal lobar degeneration, and progressive supranuclear palsy.[46,54–56]

Neuropathological alterations associated with behavioral changes in dementia syndromes also involve the frontal lobes and subcortical structures disproportionately. The frontal variant of Alzheimer's disease (Chapter 3) has a greater burden of neurofibrillary tangles in the frontal lobe than patients without evidence of frontal dysfunction. These patients exhibit more executive abnormalities and agitation.[33,34] Frontotemporal lobar degeneration (Chapter 7) with marked behavioral changes is characterized by prominent involvement of frontal lobes and frontal subcortical circuits.

Degenerative dementias are proteinopathies and the type of protein accumulated determines the clinical features (phenotype) of the disorder (Chapter 9). Specific cell populations are differentially vulnerable to aggregation of protein types, creating regional patterns of cell loss and manifesting as distinguishable clinical syndromes. Conditions characterized by abnormalities of tau protein metabolism (frontotemporal lobar degenerations, progressive supranuclear palsy, corticobasal degeneration) affect the frontal and frontal-subcortical circuits and have characteristic behavioral changes. Diseases featuring abnormalities of alpha-synuclein protein metabolism (Parkinson's disease, dementia with Lewy bodies, multiple system atrophies) have preferential effects on subcortical (brain stem, basal ganglia) and limbic system structures and are associated with neuropsychiatric symptoms (Chapter 9). Disorders with prominent beta-amyloid accumulation exhibit predominant posterior hemispheric involvement.

Neurotransmitter deficits are present in most dementia syndromes (Table 1.2). Cholinergic, noradrenergic, serotonergic, and dopaminergic deficits contribute to the cognitive, behavioral, and motor abnormalities of patients with dementia. Modulatory transmitter deficits involving acetylcholine, norepinephrine, and serotonin are implicated in the pathophysiology of behavioral changes in Alzheimer's disease and related dementias.[57–59] Depression has been linked to deficits in norepinephrine and serotonin, and psychosis to dopaminergic and serotonergic abnormalities. Deficits in acetylcholine are implicated in a variety of behavioral changes (Chapter 9). Behavioral changes in dementias may result from histological or biochemical changes.

Dementias with mixed pathologies are common. The combination of Alzheimer-type pathology and cerebrovascular disease is particularly common, and when both are present the resulting dementia syndrome is more severe than when either pathological change is present independently.[60,61] Combinations of Alzheimer-type and Lewy body pathology are also common. Combined pathology may contribute to psychopathology. In patients with Alzheimer's disease and frontal lobe ischemic injury depressive symptoms are more likely.[62]

Behavioral symptoms in dementia patients result from interruption of neural circuits. Two primary circuits are implicated: 1) frontal-

Table 1.2 Neurotransmitter deficits in patients with dementias

Diagnosis	*Transmitter deficit*
Alzheimer's disease	Cholinergic
	Serotonergic
	Noradrenergic
Parkinson's disease with dementia	Cholinergic
	Serotonergic
	Noradrenergic
	Dopaminergic
Dementia with Lewy bodies	Cholinergic
	Serotonergic
	Noradrenergic
	Dopaminergic
Frontotemporal lobar degeneration	Serotonergic
Vascular dementia	Variable cholinergic
	Variable dopaminergic
	Variable serotonergic
Progressive supranuclear palsy	Cholinergic (post-synaptic)
	Dopaminergic
Corticobasal degeneration	Dopaminergic
Multiple system atrophy	Dopaminergic
Prion diseases	Variable

subcortical circuits;[12] 2) the limbic system.[63] The modular organization of the neocortex gives rise to neurobehavioral disorders with localizing signature syndromes such as the aphasias, apraxias, and agnosias. The parallel organization of the limbic and frontal-subcortical systems link structures in integrated circuitry; disruption of any member of the circuit may give rise to symptoms of circuit dysfunction.[64] Thus highly localizing signature syndromes are not characteristic of these neural systems and similar symptoms may occur with dysfunction of several member structures within the circuit. Neocortical abnormalities produce instrumental defects such as aphasia and agnosia; limbic and frontal-subcortical disturbances produce fundamental defects involving emotion and motivation (Table 1.3).

Table 1.3 Contrasting features of instrumental and fundamental functions

Instrumental	Fundamental
Functions	
• Language, praxis, gnosis	• Emotion, motivation, executive function
Clinical syndromes	
• Signature syndromes from focal lesions	• Circuit-related syndromes; lesions of any site in the circuit produce similar symptoms
• Aphasia, apraxia, agnosia	• Executive dysfunction, apathy, disinhibition
Organization	
• Cortical modules	• Frontal-subcortical circuits
	• Limbic system
Transmitters	
• Intrinsic	• Modulatory
• GABA, glutamate, aspartate	• Acetylcholine, dopamine, serotonin, norepinephrine
Treatment	
• Cholinergic (modifies intrinsic transmitter activity)	• Cholinergic, SSRIs, adrenergic agents (TCAs, stimulants), dopaminergic agents

GABA, γ-aminobutyric acid; SSRI, selective serotonin reuptake inhibitor; TCA, tricyclic antidepressant.

Treatment of neuropsychiatric symptoms in dementias

There are four dimensions to treating patients with dementias (Chapter 10): treatment with disease-modifying agents, treatment using transmitter replacement strategies, use of psychotropic agents to reduce neuropsychiatric symptoms, and establishing an alliance with the caregiver to reduce caregiver stress and develop nonpharmacologic treatment strategies for behavioral management.

Treatments may exert their effects on behavioral symptoms through two mechanisms: 1) reduction of existing symptoms and 2) reductions in the rate of emergence of new symptoms. Since behavioral symptoms tend to emerge over time in the course of progressive dementing diseases, the amelioration of the rate at which new symptoms appear is an important treatment benefit.

A few disease-modifying therapies have been shown to be useful in dementing disorders. Vitamin E and selegiline reduce the rate of functional decline in patients with Alzheimer's disease.[65] Patients treated with both agents concomitantly have a reduced emergence of psychopathology compared with patients treated with placebo or with either agent alone. This suggests that disease-modifying therapies may reduce the rate of occurrence of new psychopathological symptoms.

Transmitter replacement therapies have been shown to reduce behavioral symptoms in patients with Alzheimer's disease and may have psychotropic effects in other dementia syndromes.[66] Cholinesterase inhibitors reduce apathy and visual hallucinations and in some studies have had effects on delusions, depression, anxiety, disinhibition, and aberrant motor behavior (pacing, rummaging, etc.). The beneficial behavioral response following treatment with cholinesterase inhibitors appears to be mediated through orbitofrontal and dorsolateral and prefrontal regions, areas implicated in mediating in psychopathological symptoms in dementia.[67] Cholinesterase inhibitors appear to both decrease existing behaviors and reduce emerging behaviors. Cholinesterase inhibitors have been shown to have beneficial behavioral effects in dementia with Lewy bodies, Parkinson's disease with dementia, and vascular dementia (Chapters 4, 6 and 7) as well as Alzheimer's disease.

Serotonergic and noradrenergic compounds have been used to treat depression in patients with Alzheimer's disease and other dementing disorders.[11,68] Serotonergic agents may reduce psychosis and agitation (Chapter 10).

Treatment with psychotropic agents appears to ameliorate many behavioral disturbances in patients with dementias, although few controlled trials have been conducted in these populations. Atypical antipsychotic agents have been shown to reduce psychosis and agitation in patients with Alzheimer's disease.[69–71] Antidepressants reduced depressive mood alterations in some trials involving patients with Alzheimer's disease[11,68] Patients with dementing disorders may have different dosage requirements, response profiles, and adverse effect sensitivities compared with patients with idiopathic psychiatric disorders, and clinical trials conducted specifically in defined populations to delineate rational use of psychotropic medications in these populations are required.

Developing a successful relationship with the caregiver is a critical aspect of the treatment of patients with dementia (Chapter 10). Dementing disorders have effects on the entire family unit, not just on the patients harboring the brain disease. Effective intervention depends on addressing the multiple facets of this caregiving unit in addition to developing therapeutic strategies for the brain disease. Caregivers experience burden and distress and develop stress-related illnesses. Stress can be reduced through support groups, educational strategies, and encouraging the caregivers to integrate friends and other family members into caregiving roles. Local chapters of the Alzheimer's Association or Alzheimer's Disease International provide support services for patients and caregivers and can refer the patient and family to other community services. Caregivers provide most of the care received by patients and instruction in nonpharmacologic management strategies can assist in reducing behavioral disturbances. Caregivers are frequently responsible for administering any medications prescribed, and ensuring that they understand the expected effects, administration regimen, and potential side effects is an important aspect of the pharmacotherapy of patients with dementia.

An integrated neurobiology of behavioral changes in dementia

Behavior is the integrated product of a complex interaction between the emotional and cognitive function of the individual in the context of

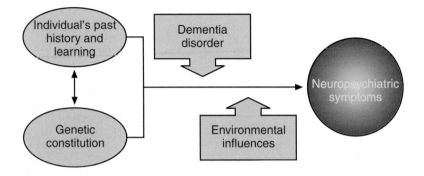

Figure 1.9 *An integrated model of neuropsychiatric symptoms reflecting the individual's past history and learning, their genetic constitution, the effects of the dementing disorder, and environmental influences.*

ongoing environmental influences. The individual's cognitive and emotional function are themselves produced by an interaction between the person's past history and learning and their genetic constitution (Figure 1.9).[72] A comprehensive and integrated view of an individual's behavior and the neuropsychiatric symptoms occurring in the course of dementing disorders requires consideration of genetic elements that determine personality, emotional growth, and cognitive development; the individual's personal, social, and cultural history learned over the lifetime; the effects of the dementing disorder producing regional cellular dysfunction and transmitter abnormalities; and ongoing environmental influences (Chapter 9). The summary outcome of these interactive components produce the neuropsychiatric symptom complexes evidenced by an individual patient. This lifespan approach emphasizes that form and content of late-life disorders reflect, in part, the lifetime experiences of the individual.

References

1. American Psychiatric Association. *Diagnostic and Statistical Manual of Mental Disorders: DSM-IV,* 4th edn. Washington, DC: American Psychiatric Association, 1994.

2. World Health Organization. *World Atlas of Ageing.* Kobe, Japan: World Health Organization, Centre for Health Development, 1998.
3. Malmgren R. Epidemiology of aging. In: Coffey CE, Cummings JL (eds) *Textbook of Geriatric Neuropsychiatry.* Washington, DC: American Psychiatric Press, 2000:17–33.
4. Jorm AF. Cross-national comparisons of the occurrence of Alzheimer's and vascular dementias. *Eur Arch Psychiatry Clin Neurosci* 1991;240:218–22.
5. Dyer C, Pavlik VN, Murphy K et al. The high prevalence of depression and dementia in elder abuse or neglect. *J Am Geriatr Soc* 2000;48:205–8.
6. Yaffe K, Fox P, Newcomer R et al. Patient and caregiver characteristics and nursing home placement in patients with dementia. *JAMA* 2002;287:2090–7.
7. Nourhashemi F, Andrieu S, Sastres N et al. Descriptive analysis of emergency hospital admissions of patients with Alzheimer disease. *Alzheimer Dis Assoc Disord* 2001;15:21–5.
8. Draper B, Brodaty H, Low L-F et al. Self-destructive behaviors in nursing home residents. *J Am Geriatr Soc* 2002;50:354–8.
9. Mega MS, Cummings JL, Fiorello T et al. The spectrum of behavioral changes in Alzheimer's disease. *Neurology* 1996;46:130–5.
10. Aarsland D, Larsen JP, Lim NG et al. Range of neuropsychiatric disturbances in patients with Parkinson's disease. *J Neurol Neurosurg Psychiatry* 1999;67:492–6.
11. Lyketsos CG, Steinberg M, Tschanz JT et al. Mental and behavioral disturbances in dementia: findings from the Cache County Study on Memory in Aging. *Am J Psychiatry* 2000;157:708–14.
12. Cummings JL, Mega M, Gray K et al. The Neuropsychiatric Inventory: comprehensive assessment of psychopathology in dementia. *Neurology* 1994;44:2308–14.
13. Chui HC, Lyness SA, Sobel E et al. Extrapyramidal signs and psychiatric symptoms predict faster cognitive decline in Alzheimer's disease. *Arch Neurol* 1994;51:676–81.
14. Mortimer JA, Ebbitt B, Jun S et al. Predictors of cognitive and functional progression in patients with probable Alzheimer's disease. *Neurology* 1992;42:1689–96.
15. Paulsen JS, Salmon DP, Thal LJ et al. Incidence of and risk factors for hallucinations and delusions in patients with probable AD. *Neurology* 2000;54:1965–71.
16. Stern Y, Albert M, Brandt J et al. Utility or extrapyramidal signs and psychosis as predictors of cognitive and functional decline, nursing home admission, and death in Alzheimer's disease: prospective analyses from the Predictors Study. *Neurology* 1994;44:2300–7.
17. Wilson RS, Gilley DW, Bennett DA et al. Hallucinations, delusions and cognitive decline in Alzheimer's disease. *J Neurol Neurosurg Psychiatry* 2000;69:172–7.
18. Starkstein SE, Mayberg JS, Preziosi TJ et al. Reliability, validity and clinical correlates of apathy in Parkinson's disease. *J Neuropsychiatry Clin Neurosci* 1992;4:134–9.
19. Lyketsos CG, Breitner JC, Rabins PV. An evidence-based proposal for the classification of neuropsychiatric disturbance in Alzheimer's disease. *Int J Geriatr Psychiatry* 2001;16:1037–42.

20. Frisoni GB, Rozzini L, Binetti G *et al.* Behavioral syndromes in Alzheimer's disease: description and correlates. *Dement Geriatr Cogn Disord* 1999;10:130–8.
21. Hope T, Keene J, Fairburn C *et al.* Behaviour changes in dementia 2: are there behavioural syndromes? *Int J Geriatr Psychiatry* 1997;12:1074–8.
22. Peterson RC, Smith GE, Waring SC *et al.* Mild cognitive impairment. *Arch Neurol* 1999;56:303–8.
23. Jost BC, Grossberg GT. The evolution of psychiatric symptoms in Alzheimer's disease: a natural history study. *J Am Geriatr Soc* 1996; 44:1078–81.
24. Marin DB, Green CR, Schmeidler J *et al.* Noncognitive disturbances in Alzheimer's disease: frequency, longitudinal course and relationship to cognitive symptoms. *J Am Geriatr Soc* 1997;45:1331–8.
25. Li Y-S, Meyer JS, Thornby J. Longitudinal follow-up of depressive symptoms among normal versus cognitively impaired elderly. *Int J Geriatr Psychiatry* 2001;16:718–27.
26. Farber NB, Rubin EH, Newcomer JW *et al.* Increased neocortical neurofibrillary tangle density in subjects with Alzheimer's disease and psychosis. *Arch Gen Psychiatry* 2000;57:1165–73.
27. Bylsma FW, Folstein M, Devanand DP *et al.* Delusions and patterns of cognitive impairment in Alzheimer's disease. *Neuropsychiatry Neuropsychol Behav Neurol* 1994;7:98–103.
28. Flynn FG, Cummings JL, Gornbein J. Delusions in dementia syndromes: investigation of behavioral and neuropsychological correlates. *J Neuropsychiatry Clin Neurosci* 1991;3:364–70.
29. Jeste DV, Wragg RE, Salmon DP *et al.* Cognitive deficits of patients with Alzheimer's disease with and without delusions. *Am J Psychiatry* 1992; 149:184–9.
30. Lopez OL, Becker JT, Brenner RP. Alzheimer's disease with delusions and hallucinations: neuropsychological and electroencephalophic correlates. *Neurology* 1991;41:906–12.
31. Migliorelli R, Petracca G, Teson A *et al.* Neuropsychiatric and neuropsychological correlates of delusions in Alzheimer's disease. *Psychol Med* 1995; 25:505–13.
32. Chen ST, Sultzer DL, Hinkin CH *et al.* Executive dysfunction in Alzheimer's disease: association with neuropsychiatric symptoms and functional impairment. *J Neuropsychiatry Clin Neurosci* 1998;10:426–32.
33. Johnson JK, Head E, Kim R *et al.* Clinical and pathological evidence for a frontal variant of Alzheimer's disease. *Arch Neurol* 1999;56:1233–39.
34. Tekin S, Mega MS, Masterman DL *et al.* Orbitofrontal and anterior cingulate cortex: neurofibrillary tangle burden is associated with agitation in Alzheimer's disease. *Ann Neurol* 2001;49:355–61.
35. Tekin S, Fairbanks LA, O'Connor S *et al.* Activities of daily living in Alzheimer's disease: neuropsychiatric, cognitive, and medical illness influences. *Am J Geriatr Psychiatry* 2001;9:81–6.
36. Forsell Y, Winblad B. Major depression in a population of demented and nondemented older people: prevalence and correlates. *J Am Geriatr Soc* 1998; 46:27–30.

37. Hargrave R, Reed B, Mungas D. Depressive syndromes and functional disability in dementia. *J Geriatr Psychiatry Neurol* 2000;13:72–7.

38. Kuzis G, Sabe L, Tiberti C *et al*. Cognitive functions in major depression and Parkinson's disease. *Arch Neurol* 1997;54:982–6.

39. Troster AI, Paulo AM, Lyons KE *et al*. The influence of depression on cognition in Parkinson's disease: a pattern of impairment distinguishable from Alzheimer's disease. *Neurology* 1995;45:672–6.

40. Troster AI, Stalp LD, Paolo AM *et al*. Neuropsychological impairment in Parkinson's disease with and without depression. *Arch Neurol* 1995;52:1164–9.

41. Devanand DP, Jacobs DM, Tang M *et al*. The course of psychopathologic features in mild to moderate Alzheimer's disease. *Arch Gen Psychiatry* 1997; 54:257–63.

42. Levy ML, Cummings JL, Fairbanks LA *et al*. Longitudinal assessment of symptoms of depression, agitation, and psychosis in 181 patients with Alzheimer's disease. *Am J Psychiatry* 1996;153:1438–43.

43. Cadieux NL, Greve KW. Emotion processing in Alzheimer's disease. *J Int Neuropsychol Soc* 1997;3:411–19.

44. Roberts VJ, Ingram SM, Lamar M *et al*. Prosody impairment and associated affective and behavioral disturbances in Alzheimer's disease. *Neurology* 1996;47:1482–88.

45. Levy ML, Miller BL, Cummings JL *et al*. Alzheimer disease and frontotemporal dementias: behavioral distinctions. *Arch Neurol* 1996;53:687–90.

46. Litvan I, Mega MS, Cummings JL *et al*. Neuropsychiatric aspects of progressive supranuclear palsy. *Neurology* 1996;47:1184–9.

47. Litvan I, Cummings J, Mega M. Neuropsychiatric features of corticobasal degeneration. *J Neurol Neurosurg Psychiatry* 1998;65:717–21.

48. Kaufer DI, Cummings JL, Christine D *et al*. Assessing the impact of neuropsychiatric symptoms in Alzheimer's disease: the Neuropsychiatric Inventory Caregiver Distress Scale. *J Am Geriatr Soc* 1998;46:210–15.

49. Hirono N, Mega MS, Dinov ID *et al*. Left frontotemporal hypoperfusion is associated with aggression in patients with dementia. *Arch Neurol* 2000; 57:861–6.

50. Kotrla KJ, Chacko RC, Harper RG *et al*. SPECT findings on psychosis in Alzheimer's disease. *Am J Psychiatry* 1995;152:1470–5.

51. Mega MS, Lee L, Dinov ID *et al*. Cerebral correlates of psychotic symptoms in Alzheimer's disease. *J Neurol Neurosurg Psychiatry* 2000;69:167–71.

52. Starkstein SE, Vazquez S, Petracca G. A SPECT study of delusions in Alzheimer's disease. *Neurology* 1994;44:2055–9.

53. Sultzer DL, Mhler Me, Mandelkern MA *et al*. The relationship between psychiatric symptoms and regional cortical metabolism in Alzheimer's disease. *J Neuropsychiatry Clin Neurosci* 1995;7:476–84.

54. Blin J, Baron JC, Dubois B. Positron emission tomography study in progressive supranuclear palsy: brain hypometabolic pattern and clinicometabolic correlations. *Arch Neurol* 1990;47:747–52.

55. Craig AH, Cummings JL, Fairbanks L *et al*. Cerebral blood flow correlates of apathy in Alzheimer's disease. *Arch Neurol* 1996;53:1116–20.

56. Migneco O, Benoit M, Koulibaly PM *et al*. Perfusion brain SPECT and statisti-

cal parametric mapping analysis indicate that apathy is a cingulate syndrome: a study of Alzheimer's disease and non-demented patients. *Neuroimage* 2001;13:896–902.

57. Lai MKP, Lai O-F, Keene J *et al*. Psychosis of Alzheimer's disease is associated with elevated muscarinic M2 binding in the cortex. *Neurology* 2001; 57:805–11.

58. Minger SL, Esiri MM, McDonald B *et al*. Cholinergic deficits contribute to behavioral disturbance in patients with dementia. *Neurology* 2000;55:1460–7.

59. Zubenko GS, Moossy J, Kopp U. Neurochemical correlates of major depression in primary dementia. Arch Neurol 1990;47:209–14.

60. Clark LM, McDonald WM, Welsh-Bohmer KA *et al*. Magnetic resonance imaging correlates of depression in early- and late-onset Alzheimer's disease. *Biol Psychiatry* 1998;44:592–9.

61. Lopez OL, Becker JT, Reynolds CF *et al*. Psychiatric correlates of MR deep white matter lesions in probable Alzheimer's disease. *J Neuropsychiatry Clin Neurosci* 1997;9:246–50.

62. Snowdon DA, Greiner LH, Mortimer JA *et al*. Brain infarction and the clinical expression of Alzheimer's disease. *JAMA* 1997;277:813–17.

63. Mega MS, Cummings JL, Salloway S *et al*. The limbic system: an anatomic, phylogenic, and clinical perspective. *J Neuropsychiatry Clin Neurosci* 1997; 9:315–30.

64. Cummings JL. Principles of neuropsychiatry: towards a neuropsychiatric epistemology. *Neurocase* 1999;5:181–8.

65. Sano M, Ernesto C, Thomas RG *et al*. A controlled trial of selegiline, alpha-tocopherol, or both as treatment for Alzheimer's disease. *N Engl J Med* 1997;336:1216–22.

66. Cummings JL. Cholinesterase inhibitors: a new class of psychotropic agents. *Am J Psychiatry* 2000;157:4–15.

67. Mega MS, Dinov ID, Lee L *et al*. Orbital and dorsolateral frontal perfusion defect associated with behavioral response to cholinesterase inhibitor therapy in Alzheimer's disease. *J Neuropsychiatry Clin Neurosci* 2000;12:209–18.

68. Taragano FE, Lyketsos CG, Mangone CA *et al*. A double-blind, randomized, fixed-dose trial of fluoxetine vs. amitriptyline in the treatment of major depression complicating Alzheimer's disease. *Psychosomatics* 1997;38:246–52.

69. Katz IR, Jeste DV, Mintzer JE *et al*. Comparison of risperidone and placebo for psychosis and behavioral disturbances associated with dementia: a randomized, double-blind trial: Risperidone Study Group. *J Clin Psychiatry* 1999;60:107–15.

70. De Deyn PP, Rabheru K, Rasmussen A *et al*. A randomized trial of risperidone, placebo, and haloperidol for behavioral symptoms of dementia. *Neurology* 1999;53:946–55.

71. Street J, Clark WS, Gannon KS *et al*. Olanzapine treatment of psychotic and behavioral symptoms in patients with Alzheimer's disease in nursing care facilities: a double-blind, randomized, placebo-controlled trial. *Arch Gen Psychiatry* 2000;57:968–76.

72. Geschwind DH, Robidoux J, Alarcon M *et al*. Dementia and neurodevelopmental predisposition: cognitive dysfunction in presymptomatic subjects precedes dementia by decades in frontotemporal dementia. *Ann Neurol* 2001; 50:741–6.

chapter 2

Neuropsychiatric assessment of patients with dementia

Neuropsychiatric assessment is a critical aspect of evaluating patients with cognitive impairment. Neuropsychiatric symptoms are present in most patients with dementing disorders; profiles of neuropsychiatric symptoms have differential diagnostic value that aid in distinguishing among otherwise similar dementia syndromes; and recognition and appropriate management of neuropsychiatric symptoms are critically important in the care of patients with dementia. Neuropsychiatric assessment is integrated into a comprehensive assessment that includes review of the evolution of the current symptoms, past medical history, medications taken by the patient (prescribed and nonprescription), family history of neurologic and psychiatric illness, observation of neuropsychiatric phenomena in the course of the assessment, neurocognitive examination, and physical and neurological evaluation. Assessment of the patient as well as an interview with a knowledgable caregiver are both critical to adequately assess a cognitively impaired patient. The clinical assessment is complemented by laboratory and neuroimaging studies and in many cases by formal neuropsychological assessment. Electrophysiological studies such as electroencephalography may be useful in some cases. Most examinations contain both standardized assessments such as rating scales and mental status questionnaires as well as individualized testing determined by the specific system complex presented by each patient.

The neuropsychiatric assessment is hypothesis driven: the presenting features suggest diagnoses which are either supported or not by observations made in the course of the neurocognitive and neurologic assessments. Laboratory, neuroimaging, neuropsychological, and electrophysiological tests offer further evidence for or against specific diagnostic formulations. Each encounter with a patient is a highly individualized, intense hypothesis-generating interaction. Examination of the patient also provides an opportunity to assess the patient's caregiver and the context in which care is received. Finally, the initial assessment and each encounter that follows provide an opportunity to build an alliance with patient and caregiver that is critical to ensuring quality care.

This chapter reviews the components of dementia assessment with an emphasis on the relevance of each aspect to the neuropsychiatry of the dementia syndromes. Definitions of neuropsychiatric symptoms commonly encountered in dementias are provided.

Definitions of neuropsychiatric symptoms

A wide variety of symptoms can be encountered in the course of the neuropsychiatric assessment of patients with dementia. These may be modified from their appearance in typical idiopathic psychiatric disorders by the presence of cognitive impairment and the simultaneous occurrence of multiple neuropsychiatric symptoms.

Affect refers to the pattern of observable behaviors that is typically the expression of the individual's subjectively experienced feeling state or emotion.[1] Affect is revealed through movements, gestures, facial expression, and voice inflection. Examples of affect include the observed manifestations of anxiety, depression, elation, irritability, perplexity, and suspiciousness.[2] In addition, affect may be labile with abnormal variability manifested by repeated and rapid shifts in affective expression; blunted with a significant reduction in the intensity of emotional expression; incongruous, wherein the emotion expressed is not in keeping with the underlying emotion or disproportionate to the emotional experience; or constricted, as evidenced by a reduction in the range or intensity of affective expression. *Mood* (the subjectively experienced emotion) and affect are typically congruent but in neurological disorders such as pseudobulbar palsy affect may be out of proportion to or at variance with the experienced emotion.

Agitation refers to excessive motor activity associated with a feeling of inner tension.[1] The forms of agitation requiring management in dementia syndromes include physical aggression with hitting, shoving, and threatening behavior; verbal aggression with shouting and cursing; and active resistance to care, making it impossible for caregivers to dress, bathe, feed, toilet, or otherwise assist the patient. Some classifications of agitation include less severe behavioral changes including pacing, fidgeting, wringing of the hands, pulling of the clothes, repeatedly asking questions, and inability to sit still. These more benign behaviors do not correlate with aggressive agitation when assessed with rating scales and are mediated by different pathophysiological mechanisms.

Anxiety is characterized by excessive and unjustified apprehension, feelings of foreboding, and thoughts of impending doom. Patients are irritable, tense, and have difficulty concentrating. Autonomic disturbances are common and include sweating, palpitations, gastrointestinal distress (nausea, diarrhea), shortness of breath, dry mouth, lightheadedness, and frequent urination.[1,3] An action tremor, exaggerated startle response, and restlessness with frequent shifting of posture, pacing, and fidgeting are common motor expressions of anxiety.

Apathy is common in many dementing disorders (Chapter 9). Apathy consists of lack of motivation with diminished goal-directed behavior, reduced goal-directed cognition, and decreased emotional engagement (Box 2.1).[4] Apathy is not attributable to diminished level of consciousness.[5] While apathy may accompany depression, it is often an independent manifestation of brain dysfunction.[6] Apathy is commonly accompanied by evidence of executive dysfunction.[7] There may be many contributing factors to apathy in patients with dementia; reduced function of the anterior cingulated cortex and related subcortical structures appears to be the primary determinant of the occurrence of apathetic behavior (Chapter 9).

Delusions are false beliefs based on incorrect inferences about external reality that are firmly held despite evidence to the contrary.[1] Delusions

Box 2.1 Criteria for the syndrome of apathy[4]

- Lack of motivation that is not attributable to intellectual impairment, emotional distress, or diminished level of consciousness (drowsiness and/or diminished attentional capacity)
- Lack of motivation, relative to the patient's previous level of functioning or the standards of his or her age and culture, as evidenced by all three of the following:
  - Diminished goal-directed overt behavior as indicated by:
    - lack of productivity
    - lack of effort
    - lack of time spent in activities of interest
    - lack of initiative or perseverance
    - behavioral compliance or dependency on others to structure activity
    - diminished socialization or recreation
  - Diminished goal-directed cognition as indicated by:
    - lack of interests, lack of interest in learning new things, lack of interest in new experiences
    - lack of concern about one's personal, health, or functional problems
    - diminished importance or value attributed to such goal-related domains as socialization, recreation, productivity, initiative, perseverance, curiosity
  - Diminished emotional concomitants of goal-directed behavior as indicated by:
    - unchanging affect
    - lack of emotional responsivity to positive or negative events
    - euphoric or flat affect
    - absence of excitement or emotional intensity
- Lack of motivation is not attributable to intellectual impairment, emotional distress, or diminished level of consciousness. When lack of motivation is attributable to intellectual impairment, emotional distress, or diminished level of consciousness (drowsiness or diminished attention), then apathy is a symptom of some other syndrome such as dementia, delirium, or depression
- Emotional distress is absent or is insufficient to account for the lack of motivation

in patients with dementia are commonly persecutory involving beliefs of theft of property, burglary, and infidelity. Delusional misidentification syndromes such as the Capgras syndrome are also common. Table 2.1 provides a list of delusions that may be encountered in patients with dementia syndromes. In idiopathic psychotic disorders such as schizophrenia, delusions are commonly accompanied by evidence of a thought disorder, but such abnormalities are either unusual or difficult to recognize in the patient with substantial cognitive changes. Hallucinations (defined below) may accompany delusions in patients with dementia. Grandiose delusions seen in patients with bipolar illness or bizarre and religious delusions observed in patients with schizophrenia or mood disorders are unusual in patients with dementia.

Depression is a mood disorder characterized by sadness or an inability to experience pleasure (anhedonia) and manifested by sadness or statements and feelings of worthlessness, hopelessness, helplessness, or inappropriate guilt; recurrent thoughts of death, diminished ability to think or concentrate, increased fatigue and loss of energy. Insomnia or psychomotor agitation or retardation may accompany the depression syndrome.[1,3] Motoric manifestations of depression include diminished interactiveness, facial immobility, postural slumping, delayed or shortened verbal responsiveness, slowed movement, and reduced spontaneity.[8] Depression can be difficult to identify in patients with dementing disorders. Cognitive disturbances, abnormalities of sleep and appetite, psychomotor retardation, and apathetic disinterest in usually pleasurable activities may occur in dementia syndromes without accompanying mood abnormalities. Reliance on these aspects of the depression syndrome for recognition of a mood disorder may lead to overdiagnosis. Subjective aspects of depression including manifestations of sadness and statements regarding helplessness, hopelessness, and worthlessness may be better guides to the existence of a depression syndrome in cognitively impaired patients. When cognitive impairment is severe, the clinician may be forced to rely on symptoms that are less cognitively mediated.

There are many complex interactions between dementia and depression and assessment of past and present depression is critical when evaluating patients with dementia. A past history of depression may be a

Table 2.1 Delusional beliefs encountered in patients with dementia

Syndrome	Content
Othello syndrome	Delusional jealousy
Parasitosis	Delusion of infestation
Lycanthropy	Werewolfism
de Clerambault's syndrome	Belief that an individual of higher social stature is in love with one (also called erotomania)
Incubus	Phantom lover (male)
Succubus	Phantom lover (female)
Picture sign	Belief that individuals on the television are present in the house
Koro	One's genitals are withdrawing into the abdomen
Dorian Gray syndrome	One is not aging
Capgras syndrome	Others are not who they claim to be or have been replaced by identical-appearing imposters
Fregoli's syndrome	A persecutor assumes the appearance of others
Intermetamorphosis syndrome	Those in one's environment look like one's enemies
Heutoscopy	Seeing oneself
Doppelganger	One has a double
One's house is not one's home	The place one is living is not the home
Abandonment	An individual is going to be abandoned or placed in an institution by their caregivers
Theft, burglary	Delusion that one's things are being stolen or that one's home is being burglarized
Phantom boarders	Unwelcome guests are living in the home
Conspiracy	Others are plotting against one
Reduplication	There are multiple versions of one's spouse or other person (often accompanies Capgras syndrome in dementia)
Infidelity	One's spouse is having an affair
Poverty	Belief that one has no or inadequate financial resources

risk factor for the occurrence of Alzheimer's disease or for the occurrence of depression as one of the manifestations of Alzheimer's disease or Parkinson's disease. Depression itself may produce a cognitive impairment syndrome known as the dementia syndrome of depression. This can be difficult to distinguish from late onset dementing disorders with depression as a symptom. Depression with dementia may be a prodromal state heralding the occurrence of a dementing disorder.[9] Depression may also be the initial manifestation of a recognizable dementing disorder. Once present, depression may exacerbate cognitive and functional disturbances in patients with dementia.

Disinhibition is a syndrome characterized by inappropriate social and interpersonal interactions. Patients are impulsive and make tactless and often lewd comments; they disregard the usual conventions of social behavior and may touch others inappropriately. They can often verbalize the socially appropriate behaviors but do not incorporate this knowledge into their behavior. Disinhibition is characteristic of dysfunction of orbitofrontal cortex and related subcortical systems and is observed in patients with frontotemporal lobar degeneration (Chapter 7) and in some patients with the frontal variant of Alzheimer's disease (Chapter 3), vascular dementia (Chapter 6), and Creutzfeldt-Jakob disease (Chapter 8).

Elation refers to an elevated mood with excessive positive feelings, happiness, and overconfidence. Elation is a relatively rare occurrence in patients with dementia syndromes but may occur in conjunction with disorders affecting the orbitofrontal cortex and related subcortical structures including some extrapyramidal disorders (Chapter 5), frontotemporal lobar degeneration (Chapter 7), and Creutzfeldt-Jakob disease (Chapter 8).

Hallucinations are sensory perceptions that have the same compelling sense of reality as a veridical sensory experience but occur without stimulation of the relevant sensory organ.[1] Patients may be aware that they are having hallucinations – in which case the hallucination is not delusional – or the patient may endorse the hallucination as representative of external reality, and the belief is a delusion. Hallucinations may be unformed including flashes, shadows, or colored lights or they may be formed images with the subject seeing objects, persons, or scenes.[2] Hallucinations may involve any sensory modality including vision, hearing (auditory hallucinations), touch (tactile hallucinations), smell (olfactory hallucinations), or taste (gustatory hallucinations), but are most commonly visual in patients with dementia. Hallucinations may be mood-congruent in patients with depression-related or mania-related psychoses or they may be mood-incongruent. Hallucinations are particularly common in patients with dementia with Lewy bodies (Chapter 4) and in patients with Parkinson's disease treated with dopaminergic agents (Chapter 5). They occur less commonly in other dementing disorders. Ocular disorders with diminished vision may cause or contribute to the occurrence of visual hallucinations.

Illusions are misinterpretations of external visual stimuli. Illusions are distinguished from hallucinations in that they are distorted perceptions rather than spontaneous abnormal perceptions. Commonly described illusions include micropsia (objects and their environment appear too small or distant), macropsia (objects and their environment appear too large), or metamorphopsia (objects appear distorted). Hallucinations and illusions occur in the same patient populations.

Mania refers to a mood disorder characterized by a persistently elevated expansive or irritable mood. Typical features include inflated self-esteem or grandiosity, diminished need for sleep, increased talkativeness, pressure of speech, flight of ideas and racing thoughts, distractibility, increased activity or psychomotor agitation, and excessive involvement in pleasurable activities that have a high possibility of painful consequences.[1] *Hypomania* is a less severe or more brief syndrome with similar manifestations. Mania and hypomania are relatively unusual in dementia but may occur with dysfunction of the orbitofrontal cortex in patients with vascular dementia (Chapter 6), frontotemporal lobar degeneration (Chapter 7), or Creutzfeldt-Jakob disease (Chapter 8).

Obsessional, compulsive, and repetitive symptoms may occur in patients with dementia. The presence of cognitive impairment often makes it impossible to establish whether the symptoms are 'ego dystonic' or 'ego syntonic' as required for the diagnosis of idiopathic obsessive-compulsive disorder. The patients exhibit patterns of recurrent thoughts or vocalizations, perform repetitive acts, or engage in repetitious purposeless behavior. True rituals may be observed in occasional patients with parkinsonian syndromes (Chapter 5) and patients with frontotemporal lobar degeneration (Chapter 7).

Sexual behavior changes are common in patients with dementia syndromes and are most frequently represented by decreased engagement in sexual activity. Occasional dementia syndromes may evolve through a phase including symptoms of the Kluver-Bucy syndrome manifested by increased or altered sexual activity. The *Kluver-Bucy syndrome* is comprised of emotional placidity, hypermetamorphosis (compulsory exploration of high stimulus items in the environment), hyperorality (a tendency to place items in the mouth), dietary alterations, and altered sexual behavior.[3] Dementia syndromes that may produce the Kluver-Bucy syndrome are listed in Box 2.2.

Table 2.2 provides a summary of neuropsychiatric symptoms and the dementia syndromes that most commonly manifest these neuropsychiatric abnormalities.

Box 2.2 Dementias that may cause the Kluver-Bucy syndrome

Post-encephalitic syndromes after herpes encephalitis
Trauma
Alzheimer's disease
Frontotemporal lobar degenerations
Adrenoleukodystrophy
Delayed, post-anoxic leukoencephalopathy
Bilateral temporal lobe stroke
Post-traumatic encephalopathy
Paraneoplastic limbic encephalitis
Hypoglycemia
Toxoplasmosis

Table 2.2 Dementias that commonly manifest specific neuropsychiatric disorders*

Neuropsychiatric disorder	Dementia
Depression	• Alzheimer's disease • Parkinson's disease • Vascular dementia • Corticobasal degeneration • Dementia with Lewy bodies
Hallucination	• Dementia with Lewy bodies • Parkinson's disease after treatment with dopaminergic agents • Vascular dementia if infarcts involve the visual system
Delusions	• Dementia with Lewy bodies • Alzheimer's disease • Parkinson's disease after treatment with dopaminergic agents
Apathy	• Progressive supranuclear palsy • Frontotemporal dementia • Dementia with Lewy bodies • Alzheimer's disease • Vascular dementia
Disinhibition	• Frontotemporal dementia
Agitation/aggression	• Alzheimer's disease • Dementia with Lewy bodies • Frontotemporal dementia
REM sleep behavior disorder	• Dementia with Lewy bodies • Parkinson's disease

*A few patients with other types of dementia may manifest these symptoms; the table comprises dementias in which the symptoms are prominent.
REM, rapid eye movement.

History of presenting features

Dementia syndromes have characteristic temporal profiles. Patients with neurodegenerative disorders such as Alzheimer's disease, dementia with Lewy bodies, and frontotemporal lobar degenerations have a gradually progressive course. Extrapyramidal syndromes such as Parkinson's disease typically begin with evidence of motor system dysfunction and manifest cognitive and behavioral changes later in the clinical course. Conversely, patients with dementia with Lewy bodies typically begin with visual hallucinations, fluctuating cognition, or cognitive abnormalities, and progress to include evidence of extrapyramidal dysfunction. Fluctuating cognition is highly characteristic of dementia with Lewy bodies (Chapter 4) and is less evident in most other dementing disorders. Vascular dementia (Chapter 6) is often characterized by an abrupt onset or periods of sudden cognitive decline (stepwise deterioration). Frontotemporal lobar degeneration (Chapter 7) is marked by onset of behavioral changes (apathy, disinhibition) followed later by cognitive deterioration. Rapid progression is characteristic of Creutzfeldt-Jakob disease (Chapter 8), where patients frequently progress from onset to death in less than 12 months.

Age of onset can also be of assistance in differential diagnosis. Patients with frontotemporal lobar degenerations typically have onset of their illness in the sixth decade and these disorders do not become increasingly common with advancing age. This contrasts with typical sporadic Alzheimer's disease which usually has its onset in the seventh or eighth decade of life and is more frequent with each advancing decade of life. Nearly any dementia syndrome may present with behavioral abnormalities as the first manifestation. However, this is the typical pattern in the frontotemporal dementias (Chapter 7), where behavioral changes such as apathy and disinhibition commonly predate substantive cognitive abnormalities.

Past medical history

A review of the past medical history may provide additional insight into the etiology of the dementia syndrome. Patients with vascular dementia commonly have predisposing risk factors for stroke including hypertension, diabetes, hypercholesterolemia, heart disease such as atrial fibrillation, cigarette smoking, or obesity.

Risk factors for Alzheimer's disease that may be elicited when reviewing the individual's past medical history include a history of head trauma and hypercholesterolemia (Chapter 3).

Excessive use of alcohol or other substances of abuse can produce cognitive impairment and a substance use history should be included in the neuropsychiatric assessment.

Review of medications

A careful review of both prescribed medication, agents purchased without a prescription, and nutraceuticals (dietary supplements and herbal remedies) is an important component of the neuropsychiatric assessment. Medication toxicity may cause depression or delirium, exacerbating cognitive abnormalities. Administration of dopaminergic agents may be associated with the onset of hallucinations, delusions, elation, or hedonistic homeostatic dysregulation disorder (Chapter 5).

Family history

Review of illnesses that have occurred in other family members, particularly in first degree relatives, may provide critically important neuropsychiatric information. Approximately 40% of patients with frontotemporal lobar degenerations have a family history of autosomal dominant inheritance (Chapter 7). A small number of families with autosomal dominant Alzheimer's disease have been described and the occurrence of Alzheimer's disease in the patient's family represents a risk for the occurrence of the disease even in families without autosomal dominant inheritance patterns. Familial prion disorders (Chapter 8) include familial Creutzfeldt-Jakob disease, Gerstmann-Straussler-Schenker disease, and fatal familial insomnia.

Neuropsychiatric observations

Interacting with the patient provides the most important opportunity to augment the history through direct observations of neuropsychiatric phenomena. The examination should begin the moment that the patient is first encountered and continue until the visit is complete. Each behavior observed – from the response to the first cordial salutation to how the patient receives the diagnosis on completion of the interview – provides additional information on neuropsychiatric status and emotional function. Patient interactions with both the examiner and the caregiver during the course of the assessment provide additional insight. Dress, hygiene, and make-up or grooming are relevant to the patient's ability to engage in these daily activities, recognition of their social importance, or disregard for social conventions. The examiner must remember that the well-groomed and well-dressed individual may be so because of the attentive care of the caregiver.

Motor system abnormalities may be apparent in the course of the assessment including tremor, parkinsonism, hemiparesis, or myoclonus relevant to the differential diagnosis of dementia. Motor activity, gestures, facial expression, and vocal inflection also provide information relevant to the presence of anxiety, depression, elation, suspiciousness, or hallucinations.

Verbalizations provide information about dysarthria, aphasia, and thought content. Dysarthria is common in patients with vascular dementia while hypophonia is common in patients with Parkinson's disease and related parkinsonian syndromes. Aphasia is present in Alzheimer's disease, some forms of frontotemporal lobar degenerations (progressive nonfluent aphasia, semantic dementia), Creutzfeldt-Jakob disease, and vascular disease if strokes involve critical language-mediating areas.

Verbalizations also may provide evidence of delusions, obsessional thought content, or mood changes.

Observations of spontaneous speech and behavior are augmented by more probing questions relevant to neuropsychiatric symptoms. The patient's ability to respond and the type of questions appropriate will be determined by the degree of cognitive impairment evidenced by the patient. Assessment of anxiety should include questions regarding worrying, feelings of nervous tension, muscular tension, irritability, smothering feelings or difficulty getting one's breath, palpitations, dizziness, tingling of face or fingers, chest tightness, dry mouth, difficulty swallowing, sweating, trembling, hot or cold flashes, and fear of dying. Assessment of depression should include questions regarding sadness, tearfulness, self-confidence, hopefulness, interest and enjoyment in pleasurable activities, productivity, optimism about the future, social interests, energy level, sleep quality, and appetite. Questions regarding hallucinations include abnormal sensory experiences not evident to others in the same environment. Delusions can be assessed by asking questions relevant to the content provided in Table 2.1 including theft, burglary, phantom boarders, infidelity, abandonment, and replacement. In many cases, the patient may not remember the delusional phenomena even though they exhibit them outside the context of the examination. In these cases, information must be obtained from the caregiver or other observer. It is common for patients with dementia syndromes to have multiple neuropsychiatric symptoms simultaneously. Delusions, hallucinations, and agitation commonly co-occur and mood-related syndromes including depression, anxiety, and irritability are also frequent comorbid symptoms (Chapter 1).

Neurocognitive assessment

The neurocognitive assessment should include examination of five domains of cognitive behavior including attention, memory, language, visuospatial skills, and executive function. These five domains plus processing of emotional information are the elements of normal cognitive

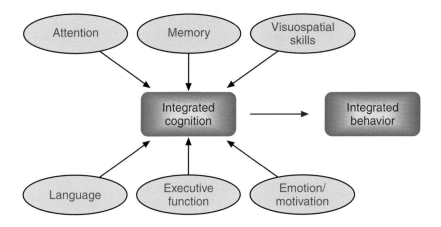

Figure 2.1 *Integrated cognition is a product of the interaction of attention, memory, visuospatial skills, language, executive function, and motivation/emotion.*

function that lead to integrated behavior (Figure 2.1). Integrated cognition is the foundation for coherent, goal-directed behavior.

Attention is the ability to focus and direct cognitive processes and to resist distraction; concentration is the ability to focus and sustain attention over a period of time.[10,11] The most elementary assessment of attention is accomplished through the digit span test. The examiner says individual digits at a rate of one per second and asks the patient to repeat the digits in exactly the same order. A normal span is seven digits plus or minus two digits. Concentration is typically assessed by a continuous performance test such as the 'A test'. In this test the examiner states a series of letters over a 30-second period. The patient is instructed to raise their hand each time the letter 'A' appears randomly in the sequence of letters. More complex tests of attention include cancellation tasks where the patient is asked to search and mark a specific letter or symbol on a page with distributed letters and symbols. Assessment of attention is critical to interpretation of other elements of the neurocognitive exam. Patients who are inattentive will exhibit disturbances in memory and executive function and possibly in other cognitive domains. In patients with dementia with Lewy bodies (Chapter 4) attention may fluctuate markedly in the course of the examination.

Memory is disturbed in nearly all patients with dementia syndromes (by definition). Two types of memory disturbances may be identified: amnestic disorders and retrieval deficit syndromes. Amnestic disorders occur in patients with medial limbic and hippocampal dysfunction such as those with Alzheimer's disease; retrieval deficit syndromes are more typical of those with frontal-subcortical circuit dysfunction. Verbal memory is assessed by asking the patient to repeat from three to 10 words. After a delay, the patient is asked to recall the words and then asked to identify unrecalled words from a list of target words (presented earlier) and foils (words not previously presented). Patients with amnestic disorders do not learn or store new information and exhibit deficits in both recall and recognition. Patients with retrieval deficit syndromes have difficulty recalling information but perform better on tasks of recognition.[12] Remote memory also is affected progressively in patients with dementia syndromes. Patients with Alzheimer's disease typically recall remote information better than more recently learned material but are no longer able to recall distant memories as the disease progresses. Patients with frontal-subcortical circuit syndromes may have difficulty recalling information but recognize it when presented in a multiple-choice fashion. The deficit is similar for all decades of personal memory. Figure 2.2 presents a classification of memory disorders and the related dementia syndromes.

Verbal output disorders include changes in articulation (dysarthria), volume (hypophonia), prosody (abnormal vocal inflection), and propositional language (aphasia). Table 2.3 presents a list of speech and language changes commonly encountered in patients with dementing disorders.

Classification of aphasias depends on assessing fluency of verbal output, comprehension, and repetition (Figure 2.3). Testing of naming, reading, writing, singing, and automatic speech (counting, reciting over-learned material) provides additional information. Fluent aphasias have relatively preserved inflection, fluency, and phrase length but have reduced semantic content and exhibit paraphasic errors. Transcortical sensory aphasia characteristic of Alzheimer's disease and semantic aphasia characteristic of frontotemporal lobar degeneration are fluent aphasias. Nonfluent aphasic syndromes have reduced verbal output with

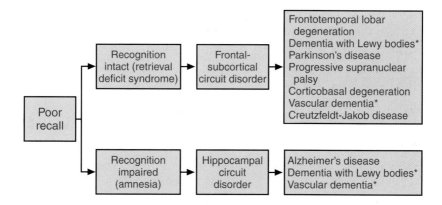

Figure 2.2 *Classification of memory disorders. Retrieval deficit syndromes have intact recognition and are associated with frontal-subcortical circuit disorders. Amnestic memory abnormalities have impaired recognition and reflect dysfunction of the medial limbic hippocampal circuit. (*Dementia with Lewy bodies and vascular dementia may exhibit either type of memory abnormality depending on the distribution of pathology.)*

short phrase lengths and reduced fluency with relative preservation of semantic content. The progressive nonfluent aphasia form of fronto-temporal lobar degeneration and the transcortical motor aphasia seen in some patients with Creutzfeldt-Jakob disease are nonfluent aphasic disorders. Fluent aphasias reflect dysfunction of the posterior left hemisphere and nonfluent aphasias reflect abnormalities of function of the anterior left hemisphere.

Language-related syndromes assessed in the course of the mental status examination include acalculia (addition, subtraction, multiplication, and division) and apraxia (the inability to carry out motor commands). Arithmetic skills may be disproportionately preserved early in the course of the frontotemporal lobar degenerations. Apraxia is disproportionately severe in patients with corticobasal degeneration (Chapter 7) and is present late in the course of patients with Alzheimer's disease (Chapter 3).

Visuospatial skills are assessed by asking the patient to copy or draw visual stimuli. Commonly the patient is asked to copy a circle, diamond, overlapping rectangles, cube, or more complex figure provided by the

Table 2.3 Speech and language changes characteristic of dementias

Dementia	Speech and language changes
Alzheimer's disease	Anomia progressing to transcortical sensory aphasia; echolalia and palilalia late in course
Frontotemporal lobar degenerations	
Frontotemporal dementia	Dysprosody common with lack of inflection of speech
Semantic dementia	Semantic anomia progressing to Wernicke-type aphasia and early mutism
Progressive nonfluent aphasia	Broca or transcortical motor-type aphasia
Dementia with Lewy bodies	Anomia progressing to transcortical sensory aphasia
Creutzfeldt-Jakob disease	Transcortical motor aphasic (most common)
Vascular dementia	
Subcortical	Dysarthria
Cortical	Aphasia (features reflect location of infarction)
Parkinson's disease	Monotone, hypophonia
Corticobasal degeneration	Progressive nonfluent aphasia in some patients
Progressive supranuclear palsy	Pseudobulbar palsy with dysarthria; mutism in some patients

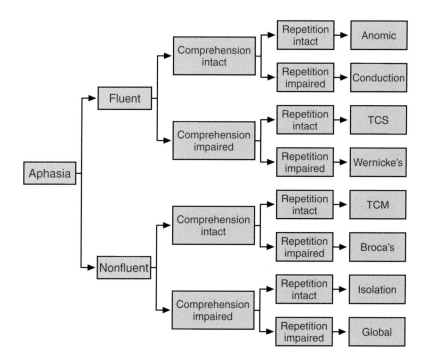

Figure 2.3 *Classification of the aphasic syndromes based on fluency, auditory comprehension, and ability to repeat verbal material. TCS, transcortical sensory aphasia; TCM, transcortical motor aphasia.*

examiner. In addition, the patient may be asked to draw the face of a clock to reflect a specified time or to draw a flower, house, or other object. Completion of a visuospatial task is dependent on attention, memory, and executive functions as well as integrity of visuospatial skills. Visual memory may be tested by asking the patient to recall the copied figures after an interval of time has elapsed. Visuospatial disturbances are most marked with dysfunction of the posterior aspects of the right hemisphere but may be seen with conditions affecting other brain areas.

Executive function is among the most difficult of functions to assess at the bedside. Executive function depends on integrating memory, emotion, and sensory input to decide on a specific action, develop a plan, create a program for execution of the plan, implement the elements of the program, monitor the outcome of the activity, adjust the plan appropriately, and decide whether to continue or alter the original activity (Figure 2.4). Assessment of this complex integrated activity is challenging. Evaluation of generative intellectual function depending on the patient's ability to generate novel information not immediately available in the environment is the basis for the assessment of executive function. *Verbal fluency* is one means of assessing generative ideation. The patient is asked to name as many animals as possible in 1 minute (or as many words as possible beginning with the letters F, A, or S in 1 minute). Normally, patients produce a word list of 12–25 animals (average 18). Patients with executive dysfunction produce fewer responses and do not systematically explore categories that would facilitate identification of class members (e.g. jungle, ocean, zoo, farm). *Perseveration* may be revealed in motor programming tasks and is evident as repetition of previous activities rather than stopping appropriately or generating new activities (Figures 2.5 and 2.6). Asking the patient to set the hands on a clock for the time 10 minutes after 11 may also reveal

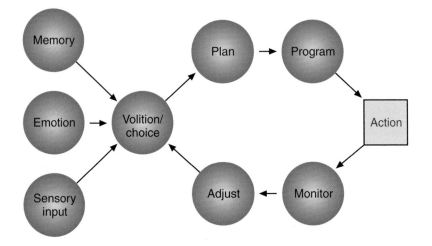

Figure 2.4 *Component neuropsychological mechanisms involved in volitional activity.*

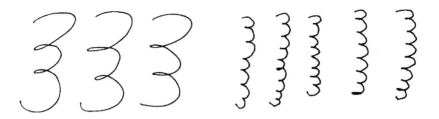

Figure 2.5 *Multiple loop test revealing perseveration (loops on the right) as the patient tries to copy the examiner's model (left).*

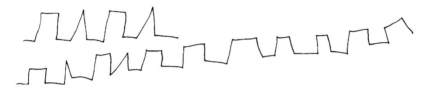

Figure 2.6 *Alternating program tests revealing perseveration (below) as the patient tries to copy the examiners model (above).*

evidence of *environmental dependency* and stimulus boundedness. Patients with executive dysfunction often place one hand on the 10 (rather than on the 2 to indicate 10 minutes after the hour) and one hand on the 11. Tests of *abstraction* (idioms and proverbs), planning, and judgment are also mediated by prefrontal regions and comprise executive activities. Insight into the integrity of these functions may be gained by asking questions about the patient's 'real life' behavior and plans. The *anti-saccade test* is another useful measure of dorsolateral-executive function. The patient is first asked to look at whichever finger the examiner moves as the examiner holds up a finger on each side of the patient's face. After this set has been attained, the patient is then asked to look away from whichever finger the examiner moves. Patients with executive dysfunction continue to look at the finger moved by the clinician. Patients with frontotemporal lobar degeneration, the frontal variant of Alzheimer's disease, dementia with Lewy bodies, subcortical vascular dementia, and Creutzfeldt-Jakob disease all exhibit substantial executive dysfunction.

Neurological examination

The neurological examination complements the other elements of the neuropsychiatric assessment. Critical elements of the exam include assessment of eye movement disturbances, motor system abnormalities, reflex changes, and abnormalities of gait.

Assessment of the cranial nerves will reveal abnormalities of extraocular movement functions, vision, and vocalization. Elderly patients frequently have some degree of reduced volitional upgaze. Distinctive supranuclear gaze palsies are evident in patients with progressive supranuclear palsy who initially manifest difficulty with volitional downgaze followed by impaired upgaze and eventually by reduced lateral and pursuit movements. Patients with vascular dementia may have visual field defects if strokes involve the geniculocalcarine radiations. Dysarthria with abnormalities of labial, lingual, or guttural movements may occur, particularly in patients with vascular dementia, and reduced voice volume is present in many patients with parkinsonian syndromes.

Motor system assessment includes examination of strength, bulk, tone, and coordination. Parkinsonism manifested by bradykinesia and rigidity is evident in some patients with frontotemporal lobar degeneration, dementia with Lewy bodies, Parkinson's disease-related parkinsonian syndromes, and Creutzfeldt-Jakob disease. Parkinson's disease has a characteristic flexed posture with a shuffling gait featuring short steps and strides. A 'lower half' parkinsonism with reduced stride length and diminished step height may occur in patients with vascular dementia produced by lacunar infarctions or diffuse white matter ischemic injury. Coordination abnormalities are evident when the cerebellum is involved in disorders such as the Gerstmann-Straussler-Scheinker type of prion disease. Spastic-type tone changes are evident in patients with upper motor neuron lesions such as those with vascular dementia or the amyotrophic lateral sclerosis form of frontotemporal lobar degeneration. Plastic or lead pipe rigidity is evident in patients with parkinsonian syndromes, while cogwheel rigidity occurs in patients with palpable tremor.

Sensory system abnormalities are less common in patients with dementia and are often difficult to assess because of the cognitive disturbances. Patients with vascular dementia may have focal sensory syndromes such as hemisensory disturbances. Peripheral neuropathies with diminished distal sensation may occur with metabolic disorders (hypothyroidism, vitamin B12 deficiency), toxic conditions, or rare inherited metabolic dementias such as metachromatic leukodystrophy and neuroacanthocytosis.

Reflex abnormalities elicited in patients with dementia syndromes include abnormalities of muscle stretch reflexes or the appearance of primitive reflexes. Muscles stretch reflexes will be exaggerated in the limbs contralateral to the side of focal upper motor neuron lesions. A Babinski sign may be evident on the same side. Primitive reflexes including suck responses and grasp reflexes are particularly common in patients with frontal lobe dysfunction.

A neurovascular assessment with auscultation of the carotid arteries and heart may provide valuable information in patients with possible vascular dementia.

Rating scales, inventories, and mental status questionnaires

The neuropsychiatric assessment is usefully augmented by symptom rating scales, inventories, and mental status questionnaires. Standardized tests of cognition, assessments of activities of daily living, and neuropsychiatric symptom scales are available for application in the clinic. The most widely used mental status screening questionnaire is the Mini-Mental State Examination (MMSE).[13] This is a 30-item questionnaire that assesses orientation, repetition, learning, subtraction/concentration, recall, naming, repetition, comprehension (verbal and written), writing, and copying. Scores of 23 and below are typically regarded as abnormal, although this cut-off leads to under-recognition of mild degrees of cognitive change. Alterations on the MMSE are not unique to dementia and abnormal scores may be obtained by patients with amnesia, aphasia, or delirium. The MMSE lacks any assessment of executive function and will provide limited assistance in the recognition of patients with frontal or frontal-subcortical circuit disorders. The MMSE assesses areas that are most relevant to dementia of the Alzheimer type; it is particularly valuable in assessing the progression of Alzheimer's disease where patients typically decline by approximately three MMSE points per year. The Alzheimer's Disease Assessment Scale[14] is a commonly used mental status assessment that includes a larger number of items than the MMSE. This test evaluates spoken language, reading, comprehension, word finding, copying, praxis, orientation, recall, and recognition. The total possible score is 70 points. The Mattis Dementia Rating Scale (DRS) is another widely used cognitive assessment of patients with dementia and includes measures of attention, initiation and perseveration, construction, conceptualization, and memory. One advantage of the DRS is inclusion of assessments of executive function.[15]

The Frontal Assessment Battery (FAB)[16] and the Executive Interview (EXIT)[17] are relatively brief standardized assessments of executive function that may be used in the assessment of patients with dementia. Evaluation of executive dysfunction is particularly important in the context of the neuropsychiatric examination, since involvement of the frontal lobes in patients with dementia syndromes frequently correlates with an array of neuropsychiatric symptoms.

Assessment of activities of daily living is also critical in a comprehensive evaluation of patients with dementia. Activities of daily living are divided into instrumental activities such as using the telephone, shopping, housekeeping, and using transportation and basic activities including grooming, feeding, and dressing. Skills commonly used to assess activities of daily living include the Instrumental Activity of Daily Living Scale (IADL),[18] the Functional Activities Questionnaire,[19] and the Alzheimer's Disease Cooperative Study (ADCS) Activities of Daily Living Scale.[20]

Assessment of neuropsychiatric symptoms employs scales that rate one symptom such as agitation or depression, or scales that provide ratings of multiple symptoms. The Cornell Scale for depression in dementia[21] and the Geriatric Depression Scale[22] are the two rating scales most commonly used to rate depression in patients with dementia. The latter is a self-rating scale and may not yield valid results in patients with deficits in insight or advanced cognitive impairment. The Cohen-Mansfield Agitation Inventory is the instrument in most widespread use in the assessment of agitation in patients with dementia.[23] Commonly used multi-symptom rating scales include the Neuropsychiatric Inventory (NPI),[24] the BEHAVE-AD,[25] and the Behavior Rating Scale for Dementia.[26]

The NPI is a scripted interview of caregivers providing ratings of 10 behaviors common in dementia syndromes: delusions, hallucinations, agitation, anxiety, depression, irritability, apathy, disinhibition, euphoria and aberrant motor behavior. Caregivers rate the frequency and severity of behavior present in the past month. They also assess their own distress in response to their patient's behavior. Data from NPI studies relevant to dementing diseases are presented in Chapters 3–7.

Measurement of the patient's quality of life is an important area of assessment. Neuropsychiatric symptoms, particularly mood alterations, influence perceived quality of life. Adequate management of neuropsychiatric symptoms may substantially improve the life quality of both patient and caregiver. Several quality of life measures have been developed for use in dementia.[27,28]

Assessment of the caregiver is an integral component of caring for a patient with dementia. This is done informally in the course of the interview and can be done formally with the use of rating scales. Burden scales[29] provide a numerical measure of the degree to which caregivers feel burdened by their caregiving role. In addition, some patient rating scales such as the Neuropsychiatric Inventory[24] and the Revised Memory and Behaviors Problem Checklist[30] have integrated caregiver measures that assess the response to patient symptoms as part of the standardized interview.

Neuropsychological assessment

Neuropsychological assessment is useful as part of the neuropsychiatric evaluation of patients with dementia. Neuropsychological evaluations utilize standardized instruments that typically have age- and education-based norms, allowing more secure differentiation of normal and abnormal than many bedside assessments.[31] Neuropsychological evaluation also provides information on general neuropsychological functioning that is typically impossible with bedside examinations. Neuropsychological tests provide insight into premorbid intellectual function, since some measures are more affected by dementing illness than others, and those that 'hold' allow an estimation of cognitive function prior to the onset of cognitive decline. The pattern of neuropsychological deficits may assist in differential diagnosis of dementia syndromes.

Table 2.4 provides a list of neuropsychological tests commonly used in neuropsychological evaluation.[32] The five domains of cognitive function assessed at the bedside (attention, memory, language, visuospatial skills, executive function) are also assessed in the course of neuropsychological evaluation. In addition, neuropsychological testing can provide a standardized assessment of general intellectual function and psychomotor speed.

General intellectual function is assessed with the Wechsler Adult Intelligence Scale-Revised or Ravens Coloured Progressive Matrices. Language is often assessed with the Boston Naming Test, Boston Diagnostic Aphasia Examination, Token Test, and the National Adult Reading Test. A variety of memory tests valuable in assessing dementia patients have been devised including the Rey Auditory Verbal Learning Test, California Verbal Learning Test, Wechsler Memory Scale, Paired Associate Learning, Fuld Object-Memory Test, and Buschke Selective Reminding Test. Delayed Recall of the Rey-Osterreith Complex Figure provides an assessment of nonverbal memory. Visuospatial skills are evaluated with the Rey-Osterreith Complex Figure (copy), Test of Line Orientation, Hooper Visual Organization Test, or Embedded Figures Test. Tests of executive function include verbal fluency, nonverbal or figural fluency, Trail Making Tests (A, B), Wisconsin Card Sort Test, Stroop Color-Word

Table 2.4 Components of a neuropsychological evaluation applicable to dementia

Function	Test employed*
General intellectual function	• Wechsler Adult Intelligence Scale-Revised (WAIS-R) • Ravens Progressive Matrices
Language	• Boston Naming Test • Boston Diagnostic Aphasia Examination • Token test • National Adult Reading Test (NART)
Memory	• Rey Auditory Verbal Learning Test • California Verbal Learning Test • Wechsler Memory Scale (WMS) • Paired Associate Learning • Fuld Object-Memory Test • Buschke Selective Reminding Test • Rey-Osterreith Complex Figure (delayed recall)
Visuospatial skills	• Rey-Osterreith Complex Figure • Hooper Visual Organization Test • Embedded Figures Test • Judgment of Line Orientation
Executive function	• Verbal fluency • Nonverbal fluency • Trail making tests (A, B) • Wisconsin Card Sort Test • Stroop Color-Word Test • Porteus mazes • Consonant trigrams • Digit-symbol test • Letter cancellation • Tower of Hanoi test
Motor function	• Finger tapping • Grooved pegboard

*Not all tests in each category are used.

Test, Porteus mazes, consonant trigrams, digit-symbol test, letter cancellation, or the Tower of Hanoi Test. Motor functions can be assessed with finger tapping and the grooved pegboard. Patients with more advanced cognitive dysfunction cannot meaningfully participate in any of these tests, and neuropsychological assessment is most useful when patients have MMSE scores of 15 or above.

Executive function is a particularly important area to evaluate in the course of assessing patients with neuropsychiatric symptoms. Dysfunction of the frontal lobes frequently produces both executive abnormalities and behavioral disturbances. Table 2.5 lists executive function tests as they relate to individual components of volitional activities.

Laboratory assessment

No dementia syndrome has a diagnostic laboratory test except for the very small number of patients with autosomal dominant Alzheimer's disease or autosomal dominant frontotemporal dementia where a causative mutation can be identified. In this small group of patients a definitive laboratory test is available. Outside of this rare circumstance, laboratory assessment of patients with dementia is targeted primarily on excluding common comorbid conditions, or generating information supportive of specific diagnoses.[33] Hypothyroidism and vitamin B12 deficiency can both cause dementia in the elderly and exacerbate dementias due to other disorders. Screening for these two conditions should be performed routinely as part of the dementia assessment.[33] A complete blood count, serum electrolytes, blood sugar, blood urea nitrogen (BUN), and liver function tests are useful for screening for physical illness in many elderly patients. Other tests such as serological tests for syphilis, acquired immunodeficiency syndrome (AIDS), and other infections should be tested when circumstances suggest that one of these infections may play a role in the dementia syndrome. Serum levels of medications may assist in determining whether medication toxicity is contributing to cognitive decline. Patients with unexplained vascular dementia should be evaluated with erythrocyte sedimentation rate,

Table 2.5 Executive function tests as they relate to individual components of volitional activities

Frontal function	Assessment	Abnormality
Volition	WCST; odd-man-out; Theory of Mind; proverbs; judgment	Poor judgment; lack of empathy; impaired insight
Plan	Fluency (verbal and nonverbal); Stroop Color-Word Test; Complex Figure tests; Tower tests	Reduced verbal and nonverbal fluency; poor strategy; inability to adjust to novelty; reduced working memory
Program	Alternating programs; reciprocal programs	Impaired programming
Implement	WCST; multiple loops; environmental dependency tests; fluency (verbal and nonverbal)	Reduced initiation; utilization behavior; imitation behavior; reduced fluency
Monitor	Cancellation tests; go/no go; mazes; Stroop Color-Word Test; anti-saccade test	Inability to withhold responses; impaired attention; distractibility; intrusions
Adjust	WCST; judgment	Perseveration; reduced response to feedback

serum cholesterol and lipid levels, sickle cell screening test, serum fibrinogen level, coagulation factor abnormalities, or anti-phospholipid and anti-cardiolipin antibodies.[34]

Neuroimaging

Neuroimaging has assumed an increasingly important role in the diagnosis and differential diagnosis of dementia syndromes. Structural imaging (computerized tomography (CT) and magnetic resonance imaging (MRI)) are recommended as a routine part of the dementia assessment.[33] CT may reveal hydrocephalus, generalized atrophy, or focal atrophy in syndromes such as frontotemporal lobar degeneration. Large strokes may be evident and subcortical white matter injury may be demonstrated as increased periventricular lucency. MRI is more sensitive to vascular changes than CT and provides better delineation of structural changes in the brain. MRI is particularly sensitive to ischemic brain injury and increased signal on the T2-weighted image will be evident in areas of ischemic injury.

Functional neuroimaging with single photon emission computerized tomography (SPECT) or positron emission tomography (PET) can provide valuable differential diagnostic information. SPECT and O^{15}-PET measure cerebral blood flow; fluorodeoxyglucose (FDG) PET provides a measure of brain-glucose metabolism. Compared with normal elderly individuals, patients with Alzheimer's disease have diminished metabolism or blood flow in the parietal regions bilaterally. Individuals with frontotemporal dementia have decreased frontal and anterior lobe function; and persons with dementia with Lewy bodies have greater reductions in occipital function than is typical in Alzheimer's disease[35,36] (Figure 2.7).

Other forms of neuroimaging such as functional MRI (fMRI) and magnetic resonance spectroscopy are not routinely applied in the assessment of dementia. They provide research-level information and may eventually be incorporated more commonly into the assessment of patients with dementia.

Electroencephalography (EEG) is not recommended as part of the routine assessment of patients with dementia. However, in specific circumstances EEG can be valuable in differential diagnosis. Patients with Creutzfeldt-Jakob disease (Chapter 8) may exhibit striking periodic polyspike and wave discharges that are rare in other dementia syndromes.

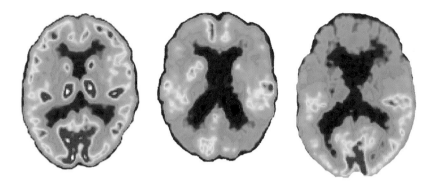

Figure 2.7 *Fluorodeoxyglucose positron emission tomogram (FDG PET) of a normal elderly individual (left), patient with Alzheimer's disease (middle), and patient with frontotemporal lobar degeneration (right) revealing parietal hypometabolism in Alzheimer's disease and frontal hypometabolism in frontotemporal lobar degeneration. (Image courtesy of J Felix and A Toga, Laboratory of Neuroimaging, UCLA School of Medicine.)*

Nerve conduction studies may be useful in aiding identification of peripheral neuropathies in patients with rare dementia syndromes that occur in conjunction with peripheral neuropathic disturbances (e.g. metachromatic leukodystrophy, neuroacanthocytosis).

Cerebrospinal fluid studies

Routine cerebrospinal fluid (CSF) studies are normal in patients with Alzheimer's disease and most other dementing illnesses. The 14-3-3 protein is elevated in patients with Creutzfeldt-Jakob disease (Chapter 8).[37,38] This protein is rarely found in other dementing disorders. Decreased levels of CSF beta-amyloid protein and increased levels of tau protein are characteristic of Alzheimer's disease.[39,40] When used together, the tests provide a diagnostic sensitivity of 85% and a specificity of 85% for the diagnosis of Alzheimer's disease.[41] Characteristic changes in other dementing illnesses such as dementia with Lewy bodies or frontotemporal dementia have not been described. Routine sampling of CSF as part of the dementia assessment is not warranted.

Synthesis

A final diagnosis rests on a synthesis of information derived from the history; neuropsychiatric, neurocognitive, and neurologic examinations; laboratory tests; and neuroimaging. Sufficient information will be obtained to provide an accurate diagnosis in most cases. In some circumstances, however, longitudinal observation with repeated examination or initiating treatment and monitoring the therapeutic benefit will be required before a diagnosis can be achieved. In all cases, periodical assessment is warranted to identify emerging neuropsychiatric symptoms as well as deterioration in cognition and function. Routine reassessment of the caregiver is required to identify signs of increasing stress and burden.

References

1. American Psychiatric Association. *Diagnostic and Statistical Manual of Mental Disorders: DSM-IV*, 4th edn. Washington, DC: American Psychiatric Association, 1994.
2. World Health Organization. *Schedules for Clinical Assessment in Neuropsychiatry: Version 2 Glossary*. Geneva: World Health Organization, 1993–1994.
3. Cummings JL, Trimble MR. *Concise Guide to Neuropsychiatry and Behavioral Neurology*. Washington, DC: American Psychiatric Association, 2002.
4. Marin RS. Apathy: a neuropsychiatric syndrome. *J Neuropsychiatry Clin Neurosci* 1991;3:243–54.
5. Marin RS. Differential diagnosis and classification of apathy. *Am J Psychiatry* 1990;147:22–30.
6. Levy ML, Cummings JL, Fairbanks LA et al. Apathy is not depression. *J Neuropsychiatry Clin Neurosci* 1998;10:314–19.
7. Kuzis G, Sabe L, Tiberti C et al. Neuropsychological correlates of apathy and depression in patients with dementia. *Neurology* 1999;52:1403–7.
8. Parker G, Hadzi-Pavlovic D. Development and structure of the CORE system. In: Parker G (ed) *Melancholia: A Disorder of Movement and Mood*. Cambridge, UK: Cambridge University Press, 1996: 82–129.
9. Alexopoulos GS, Meyers BS, Young RC et al. The course of geriatric depression with reversible dementia: a controlled study. *Am J Psychiatry* 1993; 150:1693–9.
10. Trzepacz PT, Baker RW. *The Psychiatric Mental Status Examination*. New York: Oxford University Press, 1993.
11. Strub RL, Black FW. *The Mental Status Examination in Neurology*, 3rd edn. Philadelphia: FA Davis, 1977.
12. Cummings J, Mega M. *Neuropsychiatry and Clinical Neuroscience*. New York: Oxford University Press.

13. Folstein MF, Folstein SE, McHugh PR. 'Mini-Mental State': a practical method for grading the cognitive state of patients for the clinician. *J Psychiatr Res* 1975;12:189–98.
14. Rosen WG, Mohs RC, Davis KL. A new rating scale for Alzheimer's disease. *Am J Psychiatry* 1984;141:1356–64.
15. Mattis S. *Dementia Rating Scale (DRS)*. Psychological Assessment Resources: Odessa, FL, 1988.
16. Dubois B, Slachevsky A, Litvan I *et al*. A frontal assessment battery at bedside. *Neurology* 2000;55:1621–6.
17. Royall DR, Mahurin RK, Gray KF. Bedside assessment of executive cognitive impairment: the Executive Interview. *J Am Geriatr Soc* 1992;40:1221–6.
18. Lawton MP, Brody EM. Assessment of older people: Self-maintaining and instrumental activities of daily living. *Gerontologist* 1969;9:179–86.
19. Pfeffer RI, Kurosaki TT, Harrah CH *et al*. Measurement of functional activities in older adults in the community. *J Gerontol* 1992;37:323–9.
20. Galasko D, Bennett DA, Sano K *et al*. An inventory to assess activities of daily living for clinical trials in Alzheimer's disease. *Alzheimer Dis Assoc Disorders* 1997;11:S33–S39.
21. Alexopoulos GS, Abrams RC, Young RC *et al*. Cornell Scale for depression in dementia. *Biol Psychiatry* 1988;23:271–84.
22. Yesavage JA, Brink TL, Rose TL *et al*. Development and validation of a geriatric depression screening scale: a preliminary report. *J Psychiatr Res* 1983;17:37–49.
23. Cohen-Mansfield J. Agitated behaviors in the elderly II. Preliminary results in the cognitively deteriorated. *J Am Geriatr Soc* 1986;34:722–7.
24. Cummings JL, Mega M, Gray K *et al*. The Neuropsychiatric Inventory: comprehensive assessment of psychopathology in dementia. *Neurology* 1994; 44:2308–14.
25. Reisberg B, Borenstein J, Salob SP *et al*. Behavioral symptoms in Alzheimer's disease: phenomenology and treatment. *J Clin Psychiatry* 1987;48:9–15.
26. Tariot PN, Mack JL, Patterson MB *et al*. The Behavior Rating Scale for dementia of the consortium to establish a registry for Alzheimer's disease. *Am J Psychiatry* 1995;152:1349–57.
27. Blau TH. Quality of life, social indicators, and criteria of change. *Professional Psychology* 1977:464–73.
28. Logsdon RG, Gibbons LE, McCurry SM *et al*. Quality of life in Alzheimer's disease: patient and caregiver reports. In: Albert SM, Logsdon RG (eds) *Assessing Quality of Life in Alzheimer's Disease*. New York: Springer Publishing Company, 2000: 17–30.
29. Zarit SH, Reever KE, Bach-Peterson J. Relatives of the impaired elderly: correlates of feeling of burden. *Gerontologist* 1980;20:649–55.
30. Teri L, Truax P, Logsdon R *et al*. Assessment of behavioral problems in dementia: the revised memory and behavior problems checklist. *Psychol Aging* 1992;7(4):622–31.
31. Therapeutics and Technology Assessment Subcommittee of the American Academy of Neurology. Assessment: Neuropsychological testing of adults. Considerations for neurologists. *Neurology* 1996;47:592–9.

32. Lezak MD. *Neuropsychological Assessment*. New York: Oxford University Press, 1995.
33. Knopman DS, DeKosky ST, Cummings JL *et al*. Practice parameter: diagnosis of dementia (an evidence-based review). Report of the Quality Standards Subcommittee of the American Academy of Neurology. *Neurology* 2001; 56:1143–53.
34. Adams HP Jr, del Zoppo GJ, von Kummer R. Management of stroke: a practical guide for the prevention, evaluation and treatment of acute stroke. Caddo, OK: Professional Communications, 1998.
35. Silverman D, Small GW, Chang CY *et al*. Positron emission tomography in evaluation of dementia: regional brain metabolism and long-term outcome. *JAMA* 2001;286:2120–7.
36. Steinling M, Defebvre L, Duhamel A *et al*. Is there a typical pattern of brain SPECT imaging in Alzheimer's disease? *Dement Geriatr Cogn Disord* 2001; 12:371–8.
37. Hsich G, Kenney K, Gibbs CJ *et al*. The 14-3-3 brain protein in cerebrospinal fluid as a marker for transmissible spongiform encephalopathies. *N Engl J Med* 1996;335:924–30.
38. Zerr I, Bodemer M, Gefeller O *et al*. Detection of 14-3-3 protein in the cerebrospinal fluid supports the diagnosis of Creutzfeldt-Jakob disease. *Ann Neurol* 1998;43:32–40.
39. Motter R, Vigo-Pelfrey C, Kholodenko D *et al*. Reduction of β-amyloid peptide$_{42}$ in the cerebrospinal fluid of patients with Alzheimer's disease. *Ann Neurol* 1995;38:643–8.
40. Vigo-Pelfrey C, Seubert P, Barbour R *et al*. Elevation of microtubule-associated protein tau in the cerebrospinal fluid of patients with Alzheimer's disease. *Neurology* 1995;45:788–93.
41. Hulstaert F, Blennow K, Ivanoiu A *et al*. Improved discrimination of AD patients using B-amyloid$_{(1-42)}$ and tau levels in CSF. *Neurology* 1999; 52:1555–62.

chapter 3

Alzheimer's disease

Alzheimer's disease (AD) is a progressive neurodegenerative disorder with cognitive, behavioral, and functional abnormalities. The disease is increasingly common as individuals age and typically lasts a decade from onset to death. As the world's population ages the number of individuals with AD is rising dramatically (Chapter 1).

Box 3.1 provides criteria for a diagnosis for definite, probable, or possible AD.[1] A diagnosis of *definite AD* requires that the patient meet clinical criteria for probable AD while living and have histopathologic evidence of AD at autopsy or from a cerebral biopsy. Most investigators would now allow a diagnosis of definite AD in an individual who meets clinical criteria for probable AD and has one of the identified causative mutations (described below). *Probable AD* requires that a dementia syndrome is established by clinical examination, documented by mental status questionnaire, and confirmed by neuropsychological testing. Onset of the disorder is between 40 and 90 years of age. There must be deficits in memory and at least one other cognitive function. The memory and cognitive deficits must worsen over time and be present for a minimum of 6 months. The patient must not be delirious at the time of the assessment. There must be an absence of another disorder capable of producing a dementia syndrome. *Possible AD* is diagnosed when there is a systemic disorder or second brain disease capable of producing a dementia, but not thought to be the cause of the current dementia. Alternatively, possible AD is diagnosed when there is gradually progressive decline in a single intellectual function (e.g. loss of memory or language) in the absence of any other identifiable cause. The inter-rater reliability both within nations and in cross-national studies is acceptable with 65–75% agreement.[2,3] The diagnostic accuracy rate of the criteria varies from 85% to 95% and is somewhat better in academic medical centers than in community settings.[4–6]

Box 3.1 Criteria for definite, probable, and possible Alzheimer's disease (AD)

Definite AD
• Clinical criteria for probable AD
• Histopathological evidence of AD (autopsy or biopsy)

Probable AD
• Dementia established by clinical examination and documented by mental status questionnaire
• Dementia confirmed by neuropsychologic testing
• Deficits in two or more areas of cognition
• Progressive worsening of memory and other cognitive functions
• No disturbance of consciousness
• Onset between ages 40 and 90
• Absence of systemic disorders or other brain diseases capable of producing a dementia syndrome

Possible AD
• Presence of a systemic disorder or other brain disease capable of producing dementia but not thought to be the cause of the dementia
• Gradually progressive decline in a single intellectual function in the absence of any other identifiable cause (e.g. memory loss or aphasia)

Unlikely AD
• Sudden onset
• Focal neurologic signs
• Seizures or gait disturbance early in the course of the illness

Demographic characteristics

Alzheimer's disease accounts for 60–70% of cases of progressive cognitive impairment in aged individuals. Most studies suggest that cognitive impairment is present in 10–15% of individuals over the age of 65; AD accounts for a majority of these cases. The prevalence of AD doubles approximately every 5 years after the age of 60, increasing from a prevalence of 1% among those aged 60–64 years to up to 40% among those 85 years or older.[7] Given the aging of the global population, if effective therapy for AD is not identified, the population of AD patients will nearly quadruple in the next 50 years.[8]

A variety of risk factors increase the likelihood of developing AD. Age is the most potent of the known risks. Female gender is also a risk factor; the ratio of affected women to men is 1.2:1 to 1.5:1.[9] A history of head trauma and a low level of educational attainment are additional risks.[10,11]

Genetic risk factors for late-onset AD have been identified. The most important type of these is the apolipoprotein e4 (ApoE-4) allele. This is a cholesterol-bearing protein and the e4 of its three potential forms (e2, e3, e4) increases the likelihood of developing AD and decreases the age at onset.[12] The lifetime risk of AD for an individual without the e4 allele is approximately 10%, whereas the lifetime risk for an individual carrying at least one allele is 30%. Determining the apolipoprotein genotype cannot be regarded as a diagnostic test for AD, since some individuals who do not bear the risk allele develop the illness and some who have the allele are spared the disease.

Several causative mutations for AD have been identified. These are transmitted in an autosomal dominant fashion with complete penetrance; those inheriting the mutation will manifest the illness in the course of their lifetime. Mutations in the amyloid precursor protein gene (APP gene, chromosome 21), presenilin 1 gene (chromosome 14), or the presenilin 2 gene (chromosome 1), produce familial AD.[13,14] Inherited AD is rare, accounting for <5% of all cases. They typically begin early in life, manifesting with a dementia syndrome in the 40s or 50s.

Dementia syndrome and clinical features

The dementia syndrome of AD has characteristic clinical features including memory impairment, disturbances of visuospatial function, language abnormalities, and executive function deficits. Several variants of AD are recognized including those with disproportionate language or visuospatial manifestations, a posterior cortical atrophy form with prominent agnosia and features of Balint's syndrome (simultanagnosia, optic ataxia, 'sticky' fixation), and a frontal variant with prominent executive deficits[15] and more severe behavioral changes.

The typical memory disturbance of AD is an amnestic type of storage abnormality. Patients have difficulty recalling recently learned information and are not assisted by providing clues or a multiple-choice list from which the patient can choose the learned material. Recent memory is more impaired than remote, although remote memory deteriorates as the disease progresses. Both semantic (memory for facts) and episodic (memory for personal events) types of memory are affected; motor skill learning typically is spared.[16]

Language abnormalities in AD begin with a subtle word finding deficit and empty speech with a preference for words of indefinite reference ('thing', 'it') or circumlocutions around the specific word that cannot be identified. Testing at this stage typically reveals only a deficit in verbal fluency with a reduction in the number of items from a category (e.g. animals) that can be named in 1 minute. As the disease progresses an anomia appears, first of the lexical selection type; the patient cannot name a given object but can recognize the name from a multiple-choice list. With further progression, comprehension defects appear and the anomia may progress to a semantic type in which the patient cannot name the object and cannot choose the correct name from among choices. Repetition and reading aloud are disproportionately preserved, creating a transcortical sensory type of aphasia. In the final phases of the disease, the patient's output may be reduced to echolalia (repeating what an examiner or other individual in the environment says) and palilalia (repeating what the patients themselves say).[17]

Visuospatial deficits in AD feature a progressive decline from difficulty copying complex figures such as a cube or the Rey-Osterreith Complex Figure to an inability to copy even the most simple stimulus item such as a circle or box. Environmental disorientation, route finding difficulties, and problems with dressing are common visuospatial disturbances.

Mental status questionnaires are useful in providing a global quantification of the deficits and a means of characterizing the stage of the patient's cognitive decline. The Mini-Mental State Examination (MMSE)[18] is the most widely used mental status questionnaire of this type. It includes 30 questions assessing orientation, learning, attention, serial subtraction/attention, recall, naming, repetition, comprehension, reading, writing, and copying a complex figure. It is generally insensitive to the cognitive abnormalities present in the earliest phases of AD and also loses applicability in the final phases of the disease. It is not specific for dementia and patients with aphasia, amnesia, or delirium also perform abnormally on the MMSE. Patients of low educational level perform more poorly on the examination and scores must be adjusted appropriately. Neuropsychological testing with standardized assessment of attention, language, memory, visuospatial skills, and executive functions provides a means of quantifying the deficits of AD and aids in distinguishing patients with early impairments from normal aging.

Motor and sensory abnormalities are typically absent until the final phases of AD and abrupt onset, presence of focal neurological signs, or the occurrence of seizures or gait disturbances early in the clinical course are features that render the diagnosis of AD unlikely.[1] As the disease progresses, however, rigidity, dysphagia, and incontinence appear. Patients lose the ability to ambulate and become bedridden in the final phases of the disease. Patients with AD typically succumb to bronchitis, pneumonia, or urinary tract infections.[19]

The onset of AD is not abrupt and patients pass through a phase of mild cognitive impairment (MCI) during which they exhibit cognitive deficits that are distinguishable from normal aging, but do not meet full criteria for AD. A variety of clinical criteria for MCI have been proffered; a commonly used definition defines MCI as a syndrome in which the patient or caregiver voices complaints about the patient's memory, there is a deficit in recalling new information demonstrated by neuropsychological testing, there are no significant deficits in other cognitive domains, and the patient has no disturbances in activities of daily living.[20] Patients progress to diagnosable AD from the MCI condition at a rate of approximately 15% per year. Thus, about half of the patients followed for 3 years will have converted from MCI to AD. Not all cases of MCI progress to AD.

Neuroimaging

The use of neuroimaging in the assessment of patients with dementia is described in Chapter 2. In the evaluation of patients with suspected AD, structural imaging with computerized tomography (CT) or magnetic resonance imaging (MRI) commonly reveals mild to severe cortical atrophy. Structural imaging may also reveal comorbid pathology such as cerebrovascular disease or, rarely, alternative causes of dementia such as hydrocephalus.

Functional neuroimaging with single photon emission computed tomography (SPECT) or fluorodeoxyglucose positron emission tomography (FDG PET) usually demonstrates global hypoperfusion or hypometabolism that is most marked in the parietal lobes bilaterally.[21] Patients with a variety of types of behavioral changes (described below) have greater reductions in frontal lobe activity than those without neuropsychiatric symptoms (Figure 3.1).

Pathology and molecular biology

The current criteria for the pathologic diagnosis of AD require the presence of both neuritic plaques and neurofibrillary tangles (Box 3.2). The pathologic diagnosis is confirmed when there are frequent neuritic plaques using the criteria developed by the Consortium to Establish a Registry for Alzheimer's Disease (CERAD)[22] and neurofibrillary tangles in an abundance graded by the Braak and Braak approach as stage V–VI.[23]

a   b

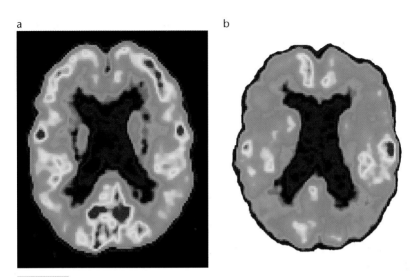

Figure 3.1 Positron emission tomogram of patient with AD and few behavioral symptoms (a) and of patient with apathy, agitation and delusions (b) showing greater frontal involvement in the patient with behavioral disturbances (images courtesy of J Felix, Laboratory of Neuroimaging, UCLA School of Medicine).

Box 3.2 Criteria for the neuropathologic diagnosis of Alzheimer's disease

The following categories are recommended to provide an estimate of the likelihood that Alzheimer's disease pathological changes underlie dementia:

- High likelihood: the presence of both neuritic plaques and neurofibrillary tangles in neocortex (i.e. a frequent neuritic plaque score according to CERAD (Consortium to Establish a Registry for Alzheimer's Disease) and a Braak and Braak stage V/VI
- Intermediate likelihood: moderate neocortical neuritic plaques and neurofibrillary tangles in limbic regions (i.e. CERAD moderate and Braak and Braak stage III/IV)
- Low likelihood: neuritic plaques and neurofibrillary tangles in a more limited distribution and/or severity (i.e. CERAD infrequent and Braak and Braak stage I/II)

(From the National Institute on Aging and Reagan Institute Working Group on Diagnostic Criteria for the Neuropathological Assessment of Alzheimer's Disease)

Neuritic plaques (Figure 3.2) have a central core of amyloid protein surrounded by astrocytes, microglia, and dystrophic neurites containing paired helical filaments.[24,25] Apolipoprotein E and acute phase reactants indicative of an inflammatory response are also present. Neuritic plaque densities are highest in the temporal and occipital lobes, intermediate in the parietal lobes, and lowest in the frontal and limbic cortex[26] (Figure 3.3). Beta-amyloid similar to that found in plaques is deposited in leptomeningeal and superficial cortical vessels thus producing an amyloid angiopathy.[27]

Neurofibrillary tangles (Figure 3.4) are the second major histopathological feature of AD. They are comprised of paired helical filaments of abnormally phosphorylated tau protein. These filaments disrupt normal intracellular transport and result in cell death. They are most likely to form in large pyramidal cells. They begin in transentorhinal cortex progressing to other limbic cortical regions and finally reach the neocortex in the most advanced phases of the illness[23,26,28] (Figure 3.5).

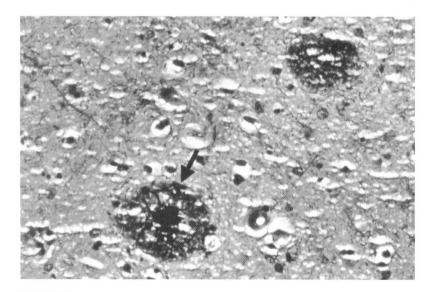

Figure 3.2 *Neuritic plaque (magnification 435 × 220; Bielschowsky stain) (courtesy of H Vinters, MD, Neuropathology, UCLA School of Medicine).*

Neuritic plaques

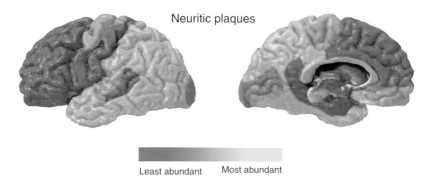

Least abundant   Most abundant

Figure 3.3 *Distribution of neuritic plaques. Reproduced with permission from: Cummings JL, Cole G. Alzheimer's disease. JAMA 2002;287:2335–8 (image courtesy of J Felix, Laboratory of Neuroimaging, UCLA School of Medicine).*

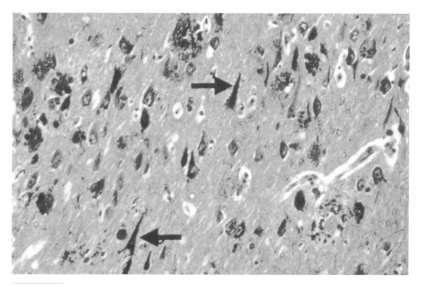

Figure 3.4 *Neurofibrillary tangle (435 × 220; Bielschowsky stain) (courtesy of H Vinters, MD, Neuropathology, UCLA School of Medicine).*

In addition to the two classical histopathological features, the brains of patients with AD also feature a reduction in synaptic density, loss of neurons, and granulovacuolar degeneration in hippocampal neurons. Neuronal loss in the nuclei responsible for maintenance of transmitter systems results in a reduction in several major neurotransmitters. Cell

Neurofibillary tangles

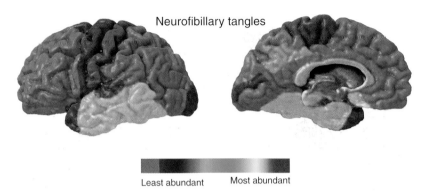

Least abundant   Most abundant

Figure 3.5 *Distribution of neurofibrillary tangles. Reproduced with permission from: Cummings JL, Cole G. Alzheimer's disease. JAMA 2002;287:2335–8 (figure courtesy of J Felix, Laboratory of Neuroimaging, UCLA School of Medicine).*

loss in the nucleus basilis leads to deficits in cortical synthesis of acetylcholine; reduction of cells in the locus ceruleus leads to a deficiency in norepinephrine; and neuronal loss in the raphe nuclei produces a serotonergic deficit.[24,29] Figure 3.6 shows the regional intensity of the cholinergic deficit in AD.

The distribution of plaques, tangles, and cell loss in the neocortex suggests that instrumental deficits such as aphasia and visuospatial abnormalities are attributable primarily to plaque formation and related cellular abnormalities. Neurofibrillary tangles contribute to the memory disturbance and the neuropsychiatric symptoms of the illness, while transmitter deficits – particularly the deficiency in acetylcholine – play a role in both cognitive and behavioral changes.

Cerebrovascular disease commonly co-occurs with AD. Up to 25% of patients clinically identified with AD may have concomitant infarctions or ischemic injury at autopsy.

Studies in the molecular biology of AD have provided substantial insights into the underlying pathophysiological process. Amyloid precursor protein (APP) is metabolized by a variety of intracellular proteases. Beta-secretase cleaves APP at an extracellular site just beyond the cell membrane; gamma-secretase cleaves APP in the transmembrane portion of the protein[28,31] (Figure 3.7). These cleavages result in the production of the beta-amyloid peptide, and these peptide molecules form

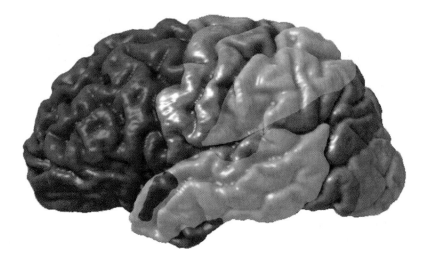

Figure 3.6 *Cortical distribution of the cholinergic deficit in Alzheimer's disease. Gray areas have no consistent reduction of cholinergic markers; magenta indicates reduction of 40–50%; light blue, reduction of 50–60%; purple, reduction of 60–70%; and yellow, reduction of 70–80%.[30] (Figure courtesy of J Felix, Laboratory of Neuroimaging, UCLA School of Medicine).*

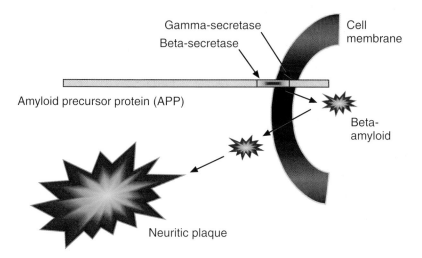

Figure 3.7 *Schematic representation of the cleavage of beta-amyloid from the amyloid precursor protein by beta-secretase and gamma-secretase to form neuritic plaques.*

protofibrils that are neurotoxic. After transport into the extracellular space, the beta-amyloid peptide aggregates to form diffuse plaques which eventually mature to neuritic plaques.[25] The accumulation of beta-amyloid may be facilitated by the ApoE 4 protein. The production of beta-amyloid initiates a series of events contributing to cell death[32] (Figure 3.8). The generation of reactive oxygen species leads to mitochondrial dysfunction and the activation of cell death programs as well as oxidation of lipids and disruption of cell membranes. This oxidative injury may provide the basis for the use of antioxidants in the treatment of AD (described below). Amyloid beta protein also leads to complement activation, recruitment of microglial cells, and exaggeration of cell death through inflammatory mechanisms.[33,34] Cholesterol enhances amyloid protein production or aggregation, and epidemiologic studies suggest that cholesterol-lowering statin drugs reduce the risk of AD.[35] The linkage between the formation of neuritic plaques and the generation of neurofibrillary tangles is not completely understood, but there is increas-

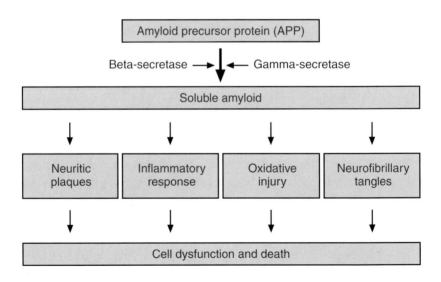

Figure 3.8 *Cascade of events beginning with amyloid precursor protein, progressing to the generation of soluble amyloid, the formation of neuritic plaques, an inflammatory response, oxidative injury, and neurofibrillary tangles that lead to cell dysfunction or neuronal death.*

ing consensus that in AD tangle formation is a product of metabolic events initiated by beta-amyloid formation. All mutations associated with AD lead to increased production of beta-amyloid and several of the modifying factors (ApoE genotype, statins, administration of anti-inflammatory drugs, etc.) appear to exert their effects through the amyloid cascade.

Neuropsychiatric symptoms

Alzheimer's disease is accompanied by a variety of neuropsychiatric disturbances. Symptoms such as apathy, dysphoria, and agitation are common, occurring in a majority of patients. Other symptoms such as euphoria are rare and aid in distinguishing patients with AD from other types of dementia syndromes including frontotemporal lobar degeneration (Chapter 7). Behavioral disturbances and neuropsychiatric symptoms are more common in the frontal variant of AD than in other subsyndromes of the disorder.[16,24]

The Neuropsychiatric Inventory (NPI)[36] has been used to provide a multi-dimensional profile of the behavioral alterations occurring in patients with AD (Figure 3.9). When the NPI is analyzed according to dementia severity, patients with more severe cognitive abnormalities are more likely to exhibit behavioral changes. Thus, as the brain disease worsens, there is a decline in cognition and the emergence of new neuropsychiatric symptoms (Figure 3.10). Multiple simultaneous symptoms are the rule in patients with AD. Patients not uncommonly simultaneously manifest agitation, psychosis, and symptoms of depression or other symptom constellations.[38] Longitudinal studies reveal that although they fluctuate somewhat, once symptoms appear they are highly likely to persist and be present on subsequent examinations.[38,39]

Factor analysis of the NPI reveals a three-factor solution including eight of the 10 subscales and accounting for 60% of the total variance. The three factors comprise a mood factor with anxiety and depression, a psychosis factor including agitation, hallucinations, delusions, and irritability, and a frontal behavior factor including disinhibition and

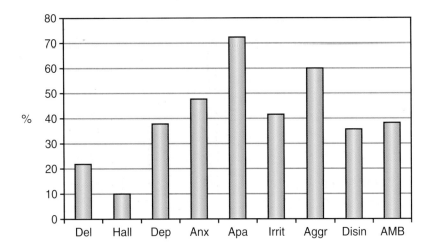

Figure 3.9 *Percent of patients with scoreable symptoms on the Neuropsychiatric Inventory (n = 50).[37] Del, delusions; Hall, hallucinations; Dep, depression; Anx, anxiety; Apa, apathy; Irrit, irritability; Aggr, aggression/agitation; Disin, disinhibition; AMB, aberrant motor behavior.*

euphoria.[40] Apathy and aberrant motor behavior did not load heavily on any single factor. Similarly, latest class analysis of the NPI suggests three groups of patients: one with few neuropsychiatric symptoms, one with a mood disorder and one with psychotic symptoms.[41] There is a correlation between the presence of psychiatric symptoms and impairment in activities of daily living. This relationship remains even after adjustment for severity of cognitive impairment.[42]

Apathy

Apathy is among the most common symptoms of AD in some investigations.[37,43–45] The apathy of AD is characterized by a lack of interest in usual activities, hobbies, and pursuits; loss of interest in social engagements and interpersonal activities such as meeting friends or spending time with family members; and loss of emotional engagement with reduced affect and diminished intimacy. Apathy is related to the severity of cognitive impairment, but cognitive changes do not account entirely for its occurrence. Likewise, depression and apathy commonly co-occur,

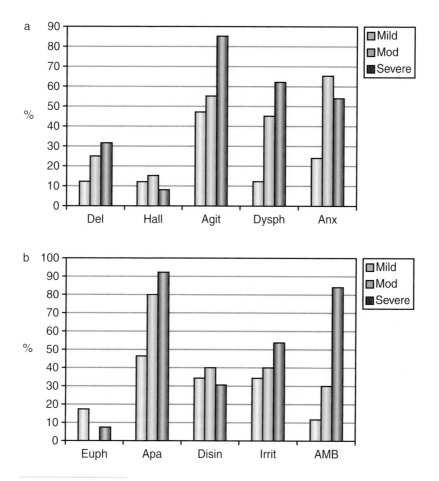

Figure 3.10a and b *Percent of patients manifesting neuropsychiatric symptoms according to disease severity. Mild, Mini-Mental State Examination (MMSE) scores 30–29; Moderate, MMSE scores 20–11; Severe, MMSE scores 10–0 (*n = 50*).[37] Del, delusions; Hall, hallucinations; Agit, agitation; Dysph, dysphoria; Anx, anxiety; Euph, euphoria; Apa, apathy; Disin, disinhibition; Irrit, irritability; AMB, aberrant motor behavior.*

but apathy can occur in the absence of depression and is not necessarily a manifestation of depression.[46] Apathy may coexist with both aberrant motor behavior such as pacing, wandering, and rummaging and with agitation since patients with apathy are not necessarily hypokinetic. Apathy has been associated with diminished executive function including set shifting and verbal fluency; these abilities are more impaired in patients with apathy than those without.[47] Apathetic patients are more functionally impaired than those without apathy.[42,48]

Cerebral blood flow and metabolism are more reduced in the frontal lobes of patients with apathy compared to those without.[49-51] The changes are most marked in the medial frontal/anterior cingulate areas.

Agitation

Agitation is another common behavioral symptom in patients with AD, occurring in approximately 70% of AD patients.[37,52] Consensus about the definition of agitation is lacking, but most definitions include aggressive, disruptive, and resistive behaviors such as threats, pushing, hitting, shouting, and cursing. Some definitions of agitation include less severe behavior such as repeatedly asking questions, pacing, and repetitive stereotyped motor behaviors.[37,53-55] Agitation has been associated with more advanced age, later onset of dementia, and more severe cognitive decline.[37,56] Most studies have found a higher prevalence of aggressive behaviors among men.[57-59] Aggression is significantly related to delusions, misidentification syndromes, activity disturbances, and diurnal behavioral abnormalities.[48,56,59,60] Executive dysfunction indicative of frontal lobe involvement is significantly greater in patients with agitation than those without.[61,62] Agitated and aggressive behaviors tend to be persistent once they have begun in the course of the illness.[39,63,64]

Neuroimaging reveals disproportionately reduced functioning in frontal and temporal regions in patients with aggression and agitation (Figure 3.11).[65,66]

There have been few studies correlating postmortem autopsy findings with agitation and aggression. Palmer and colleagues linked reduced serotonin and its metabolites in the frontal lobes of patients with AD to aggressive behaviors[67] and cholinergic deficits are also more severe in patients with agitation.[68] Dopaminergic cells in the substantia nigra are relatively better preserved in patients with more physical aggression, while the rostral locus ceruleus has greater cell loss in aggressive patients.[69,70] Histopathological studies have identified relationships between agitation and neurofibrillary tangles in the frontal lobe. The

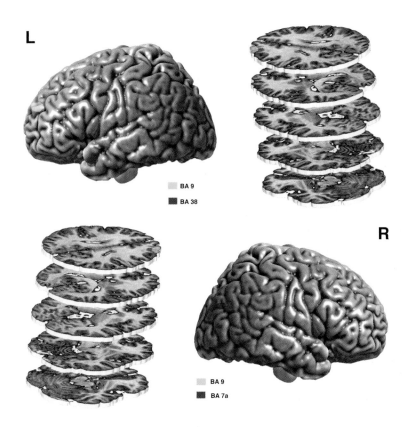

Figure 3.11 *Lateral and medial brain images demonstrating the areas of reduced cerebral blood flow in AD patients with aggression compared with those without aggression[65] (image courtesy of J Felix, Laboratory of Neuroimaging, UCLA School of Medicine).*

neurofibrillary tangle counts were higher in the orbitofrontal and anterior cingulate regions of patients with agitation compared with those without agitation (Figure 3.12).[71] There was no difference in the abundance of neuritic plaques or Lewy bodies in the two groups.

Given the neuropsychological evidence of frontal dysfunction as well as imaging and pathological evidence of disproportional involvement of the frontal lobes in patients with AD and agitation, this syndrome may be viewed as a dysregulation syndrome with a loss of ability to modulate behavior in response to environmental provocations or emotional

a   b

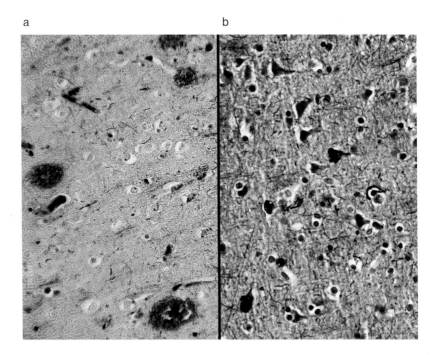

Figure 3.12 *Section of the frontal cortex from a patient without agitation (a) and with agitation (b) demonstrating more neurofibrillary tangles in the patient with agitation (400×; modified Bielschowski silver technique)[71] (reprinted with the permission of the publisher).*

disturbances arising from comorbid neuropsychiatric disorders such as psychosis or depression (Chapter 9).

Depression

The relationship between depression and AD is complex and not all research findings agree. Several studies suggest that late-onset depression is commonly present in the few years immediately preceding the onset of AD.[72,73] A remote history of depression also may confer an increased risk for AD later in life.[73] Depression symptoms are common at the onset of AD[74] and most studies concur that depressive symptoms become increasingly common with disease progression.[37] A positive family history of depressive illness is a risk factor for the occurrence of depression after the onset of AD.[75–77]

Studies of convenience samples of patients attending clinics find prevalence rates of major depression of patients with AD varying between 1.5% and 25%. Minor depression is reported in 10–30%.[78-84] Family reporters tend to overestimate the presence of depression, attributing many symptoms of dementia to a mood disorder.[85,86] Thus, the information source may affect the recorded frequency of depression in a given population of AD patients. Major depression is more persistent in longitudinal studies than minor depression.

Depression is related to other behavioral symptoms including aggressive behavior[79,87] and behaviors such as irritability/complaining and demandingness/dependency may be alternative manifestations of mood changes in patients with AD.[83] Patients with depressive symptoms manifest greater dysfunctional disability on measures of activities of daily living than patients without mood symptoms.[79,88-90] Depression tends to worsen with more cognitive impairment.[37,91]

Provisional diagnostic criteria for depression of AD modeled on those of the 4th edition of the *Diagnostic and Statistical Manual of Mental Disorders*[92] have been developed by a work group of the National Institute of Mental Health (Box 3.3).[93] Patients must exhibit either a depressed mood, decreased positive affect, or inability to experience pleasure, plus at least three of the following symptoms during the same 2-week period: depressed mood, decreased affect or pleasure in response to social contacts and usual activities, social isolation or withdrawal, disruption in appetite, disruption in sleep, psychomotor changes (e.g. agitation or retardation), irritability, fatigue or loss of energy, feelings of worthlessness, hopelessness, or excessive or inappropriate guilt, or recurrent thoughts of death or suicidal ideation, plan or attempt. The symptoms must be sufficiently severe to produce significant distress or disrupt functioning and must not occur exclusively with delirium. They must not be due to the direct effects of a substance or be better accounted for by another cause of depression.[93] These actions define a disorder which may not necessarily be severe enough to meet all criteria for a major depressive episode. This is characteristic of AD where depressive symptoms of the type described in the criteria are more common than major depressive episodes.[94,95]

Box 3.3 Provisional National Institute of Mental Health diagnostic criteria for depression of Alzheimer's disease[93]

- Three (or more) of the following symptoms have been present during the same 2-week period and represent a change from previous functioning: at least one of the symptoms is either (1) depressed mood or (2) decreased positive affect or pleasure

  Note: Do not include symptoms that, in your judgment, are clearly due to a medical condition other than Alzheimer's disease, or are a direct result of non-mood-related dementia symptoms (e.g. loss of weight due to difficulties with food intake)

- Clinically significant depressed mood (e.g. depressed, sad, hopeless, discouraged, tearful)
- Decreased positive affect or pleasure in response to social contacts and usual activities
- Social isolation or withdrawal
- Disruption in appetite
- Disruption in sleep
- Psychomotor changes (e.g. agitation or retardation)
- Irritability
- Fatigue or loss of energy
- Feelings of worthlessness, hopelessness, or excessive or inappropriate guilt
- Recurrent thoughts of death, suicidal ideation, plan or attempt
- All criteria are met for Dementia of the Alzheimer's Type (DSM-IV)
- The symptoms cause clinically significant distress or disruption in functioning
- The symptoms do not occur exclusively during the course of a delirium
- The symptoms are not due to the direct physiological effects of a substance (e.g. a drug of abuse or a medication)
- The symptoms are not better accounted for by other conditions such as major depressive disorder, bipolar disorder, bereavement, schizophrenia, schizoaffective disorder, psychosis of Alzheimer's disease, anxiety disorders, or substance-related disorder

Specify if:
- Co-occurring onset: if onset antedates or co-occurs with the AD symptoms
- Post AD onset: if onset occurs after AD symptoms

Specify:
- With psychosis of Alzheimer's disease
- With other significant behavioral signs or symptoms
- With past history of mood disorder

Quantitative EEG studies reveal increased posterior slowing in patients with AD and depression compared with AD patients without depressive mood changes.[96] Imaging studies have found a relationship between white matter intensity on MRI and the presence of depressive symptoms in patients with AD. This correlation is strongest with white matter abnormalities in the frontal lobes.[97–99] Results from functional imaging studies have been variable. There is a consistent observation that cerebral blood flow and metabolism are reduced in depressed compared with nondepressed patients with AD; regions of hypoperfusion have included frontal, temporal, and parietal areas.[68,100,101] Several studies have found that patients with AD and depression have greater cell loss in the locus ceruleus than patients without depression;[102–104] there is a corresponding reduction of norepinephrine in the cortex.[105] There is also a reduction in cortical serotonin reuptake sites in AD patients with depression compared with those without depressive symptoms.[106]

The dexamethazone suppression test (DST) is abnormal in many elderly patients with depression (failure to suppress serum cortisol levels in response to administration of exogenous dexamethazone). This test has been applied to patients with AD and found not to be useful for identifying patients with mood abnormalities. Many patients with AD exhibit abnormal DST responses whether or not mood abnormalities are present.[107–109]

Psychosis

Psychosis in AD is represented by the occurrence of delusions or hallucinations that have their onset after the appearance of the dementia syndrome, have been present at least intermittently for 1 month or longer, are severe enough to disrupt patient function, do not occur exclusively during delirium, and are not attributable to some other psychotic disorder or to a substance-induced disorder[110] (Box 3.4). The combined prevalence of delusions and hallucinations in cross-sectional studies is 40–65%; delusions account for 30–50% of psychotic phenomena, and hallucinations for 10–20%.[111–114] Typical delusions manifested by patients with AD include erroneous beliefs that others are stealing from them, a misidentification delusion similar to the Capgras syndrome in

Box 3.4 Diagnostic criteria for psychosis of Alzheimer's disease (AD)[110]

- *Presence of one (or more) of the following symptoms:*
  Visual or auditory hallucinations
  Delusions
- *Primary diagnosis*
  All the criteria for dementia of the Alzheimer type are met
- *Chronology of the onset of symptoms of psychosis vs onset of symptoms of dementia*
  There is evidence from the history that the symptoms in the delusions or hallucinations were not present continuously before the onset of the symptoms of dementia
- *Duration and severity*
  The symptom(s) in the delusions or hallucinations have been present, at least intermittently, for 1 month or longer
  Symptoms are severe enough to cause some disruption in the patient's functioning
- *Exclusion of schizophrenia and related psychotic disorders*
  Criteria for schizophrenia, schizoaffective disorder, delusional disorder, or mood disorder with psychotic features have never been met
- *Relationship to delirium*
  The disturbance does not occur exclusively during the course of a delirium
- *Exclusion of other causes of psychotic symptoms*
  The disturbance is not better accounted for by another general medical condition or direct physiological effects of a substance (e.g. a drug of abuse, a medication)

Associated features: *(specify if present)*
- With agitation: when there is evidence, from history or examination, of prominent agitation with or without physical or verbal aggression
- With negative symptoms: when prominent negative symptoms, such as apathy, affective flattening, avolition, or motor retardation, are present
- With depression: when prominent depressive symptoms, such as depressed mood, insomnia or hypersomnia, feelings of worthlessness or excessive or inappropriate guilt, or recurrent thoughts of death, are present

which the patient believes that a family member is not whom they claim to be, delusions of infidelity, and the delusion that the house in which they are living is not their home.[42,115-120] More unusual delusions in patients with AD include persistent beliefs in visitations from a deceased spouse,[121] delusions of infestation,[122] erotomania or the belief that someone of higher social position is in love with them,[123] and misidentification of the self.[124] In some cases it may be difficult to distinguish delusions from convictions resulting from memory impairment, but in most cases the distress associated with the false belief, the co-occurrence of delusions and hallucinations, and the maintenance of the belief over time help to distinguish delusions from memory disorders. Most delusional patients have several types of delusions simultaneously.[119]

Delusions become more frequent in patients in more advanced phases of the disease and are correlated with more severe dementia.[37,125] In the most advanced phases of AD, patients lose the ability to speak and in this inchoate state may be unable to verbalize paranoid and persecutory experiences. The delusions may be one etiology of agitation in these advanced patients. Patients with delusions and hallucinations experience more rapid cognitive decline although they may not have a shortened disease course.[126-131] In rare cases, delusions may be the presenting manifestations of AD.[132,133] Delusions are associated with aggression, anxiety, and purposeless behavior.[48,134-136] Correlations between specific cognitive deficits and the occurrence of delusions have varied. Individual studies have found relationships with language comprehension, naming, abstraction, memory, and verbal fluency.[136-139] Individual domains of cognitive abnormality appear to account for relatively little of the variance in the occurrence of delusional disorders in AD. Deafness may worsen psychotic symptoms.[140]

Patients with visual hallucinations are more likely to evidence auditory hallucinations, delusions, and aggressive outbursts. They have more advanced disease and are more likely to manifest extrapyramidal symptoms than patients without hallucinations.[141,142] Visual hallucinations may be exaggerated or precipitated by impaired visual acuity.[143,144]

Several studies have assessed the utility of electroencephalography (EEG) or quantified electroencephalography (QEEG) to distinguish psychotic from nonpsychotic patients with AD. Most studies have found greater EEG and QEEG slowing in patients with psychosis compared with those without delusions and hallucinations[138,145] (Figure 3.13). These differences are maintained even after adjustment for severity of cognitive impairment.

Studies using SPECT have identified differences between AD patients with and without delusions. Findings vary somewhat from study to study, but all have shown reduced perfusion in the psychotic compared with the nonpsychotic group and the regional abnormalities have been in either the frontal or temporal lobes.[146–150] Mega and colleagues[147] found lower perfusion in right and left dorsolateral prefrontal left anterior cingulate and left ventral striatal regions. There were also reductions in the left pulvinar and the dorsolateral parietal cortex bilaterally[147] (Figure 3.14). Studies using FDG PET largely confirm the observations made with SPECT. The differences between psychotic and nonpsychotic patients are in the direction of reduced metabolic activity in those with psychosis and the areas most commonly implicated are the frontal and temporal regions.[66,151,152]

Relatively few studies have investigated the relationship of psychosis to neuropathological changes at postmortem examination. Psychosis has been associated with significant increases in senile plaques in the medial temporal prosubiculum area and neurofibrillary tangles in the middle frontal cortex, and with diminished neuron counts in the parahippocampal region of the medial temporal lobe.[153,154] Patients with psychosis have a significantly greater density of neocortical neurofibrillary tangles than subjects without psychosis.[155] Relationships have been found between greater concentrations of norepinephrine in the substantia nigra and reduced concentrations of serotonin in the prosubiculum and psychosis.

An increase in M2 muscarinic cholinergic receptors is present in the frontal and temporal cortex of patients with AD and psychosis.[156] The increased abundance of these receptors suggests that they have been upregulated in response to the degenerating presynaptic cholinergic system. This change in receptor density may provide a basis for the

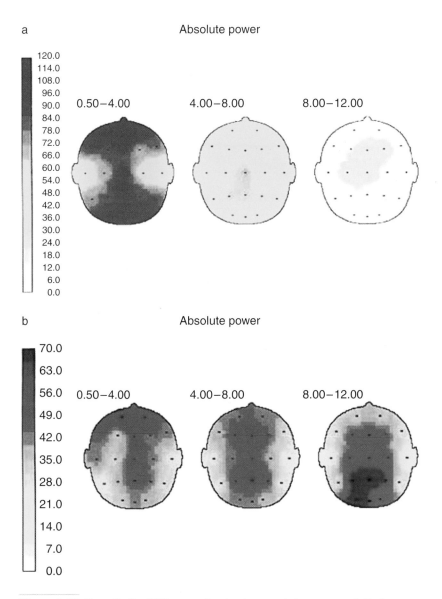

Figure 3.13 *Quantitative EEG maps showing increased slow wave activity in psychotic patients (a) compared with nonpsychotic patients (b) with AD (reprinted with the permission of the publisher).*[145]

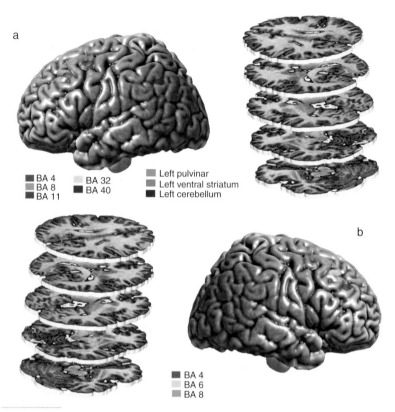

Figure 3.14 *Lateral and medial brain images demonstrating the areas of reduced cerebral blood flow in AD patients with psychosis compared with those without psychosis[147] (image courtesy of J Felix, Laboratory of Neuroimaging, UCLA School of Medicine).*

utility of cholinomimetic compounds in the treatment of behavioral disturbances in AD (described below).

Personality alterations

The concept of personality embraces a wide range of behaviors, but is viewed as a consistent response style characterizing individuals and applying to a diverse array of externally-directed behaviors and internal emotional states. A wide variety of techniques has been applied to assess personality in patients with AD. The NPI identifies several types of personality alterations such as irritability and disinhibition (Figures 3.9 and 3.10). The most consistent change observed in patients with AD is apathy and an increased passivity, as discussed above.[37,51] A similar finding emerges from the personality section of the Blessed Dementia Scale where increased passivity is reported as the most common behavioral change described by the caregivers.[157,158] Self-centered behaviors also are commonly reported in studies based on this instrument. Several investigations have used an instrument developed to measure personality alterations following dramatic brain injury where frontal lobe dysfunction is prominent. These studies show that patients with AD are more out of touch, reliant on others, childish, listless, changeable, unreasonable, lifeless, cold, irritable, and mean compared with normal elderly controls.[159–161] The NEO personality inventory has been used in a number of studies to assess patients with AD, although this instrument was not originally conceived as applicable to patients with neurologic disorders. These studies demonstrate increased neuroticism (including anxiety, hostility, depression, self-consciousness, impulsivity, and feelings of vulnerability), reduced extroversion, and reduced conscientiousness compared with normal elderly persons.[162–164] While some characteristics such as passivity are a common feature of many patients with AD, the degree of change in neuroticism is highly variable. A few studies have addressed relationships between premorbid personality and behavioral changes following the onset of AD. One examination found an association between premorbid neuroticism and the neuroticism score of the NEO personality inventory following onset of the illness.[164] Another found a relationship between premorbid neuroticism and anxiety in patients with AD.[165]

Other behavioral changes

A variety of other behavioral changes have been observed in patients with AD. *Mania* is relatively rare in AD, occurring in less than 5% of patients.[166] *Euphoria* is more common, but is still a relatively unusual mood state; it occurs in approximately 8–10% of patients.[37] Patients with euphoria have greater evidence of frontal dysfunction on neuropsychological testing and more severe reductions of frontal cerebral perfusion than patients without elation.[167]

Catastrophic reactions represent another form of mood disorder occasionally reported in patients with AD. It consists of short-lasting emotional outbursts characterized by anxiety, tears, aggressive behavior, swearing, and refusal to cooperate. It is reported in approximately 16% of patients with AD.[168] It occurs more frequently in patients with underlying irritability and depression.

Anxiety is not uncommon in AD, occurring in almost half of the patients, although the severity of the anxiety is relatively limited. Anxiety becomes more common as the disease progresses and is associated with greater disability in activities of daily living beyond what can be attributed to increasing dementia severity.[169] Anxiety is more common among patients whose disease begins before age 65.

Changes in *sexual behavior* are common in patients with AD, occurring in 80% of individuals. In 70% there is a reduced sexual involvement with an indifference to sexual activity.[170] A few patients have transient increased sexual behavior usually as a manifestation of the Kluver-Bucy syndrome.[85,171]

Patients with AD may exhibit *abnormal night-time behaviors and disrupted sleep*. At least 10% exhibit afternoon worsening of cognition or 'sundowning' and 25% have such behaviors in the evening. Fifteen percent of patients have nocturnal awakenings, sometimes with agitated behavior.[172]

Eating behaviors may change with a tendency to put too much food in the mouth at one time and overall reduction in eating, with anorexia and weight loss.

Hoarding behavior with collecting of food, garbage, newspaper, or magazines, broken items, plastic bags, old clothes, cigarette butts, and other superfluous items is seen in several types of dementia including AD. It is associated with other types of repetitive behavior.[173]

Neuropsychiatric symptoms in minimum cognitive impairment

Minimum cognitive impairment (MCI) is characterized by abnormal memory in patients who have otherwise preserved intellectual function and no disturbance of activities of daily living.[20] Minimum cognitive impairment represents a transitional state between normal aging and AD. Neuropsychiatric symptoms are common among patients with MCI. Figure 3.15 contrasts MCI patients with neuropsychiatric symptoms as demonstrated on the NPI compared with patients with early AD (MMSE score >20). Symptoms of depression and apathy are particularly common preceding the onset of diagnosable AD.[174]

Processing of emotional information

Less attention has been paid to the disruption of normal processing of emotion than to the emergence of psychopathology in patients with AD. Existing studies show that there is progressive impairment of the ability to identify emotions, recognize facial emotion, and to accurately interpret emotions portrayed in drawings or in verbal descriptions of emotional situations.[175–179] Patients with greater right hemisphere involvement and more severe visual perceptual deficits exhibit greater difficulty in processing of emotional information. Figure 3.16 shows a series of facial drawings done by a patient over the course of his AD. In each case he was attempting to copy the same stimulus figure. The loss

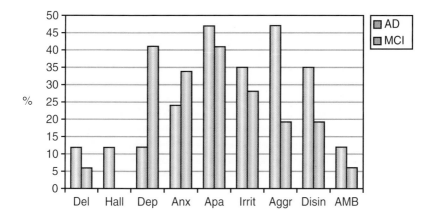

Figure 3.15 *Percent of patients with minimum cognitive impairment (MCI) and early Alzheimer's disease (AD) (MMSE score >20) with scoreable symptoms on the Neuropsychiatric Inventory (data from UCLA Alzheimer's Disease Center). (See legend to Figure 3.10 for explanation of abbreviations.)*

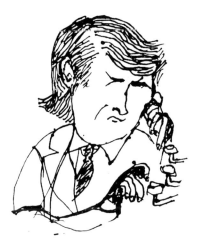

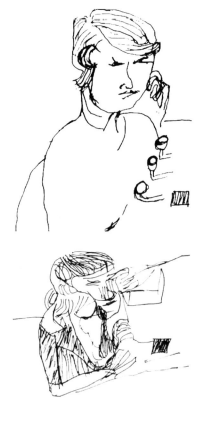

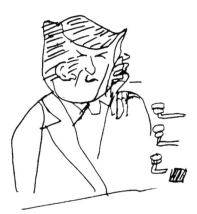

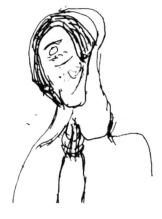

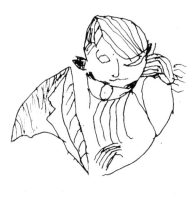

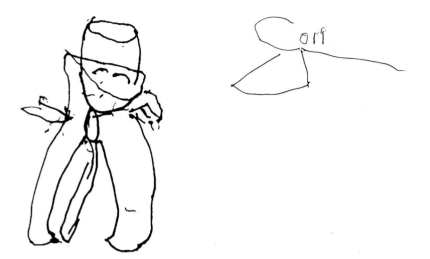

Figure 3.16 *Images of a person drawn by a patient with AD over a 3-year period and showing progressive loss of the ability to reproduce the features of the face. The patient was copying the same target figure on each occasion. The progression is from left to right beginning at the top left. The diagnosis of AD was confirmed at autopsy.*

of facial recognition and of the ability to reproduce the face is a poignant demonstration of the progressive dehumanization of the emotional environment of the AD patient.

Patients with mild to moderate AD continue to comprehend emotional inflection in spoken speech, but exhibit progressively less inflection (prosody) of their own verbal output.[180] A decline in the prosody is correlated with agitation and depressive symptoms. Patients with aprosodia have significantly higher total NPI scores as well as significantly higher scores on apathy and irritability subscales of the NPI.[181]

Behavioral genetics

Preliminary investigations have been conducted into the relationship of genetic variations to behavioral manifestations of AD. Results across studies are not always confirmatory and additional studies are needed. There is an increased risk for AD plus psychosis among family members with AD whose proband also had psychotic symptoms.[182] Studies of dopamine receptor gene polymorphisms have revealed relationships between DRD1 B2/B2 and DRD3 1/1 or 2/2 homozygotes and psychosis.[183,184] Similarly, studies of the serotonin 2A receptor gene polymorphisms reveal an over-representation of the C102 allele among AD patients exhibiting psychotic phenomena.[185,186] An association between Ser 23 allele and visual hallucinations was also identified.[185] Aggression or psychosis have been linked to the l/l polymorphism of the serotonin transporter gene[187,188] and the DRD1 B2/B2 allele, or the DRD3 polymorphism.[183,184] Hyperphagia was noted to be more common among those with the Cys23 Ser polymorphism.[185] Several investigations have found no relationship between behavioral alterations in patients with AD and the apolipoprotein E4 genotype,[189–191] although one study found an increase in psychosis among patients with advanced AD and the e4 allele, and identified an increased incidence of psychosis among AD patients bearing the e4 allele.[192,193]

Treatment

Treatment of AD has four principal components: 1) disease-modifying therapies aimed at reducing the progression of AD; 2) cholinesterase inhibitor therapy intended to improve, temporarily stabilize, or temporarily reduce the rate of decline of cognitive function; 3) psychotropic agents used to treat behavioral disturbances in neuropsychiatric symptoms; 4) working with caregivers to support their emotional needs and develop an alliance for optimal care of the patient. Each of these approaches impacts neuropsychiatric symptoms as well as cognition or disease progression.

Disease-modifying treatment

The antioxidants alpha-tocopherol (vitamin E) and selegiline are the only two agents in widespread clinical use as disease-modifying therapies. A randomized controlled trial showed that these two agents separately and in combination deferred the occurrence of major milestones in the progression of AD including death, nursing home placement, loss of activities of daily living, or progression to severe dementia.[194] The combination of agents was not superior to either agent alone for these outcomes. Behavioral effects were also seen in this study. Using the Behavioral Rating Scale for Dementia,[195] it was observed that patients on combined selegiline and vitamin E therapy had a reduction in behavioral disturbances over the course of the study, whereas those in the other three groups had an increase in behavioral abnormalities (Figure 3.17). This suggests that combined therapy with an antioxidant and a monoamine oxidase B inhibitor (selegiline) may inhibit the emergence of new behavioral disturbances and possibly reduce existing behavioral disturbances in patients with AD.

Cholinesterase inhibitors

Cholinesterase inhibitors (ChE-Is) improve cholinergic function in AD by inhibiting the destruction of intrasynaptic acetylcholine by acetyl-cholinesterase, thus increasing the synaptic residence time of acetyl-

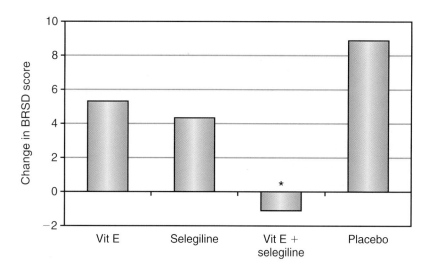

Figure 3.17 *Score changes on the Behavior Rating Scale for Dementia (BRSD) following treatment with vitamin E, selegiline, vitamin E plus selegiline, or placebo.*[195]

choline and increasing the likelihood of a signal in the postsynaptic cholinergic neuron. Four ChE-Is are generally available globally including tacrine (Cognex), donepezil (Aricept), galantamine (Reminyl), and rivastigmine (Exelon) (Table 3.1). Because of the hepatotoxicity associated with tacrine administration and the apparently equal efficacy of the other agents in the absence of substantial hepatotoxicity, tacrine is used relatively little and will not be discussed in detail here. Regulatory requirements in the USA demand that anti-dementia agents improve cognitive function and global function relative to placebo. European regulatory agencies require functional improvement in addition. Studies using a variety of outcome measures in treatment trials of ChE-Is demonstrate that, relative to placebo, these agents improve global function, enhance cognition, defer the loss of ability to perform activities of daily living, improve behavior, reduce the emergence of new behavioral disturbances, reduce dependency on the caregiver, and defer nursing home placement.[15,196–199] The available ChE-Is have similar efficacy in existing trials. They have different pharmacologic mechanisms and there is individual patient variability in response to treatments.

Donepezil is a pure acetylcholinesterase inhibitor that has a half-life of 72 hours, facilitating once daily administration. It is initiated at a dose of 5 mg daily and increased to a dose of 10 mg daily after 1 month. In addition to effects on cognition and global function[200,201] it has been shown to reduce the rate of loss of activities of daily living[198] and to improve behavior in patients with moderate to severe AD.[202] Symptoms of depression, anxiety, and apathy were improved by treatment. In a double-blind placebo-controlled trial of donepezil in patients residing in nursing homes, treatment reduced agitation.[203]

Galantamine is a ChE-I with a dual mechanism of action, inhibition of acetylcholinesterase and allosteric nicotinic receptor modulation. Galantamine is initiated at a dose of 4 mg twice daily. After 1 month it is increased to a dose of 8 mg twice daily and this is an optimal dose for many patients. Those showing no response to 16 mg or who deteriorate after continuous therapy may have their dose increased to 12 mg twice daily. Galantamine has been shown to improve global function, cognition, and activities of daily living relative to placebo.[204–206] Galantamine

Table 3.1 Pharmacologic properties of the cholinesterase inhibitors

Parameter	Donepezil (Aricept)	Galantamine (Reminyl)	Rivastigmine (Exelon)
Mechanism of action	Acetylcholinesterase inhibitor	Acetylcholinesterase inhibitor and allosteric nicotinic modulator	Acetylcholinesterase inhibitor and butyrylcholinesterase inhibitor
Class	Piperazine	Phenanthrene alkaloid	Carbamate
Reversibility	Reversible	Reversible	Pseudo-irreversible
Bioavailability	100%	80%	40%
Time to maximum serum concentration	3–5 hours	30–60 minutes	0.5–2 hours
Food delays absorption	No	Yes	Yes
Serum half-life	70–80 hours	5–7 hours	2 hours – serum 8 hours – brain
Protein binding	96%	0%	40%
Metabolism	Hepatic (CYD 2D6, 3A4)	Hepatic (CYP 2D6)	Nonhepatic
Starting dose	5 mg/day	4 mg b.i.d	1.5 b.i.d
Final dose	10 mg/day	8–12 mg b.i.d	3–6 mg b.i.d

reduces behavioral disturbances in patients who exhibit them at the time treatment is initiated (Figure 3.18) and ameliorates the emergence of new behavioral disturbances in patients who are asymptomatic at the time therapy is begun (Figure 3.19).[203,207] Beneficial effects were exhibited on the symptoms of apathy, disinhibition, anxiety, and agitation. Distress associated with behavioral changes was reduced in caregivers of patients treated with galantamine (Figure 3.20).[207]

Rivastigmine is a combined acetylcholinesterase and butyrylcholinesterase inhibitor. Rivastigmine is initiated at a dose of 1.5 mg twice daily, increased to a dose of 3 mg twice daily after 1 month, and to 4.5 mg twice daily after an additional month. Some patients may benefit additionally from a dose of 6 mg twice daily. Side effects are somewhat more common with rivastigmine than with the other ChE-Is. Patients should be titrated according to their individual tolerability. Weight loss occurs more commonly with rivastigmine than with other ChE-Is and should be monitored, particularly in women with AD. Rivastigmine has been shown to have beneficial global and cognitive effects, to reduce the rate of decline in activities of daily living, and to improve behavior.[208,209] In an open-label extension of a double-blind placebo-controlled trial,

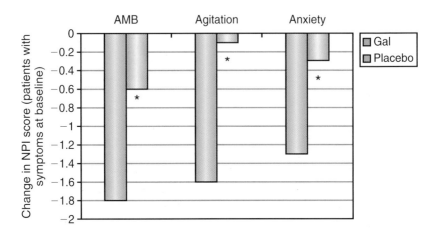

Figure 3.18 Galantamine reduced depression, anxiety, and agitation in patients exhibiting these symptoms.[207]

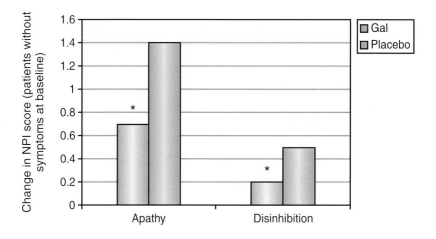

Figure 3.19 *Galantamine decreased the emergence of behaviors in patients without these symptoms before treatment.[207]*

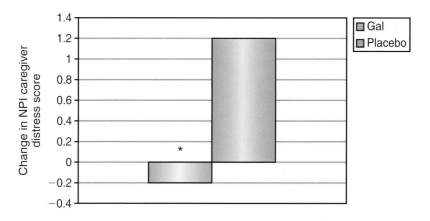

Figure 3.20 *Change in behavior-related caregiver distress score following treatment with galantamine.[207]*

rivastigmine reduced mood disturbances compared with baseline levels and reduced the expected emergence of other behavioral changes.[210]

Treatment with ChE-Is should be started as soon as the diagnosis of AD is established. Patients on long-term therapy continue to benefit from the use of these agents compared with patients not receiving cholinergic therapy, and treatment with ChE-Is should be continued until advanced phases of the disease are reached. When ChE-Is are discontinued the patient should be monitored closely for deterioration in activities of daily living, behavior, or cognition; decline in any of these functions in concert with discontinuation of therapy suggests that the patient was continuing to benefit from cholinergic enhancement strategies and treatment should be continued. These agents may also be used in other dementias with cholinergic deficits such as dementia with Lewy bodies (Chapter 4), Parkinson's disease with dementia (Chapter 5), AD with cerebrovascular disease (Chapter 6), and vascular dementia (Chapter 6).

Cholinesterase inhibitors have psychotropic properties that have emerged in most studies where patients exhibited sufficiently severe behavioral disturbances at baseline to have measurable reductions in psychopathology in the course of a treatment trial.[211] Benefits are most obvious in patients in moderate to severe phases of the disease.[202,212] Patients with more behavioral disturbances have more evidence of frontal lobe dysfunction, and comparatively reduced perfusion of orbitofrontal cortex as measured by SPECT is a predictor of the benefit from ChE-I treatment[213] (Figure 3.21).

Psychotropic agents

Table 10.1 presents the agents most commonly used to treat behavioral disturbances in patients with AD. General principles of geriatric psy-

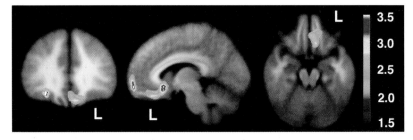

Figure 3.21 Lateral and medial brain images demonstrating the areas of reduced cerebral blood flow in AD patients who exhibited the best behavioral response (greatest reduction of behavioral symptoms) following treatment with donepezil[213] (image courtesy of M Mega and A Toga, PhD, Laboratory of Neuroimaging, UCLA School of Medicine).

chopharmacology should be applied when treating patients with AD including starting at a low dose, increasing the dose slowly, and escalating the dose until an adequate beneficial response occurs or tolerability limits further dose increases (Box 10.2). Adherence to the treatment regimen requires understanding by the caregiver as well as instruction to the patient, and both verbal and written instructions should be provided. Potential side effects of therapy should be monitored regularly and dose reductions may be attempted if symptoms are ameliorated for several months. Given the persistence of behavioral symptoms following their onset, relapse following discontinuation of medication is high, and dose reduction should be attempted cautiously.

Apathy is the most common symptom observed in AD and is typically not treated unless it is severe. Apathy often responds to treatment with ChE-Is. Treatment alternatives include methylphenidate, dextroamphetamine, and modafanil.[214]

Agitation typically is treated with antipsychotic agents or mood-stabilizing anticonvulsant compounds. Atypical antipsychotic agents are the treatment of choice for most patients. They induce less parkinsonism and tardive dyskinesia than conventional neuroleptic agents and have a larger effect size than observed in most studies of mood-stabilizing compounds.[215,216] In a controlled trial, risperidone was shown to decrease total scores on the BEHAVE-AD[121] in patients receiving 1 mg and 2 mg per day compared with those receiving placebo. Significant differences were also obtained on the aggressiveness subscale of the BEHAVE-AD at doses of 1 and 2 mg per day compared with placebo[217] (Figure 3.22). Similarly, a significant reduction in agitation as measured by the Cohen-Mansfield Agitation Inventory[54] has been found following treatment with risperidone[218] (Figure 3.23). In the course of these studies it was observed that risperidone produces significantly less adverse effects on cognitive function as measured by the MMSE than haloperidol (Figure 3.24).[218] Olanzapine, another atypical antipsychotic agent, has also been shown to reduce agitation in randomized controlled trials. Doses of 5 mg and 10 mg decreased agitation compared with placebo. The effective treatment window did not extend to 15 mg, which was no more effective than placebo[219] (Figure 3.25). Using the occupational dis-

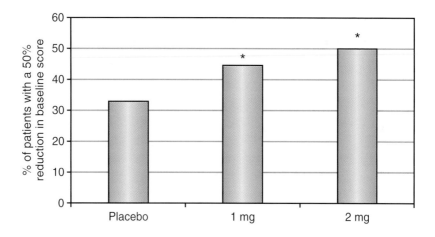

Figure 3.22 *Percent of patients with a 50% reduction in baseline score on the BEHAVE-AD following treatment with risperidone.[217]*

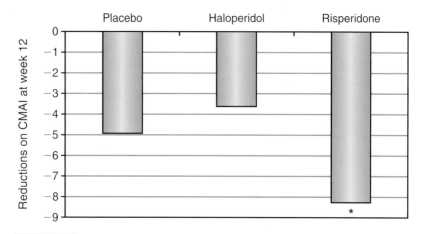

Figure 3.23 *Reduction in agitation as measured by the Cohen-Mansfield Agitation Inventory (CMAI) after 12 weeks of therapy with risperidone, haloperidol, or placebo.[218]*

ruptiveness scale of the Nursing Home Version of the Neuropsychiatric Inventory[220] patients treated with olanzapine (5 mg per day) were found to be significantly less disruptive in a residential setting than patients receiving placebo[219] (Figure 3.26). Sedation was the principal side effect

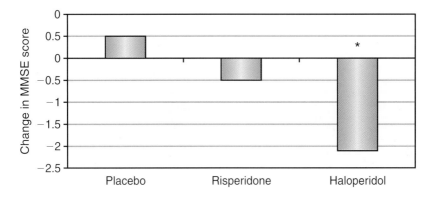

Figure 3.24 *Change in Mini-Mental State Examination (MMSE) score following treatment with placebo, risperidone, or haloperidol. There was a significant reduction in MMSE score following administration of haloperidol.*[218]

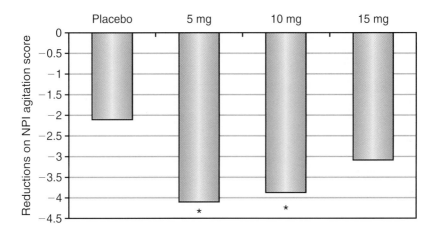

Figure 3.25 *Reductions on the Neuropsychiatric Inventory Nursing Home Version (NPI-NH) agitation subscale score following treatment with placebo or 5, 10, or 15 mg of olanzapine.*[219]

observed in the use of atypical antipsychotic agents. Extrapyramidal symptoms may occur even with atypical agents when these drugs are administered in high doses.

Conventional neuroleptic agents, such as haloperidol, also reduce

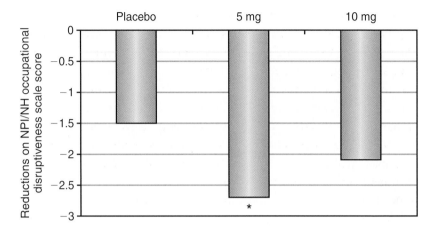

Figure 3.26 Reductions on the Neuropsychiatric Inventory Nursing Home Version
(NPI-NH) occupational disruptiveness scale score following treatment with placebo
or 5 or 10 mg of olanzapine.[219]

agitation in AD. In a meta-analysis of trials of neuroleptic therapy of
agitation, an effect size of 18% of neuroleptics over placebos was identified.[221] Doses of 2–3 mg of haloperidol produce response rates of 55–65%
(percent of patients experiencing significant reduction of symptoms)
compared with response rates of 25–35% with lower doses (not different
from placebo).[222]

Mood-stabilizing anticonvulsant agents also may be useful in reducing
agitation in patients with AD. Randomized trials with carbamazepine
show a statistically significant effect compared with placebo.[223,224] A randomized trial comparing divalproex sodium to placebo in AD patients
with agitation also showed a significantly superior effect with the active
agent.[225] Anecdotal observations suggest that topiramate, gabapentin,
and lamotrogine also have anti-agitation properties.[226–228]

Citalopram was more effective than perphenazine or placebo in reducing behavioral disturbances (psychosis and agitation) in AD patients in
a psychiatric unit.[229] Other agents that have been studied less compre-
hensively but appear to reduce agitation in AD include trazodone, propranolol, and estrogen.[230–234]

In view of the heterogeneity of neuropsychiatric disorders found in conjunction with agitation, a rational approach is to treat the obvious psychopathology with targeted psychopharmacologic agents. In most cases this will be an atypical antipsychotic agent, in others an antidepressant or angiolytic may be useful first. If a sufficient response is not obtained, an anticonvulsant may be used as adjunctive therapy (Figure 10.4). Since agitation may be a response to pain associated with a urinary tract infection, decubitus ulceration, constipation, or other physical illness, it is critical to assess the patient for the presence of treatable medical or environmental provocation before initiation of treatment with a psychotropic drug.

Psychosis is treated preferentially with atypical antipsychotics or with conventional neuroleptics if the patient does not tolerate treatment with an atypical agent or is unresponsive to it (Table 10.1). Both risperidone and olanzapine have been shown to reduce psychosis in patients with AD and delusions and hallucinations[217,219] (Figures 3.27 and 3.28). Patients treated with olanzapine for agitation had significantly less emergence of psychosis than those receiving placebo.[235] Thus atypical antipsychotics may both reduce acute symptoms and suppress emergent psychotic symptoms. Long-term treatment with olanzapine led to

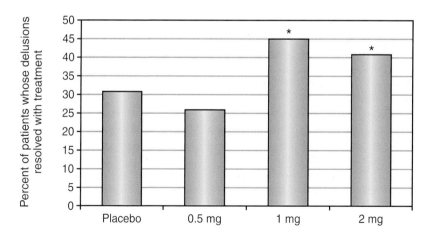

Figure 3.27 *Percent of patients whose delusions resolved with treatment (symptoms were present at baseline and not at the end of the study) with risperidone.[217]*

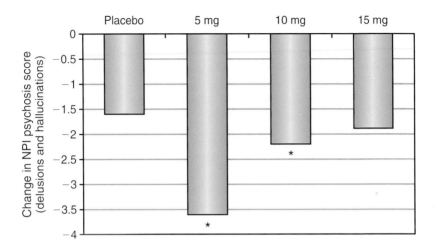

Figure 3.28 *Change in Neuropsychiatric Inventory Nursing Home Version (NPI-NH) psychosis score following treatment with 5, 10, or 15 mg of olanzapine.[219]*

further reductions in psychosis and agitation following amelioration of the acute symptom-complex.[236] Haloperidol has been shown to be an effective antipsychotic agent.[222] Open-label studies indicate that selective serotonin reuptake inhibitors may be useful in reducing symptoms of depression and psychosis in patients with AD even in the absence of concomitant therapy with an antipsychotic agent.[237,238] Antipsychotic agents with anticholinergic side effects should be avoided in the treatment of psychosis and agitation.

Some randomized controlled trials have shown no difference between placebo and an active agent in treatment of AD and depression. Depression in AD may fluctuate or spontaneously remit more than in other circumstances, making treatment effects more difficult to document.[239] However, some studies have shown antidepressant effects with selective serotonin reuptake inhibitors, tricyclic antidepressants, and monoxidase B inhibitors.[240-244] Antidepressants may have beneficial effects on activities of daily living in addition to ameliorating depressive symptoms[241] (Figure 3.29). Antidepressants with anticholinergic side effects should be avoided.

Controlled data are unavailable for treatment of other behavioral

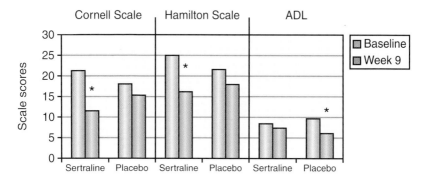

Figure 3.29 *Changes on the Cornell Scale for Depression in Dementia, the Hamilton Depression Rating Scale, and an activities of daily living (ADL) scale following treatment with sertraline.[241]*

symptoms in AD. Olanzapine reduced anxiety in AD patients with psychotic and anxiety symptoms.[245] Therapy of anxiety and insomnia should emphasize agents that are well metabolized in the elderly (Table 10.1). For severe sexual aggression in males, treatment with medroxyprogesterone or leuprolide may be considered.[246–248]

Caring for the caregiver

Neuropsychiatric symptoms are disruptive to the patient–caregiver relationship and exacerbate the burden of caring. The behavioral disturbances may precipitate institutionalization when they exceed the tolerance of the caregiver. They have also been associated with physical abuse of patients by spouses. Neuropsychiatric symptoms have been associated with depression in carers.[249] Caring for the caregiver is thus an essential part of ameliorating behavioral disturbances in patients with AD, and it is important to develop a therapeutic alliance with the caregiver to ensure adherence to medication regimens. Carers may also be trained in nonpharmacologic intervention strategies to reduce behavioral disturbances without employing medications; caregiver educational interventions have been shown to reduce the rate of institutionalization of patients with AD.[250] Family caregivers should be referred to the

Alzheimer's Association or to the local branch of the Alzheimer's Disease International for support services and guidance to local community resources.

An integrated model of pharmacologic and nonpharmacologic interventions

Following an accurate diagnosis of AD, a patient should be treated with an antioxidant and a cholinesterase inhibitor (Figure 3.30). In advanced cases family members may choose not to prolong the patient's life through use of disease-modifying agents such as antioxidants. In those with evidence of executive dysfunction and at a high risk of behavioral disturbances, a combination of selegiline and vitamin E may be superior to either agent alone. These drugs can be administered safely in conjunction with ChE-Is. If behavioral disturbances are not so urgent as to require immediate intervention with psychotropic agents, pharmacologic treatment of behavioral disorders should be deferred until the impact of the ChE-I can be assessed. If behavioral disturbances remain after ChE-I therapy has been optimized, nonpharmacologic interven-

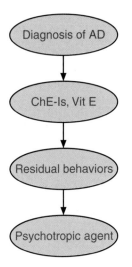

Figure 3.30 *Treatment algorithm for pharmacologic management of patients with Alzheimer's disease (ChE-Is, cholinesterase inhibitors).*

tions should be instituted, minimizing environmental provocations, and training family or professional caregivers to reassure, reorient, repeat, and redirect (the four Rs of dementia care) in an attempt to avoid use of additional psychotropic medications. If residual behavioral disturbances require pharmacologic agents then treatment with agents specifically targeted for each behavioral subtype should be employed.

References

1. McKhann G, Drachman D, Folstein M *et al*. Clinical diagnosis of Alzheimer's disease: report of the NINCDS-ADRDA Work Group* under the auspices of Department of Health and Human Services Task Force on Alzheimer's disease. *Neurology* 1984;34:939–74.
2. Baldereschi M, Amato MP, Nencini P *et al*. Cross-national interrater agreement on the clinical diagnostic criteria for dementia. *Neurology* 1994;44:239–42.
3. Farrer LA, Cupples LA, Blackburn S *et al*. Interrater agreement for diagnosis of Alzheimer's disease: the MIRAGE study. *Neurology* 1994;44:652–6.
4. Galasko D, Hansen LA, Katzman R *et al*. Clinical-neuropathological correlations in Alzheimer's disease and related dementias. *Arch Neurol* 1994; 51:888–95.
5. Kosunen O, Soininen H, Paljarvi L *et al*. Diagnostic accuracy of Alzheimer's disease: a neuropathological study. *Acta Neuropathol* 1996;91:185–93.
6. Lim A, Tsuang D, Kukull WA *et al*. Clinico-neuropathological correlation of Alzheimer's disease in a community-based case series. *J Am Geriatr Soc* 1999; 47:564–9.
7. von Strauss E, Viitanen M, De Ronchi D *et al*. Aging and the occurrence of dementia. *Arch Neurol* 1999;56:587–92.
8. Brookmeyer R, Gray S, Kawas C. Projections of Alzheimer's disease in the United States and the public health impact of delaying disease onset. *Am J Public Health* 1998;88:1337–42.
9. Gao S, Hendrie HC, Hall KS *et al*. The relationship between age, sex, and the incidence of dementia and Alzheimer disease – a meta-analysis. *Arch Gen Psychiatry* 1998;55:809–15.
10. Evans DA, Hebert LE, Beckett LA *et al*. Education and other measures of socioeconomic status and risk of incident Alzheimer disease in a defined population of older persons. *Arch Neurol* 1997;54:1399–405.
11. Guo Z, Cupples LA, Kurz A *et al*. Head injury and the risk of AD in the MIRAGE study. *Neurology* 2000;54:1316–23.
12. Seshadri S, Drachman DA, Lippa CF. Apolipoprotein E4 allele and the lifetime risk of Alzheimer's disease – what physicians know, and what they should know. *Arch Neurol* 1995;52:1074–9.
13. Hardy J. Amyloid, the presenilins and Alzheimer's disease. *Trends Neurosci* 1997;20:154–9.
14. St George-Hyslop PH. Molecular genetics of Alzheimer's disease. *Biol Psychiatry* 2000;47:183–99.

15. Cummings JL. Cognitive and behavioral heterogeneity in Alzheimer's disease: seeking the neurological basis. Response to commentaries. *Neurobiol Aging* 2000;21:845–61.

16. Zec RF. Neuropsychological functioning in Alzheimer's disease. In: Parks RW, Zec RF, Wilson RF (eds) *Neuropsychology of Alzheimer's Disease and Other Dementias*. New York: Oxford University Press, 1993: 203–80.

17. Cummings JL, Benson F, Hill MA, Read S. Aphasia in dementia of the Alzheimer type. *Neurology* 1985;35:394–7.

18. Folstein MF, Folstein SE, McHugh PR. 'Mini-Mental State': a practical method for grading the cognitive state of patients for the clinician. *J Psychiatr Res* 1975;12:189–98.

19. Beard CM, Kokmen E, Sigler C *et al*. Cause of death in Alzheimer's disease. *Ann Epidemiol* 1996;6:195–200.

20. Petersen RC, Smith GE, Waring SC *et al*. Mild cognitive impairment. *Arch Neurol* 1999;56:303–8.

21. Förstl H, Burns A. Alzheimer's disease. In: Ames D, Chiu E (eds) *Neuroimaging and the psychiatry of late life*. Cambridge, UK: Cambridge University Press, 1997: 100–21.

22. Mirra SS, Heyman A, McKeel D *et al*. The consortium to establish a registry for Alzheimer's disease (CERAD). II. Standardization of the neuropathological assessment of Alzheimer's disease. *Neurology* 1991;41:479–86.

23. Braak H, Braak E. Neuropathological staging of Alzheimer-related changes. *Acta Neuropathol* 1991;82:239–59.

24. Cummings J, Back C. The cholinergic hypothesis of neuropsychiatric symptoms in Alzheimer's disease. *Am J Geriatr Psychiatry* 1998;6:S64–S78.

25. Morris JH. Alzheimer's disease. In: Esiri MM, Morris JH (eds) *The Neuropathology of Dementia*. Cambridge, UK: Cambridge University Press, 1997: 70–121.

26. Arnold SE, Hyman BT, Flory J *et al*. The topographical and neuroanatomical distribution of neurofibrillary tangles and neuritic plaques in the cerebral cortex of patients with Alzheimer's disease. *Cerebral Cortex* 1991;1:103–16.

27. Vinters HV, Wang ZZ, Secor DL. Brain parenchymal and microvascular amyloid in Alzheimer's disease. *Brain Pathol* 1996;6:179–95.

28. Cummings JL, Vinters HV, Cole GM *et al*. Alzheimer's disease: etiologies, pathophysiology, cognitive reserve, and treatment opportunities. *Neurology* 1998;51:S2–S17.

29. Lantos P, Cairns N. The neuropathology of Alzheimer's disease. In: O'Brien J, Ames D, Burns A (eds) *Dementia* 2nd edn. London: Arnold, 2000: 443–59.

30. Palmer AM, Stratmann GC, Procter AW, Bowen DM. Possible neurotransmitter basis of behavioral changes in Alzheimer's disease. *Ann Neurol* 1988;23:616–20.

31. Selkoe DJ. Presenilins, B-amyloid precursor protein and the molecular basis of Alzheimer's disease. *Clin Neurosci Res* 2001;1:91–103.

32. Mattson MP, Pedersen WA, Culmsee C. Cellular and molecular mechanisms underlying synaptic degeneration and neuronal death in Alzheimer's disease. In: Mattson MP (ed.) *Pathogenesis of Neurodegenerative Disorders*. Totowa, NJ: Humana Press, 2001: 113–38.

33. Aisen PS, Davis KL. Inflammatory mechanisms in Alzheimer's disease: implications for therapy. *Am J Psychiatry* 1994;151:1105–13.

34. Akiyama H, Barger S, Barnum S *et al*. Inflammation and Alzheimer's disease. *Neurobiol Aging* 2000;21:383–421.

35. Simons M, Keller P, Dichgans J *et al*. Cholesterol and Alzheimer's disease: is there a link? *Neurology* 2001;57:1089–93.

36. Cummings JL, Mega M, Gray K *et al*. The Neuropsychiatric Inventory: comprehensive assessment of psychopathology in dementia. *Neurology* 1994; 44:2308–14.

37. Mega MS, Cummings JL, Fiorello T *et al*. The spectrum of behavioral changes in Alzheimer's disease. *Neurology* 1996;46:130–5.

38. Levy ML, Cummings JL, Fairbanks LA *et al*. Longitudinal assessment of symptoms of depression, agitation, and psychosis in 181 patients with Alzheimer's disease. *Am J Psychiatry* 1996;153:1438–43.

39. Devanand DP, Jacobs DM, Tang M *et al*. The course of psychopathologic features in mild to moderate Alzheimer's disease. *Arch Gen Psychiatry* 1997; 54:257–63.

40. Frisoni GB, Rozzini L, Binetti G *et al*. Behavioral syndromes in Alzheimer's disease: description and correlates. *Dementia* 1999;10:130–8.

41. Lyketsos CG, Breitner JC, Rabins PV. An evidence-based proposal for the classification of neuropsychiatric disturbance in Alzheimer's disease. *Int J Geriatr Psychiatry* 2001;16:1037–42.

42. Tekin S, Fairbanks LA, O'Connor S *et al*. Activities of daily living in Alzheimer's disease: neuropsychiatric, cognitive, and medical illness influences. *Am J Geriatr Psychiatry* 2001;9:81–6.

43. Cooper JK, Mungas D, Weiler PG. Relation of cognitive status and abnormal behaviors in Alzheimer's disease. *J Am Geriatr Soc* 1990;38:867–70.

44. Kurita A, Blass JP, Nolan KA *et al*. Relationship between cognitive status and behavioral symptoms in Alzheimer's disease and mixed dementia. *J Am Geriatr Soc* 1993;41:732–6.

45. Landes AM, Sperry SD, Strauss ME *et al*. Apathy in Alzheimer's disease. *J Am Geriatr Soc* 2001;49:1700–7.

46. Levy ML, Cummings JL, Fairbanks LA *et al*. Apathy is not depression. *J Neuropsychiatry Clin Neurosci* 1998;10:314–19.

47. McPherson S, Fairbanks L, Tiken S, Cummings JL, Back-Madruga C. Apathy and executive function in Alzheimer's disease. *J Int Neuropsychol Soc* 2002;8:373–81.

48. Rapoport MJ, van Reekum R, Freedman M *et al*. Relationship of psychosis to aggression, apathy and function in dementia. *Int J Geriatr Psychiatry* 2001; 16:123–30.

49. Craig AH, Cummings JL, Fairbanks L *et al*. Cerebral blood flow correlates of apathy in Alzheimer's disease. *Arch Neurol* 1996;53:1116–20.

50. Migneco O, Benoit M, Koulibaly PM *et al*. Perfusion brain SPECT and statistical parametric mapping analysis indicate that apathy is a cingulate syndrome: a study of Alzheimer's disease and non-demented patients. *Neuroimage* 2001; 13:896–902.

51. Galynker I, Dutta E, Vilkas N *et al*. Hypofrontality and negative symptoms in patients with dementia of Alzheimer type. *Neuropsychiatry Neuropsychol Behav Neurol* 2000;13:53–9.

52. Tractenberg RE, Weiner MF, Thal LJ. Estimating the prevalence of agitation of

community-dwelling persons with Alzheimer's disease. *J Neuropsychiatry Clin Neurosci* 2002;14:11–18.

53. Cohen-Mansfield J, Billig N. Agitated behaviors in the elderly, I. A conceptual review. *J Am Geriatr Soc* 1986;34:711–21.

54. Cohen-Mansfield J. Agitated behaviors in the elderly II. Preliminary results in the cognitively deteriorated. *J Am Geriatr Soc* 1986;34:722–7.

55. Cohen-Mansfield J, Marx MS, Rosenthal AS. A description of agitation in a nursing home. *J Gerontol* 1989;44:M77–M84.

56. Tsai SJ, Hwang JP, Yang CH *et al.* Physical aggression and associated factors in probable Alzheimer disease. *Alzheimer Dis Assoc Disord* 1996;10:82–5.

57. Eastley R, Wilcock G. Prevalence and correlates of aggressive behaviours occurring in patients with Alzheimer's disease. *Int J Geriatr Psychiatry* 1997;12:484–7.

58. Teri L, Borson S, Kiyak HA *et al.* Behavioral disturbance, cognitive dysfunction, and functional skill: prevalence and relationship in Alzheimer's disease. *J Am Geriatr Soc* 1989;37:109–16.

59. Eustace A, Kidd N, Greene E *et al.* Verbal aggression in Alzheimer's disease: clinical, functional, and neuropsychological correlates. *Int J Geriatr Psychiatry* 2001;16:858–61.

60. Aarsland D, Cummings JL, Yenner G *et al.* Relationship of aggressive behavior to other neuropsychiatric symptoms in patients with Alzheimer's disease. *Am J Psychiatry* 1996;153:243–7.

61. Chen ST, Sultzer DL, Hinkin CH *et al.* Executive dysfunction in Alzheimer's disease: association with neuropsychiatric symptoms and functional impairment. *J Neuropsychiatry Clin Neurosci* 1998;10:426–32.

62. Stewart JT, Gonzalez-Perez E, Zhu Y *et al.* Cognitive predictors of resistiveness in dementia patients. *Am J Geriatr Psychiatry* 1999;7:259–63.

63. Keene J, Hope T, Fairburn CG *et al.* Natural history of aggressive behaviour in dementia. *Int J Geriatr Psychiatry* 1999;14:541–8.

64. Hope T, Keene J, Fairburn CG *et al.* Natural history of behavioural changes and psychiatric symptoms in Alzheimer's disease. *Br J Psychiatry* 1999;174:39–44.

65. Hirono N, Mega MS, Dinov ID *et al.* Left frontotemporal hypoperfusion is associated with aggression in patients with dementia. *Arch Neurol* 2000;57:861–6.

66. Sultzer DL, Mhler Me, Mandelkern MA *et al.* The relationship between psychiatric symptoms and regional cortical metabolism in Alzheimer's disease. *J Neuropsychiatry Clin Neurosci* 1995;7:476–84.

67. Palmer AM, Stratmann GC, Procter AW *et al.* Possible neurotransmitter basis of behavioral changes in Alzheimer's disease. *Ann Neurol* 1988;23:616–20.

68. Minger SL, Esiri MM, McDonald B *et al.* Cholinergic deficits contribute to behavioral disturbance in patients with dementia. *Neurology* 2000;55:1460–7.

69. Victoroff JI, Zarow C, Mack WJ *et al.* Physical aggression is associated with preservation of substantia nigra pars compacta in Alzheimer disease. *Arch Neurol* 1996;53:428–34.

70. Matthews KL, Chen CP, Esiri MM *et al.* Noradrenergic changes, aggressive behavior and cognition in patients with dementia. *Biol Psychiatry* 2002;51:407–16.

71. Tekin S, Mega MS, Masterman DL *et al.* Orbitofrontal and anterior cingulate cortex: neurofibrillary tangle burden is associated with agitation in Alzheimer's disease. *Ann Neurol* 2001;49:355–61.

72. Devanand DP, Sano M, Tang M-X *et al*. Depressed mood in the incidence of Alzheimer's disease in the elderly living in the community. *Arch Gen Psychiatry* 1996;53:175–82.

73. Speck CE, Kukull WA, Brenner DE *et al*. History of depression as a risk factor for Alzheimer's disease. *Epidemiology* 1995;6:366–9.

74. Chen P, Ganguli M, Mulsant BH *et al*. The temporal relationship between depressive symptoms and dementia. *Arch Gen Psychiatry* 1999;56:261–6.

75. Harwood DG, Barker WW, Ownby RL *et al*. Association between premorbid history of depression and current depression in Alzheimer's disease. *J Geriatr Psychiatry Neurol* 1999;12:72–5.

76. Pearlson GD, Roos CA, Lohr WD *et al*. Association between family history of affective disorder and the depressive syndrome of Alzheimer's disease. *Am J Psychiatry* 1990;147:452–6.

77. Strauss ME, Ogrocki PK. Confirmation of an association between family history of affective disorder and the depressive syndrome in Alzheimer's disease. *Am J Psychiatry* 1996;153:1340–2.

78. Ballard C, Bannister C, Solis M *et al*. The prevalence, associations and symptoms of depression amongst dementia sufferers. *J Affect Disord* 1996;36:135–44.

79. Lyketsos CG, Steele C, Baker L *et al*. Major and minor depression in Alzheimer's disease: prevalence and impact. *J Neuropsychiatry Clin Neurosci* 1997;9:556–61.

80. Migliorelli R, Teson A, Sabe L *et al*. Prevalence and correlates of dysthymia and major depression among patients with Alzheimer's disease. *Am J Psychiatry* 1995;152:37–44.

81. Reichman WE, Coyne AC. Depressive symptoms in Alzheimer's disease and multi-infarct dementia. *J Geriatr Psychiatry Neurol* 1995;8:96–9.

82. Starkstein SE, Chemerinski E, Sabe L *et al*. A prospective longitudinal study of depression and anosognosia in Alzheimer's disease. *Br J Psychiatry* 1997;171:47–52.

83. Vida S, Des Rosiers P, Carrier L *et al*. Prevalence of depression in Alzheimer's disease and validity of research diagnostic criteria. *J Geriatr Psychiatry Neurol* 1994;7:238–44.

84. Weiner MF, Edland SD, Luszczynska H. Prevalence and incidence of major depression in Alzheimer's disease. *Am J Psychiatry* 1994;151:1006–9.

85. Burns A, Jacoby R, Levy R. Psychiatric phenomena in Alzheimer's disease, IV: Disorders of behaviour. *Br J Psychiatry* 1990;157:86–94.

86. Mackenzie TB, Robiner WN, Knopman D. Differences between patient and family assessments of depression in Alzheimer's disease. *Am J Psychiatry* 1989;146:1174–8.

87. Lyketsos CG, Steele C, Galik E *et al*. Physical aggression in dementia patients and its relationship to depression. *Am J Psychiatry* 1999;156:66–71.

88. Forsell Y, Winblad B. Major depression in a population of demented and non-demented older people: prevalence and correlates. *J Am Geriatr Soc* 1998;46:27–30.

89. Fitz AG, Teri L. Depression, cognition, and functional ability in patients with Alzheimer's disease. *J Am Geriatr Soc* 1994;42:186–91.

90. Hargrave R, Reed B, Mungas D. Depressive syndromes and functional disability in dementia. *J Geriatr Psychiatry Neurol* 2000;13:72–7.

91. Rovner BW, Broadhead J, Spencer M *et al.* Depression and Alzheimer's disease. *Am J Psychiatry* 1989;146:350–3.

92. American Psychiatric Association. *Diagnostic and Statistical Manual of Mental Disorders: DSM-IV,* 4th edn. Washington, DC: American Psychiatric Association, 1994.

93. Olin JT, Schneider LS, Katz IR *et al.* Provisional diagnostic criteria for depression of Alzheimer disease. *Am J Geriatr Psychiatry* 2002;10:129–41.

94. Purandare N, Burns A, Craig S *et al.* Depressive symptoms in patients with Alzheimer's disease. *Int J Geriatr Psychiatry* 2001;16:960–4.

95. Weiner MF, Doody RS, Sairam R *et al.* Prevalence and incidence of major depressive disorder in Alzheimer's disease: findings from two databases. *Dement Geriatr Cogn Disord* 2002;13:8–12.

96. Pozzi D, Golimstock A, Migliorelli R *et al.* Quantified electroencephalographic correlates of depression in Alzheimer's disease. *Biol Psychiatry* 1993; 34:386–91.

97. Clark LM, McDonald WM, Welsh-Bohmer KA *et al.* Magnetic resonance imaging correlates of depression in early- and late-onset Alzheimer's disease. *Biol Psychiatry* 1998;44:592–9.

98. Frisoni GB, Geroldi C. Cerebrovascular disease affects noncognitive symptoms in Alzheimer disease. *Arch Neurol* 2001;58:1939–40.

99. Lopez OL, Becker JT, Reynolds CF *et al.* Psychiatric correlates of MR deep white matter lesions in probable Alzheimer's disease. *J Neuropsychiatry Clin Neurosci* 1997;9:246–50.

100. Hirono N, Mori E, Ishii K *et al.* Frontal lobe hypometabolism and depression in Alzheimer's disease. *Neurology* 1998a;50:380–3.

101. Starkstein SE, Vazquez S, Migliorelli R *et al.* A SPECT study of depression in Alzheimer's disease. *Neuropsychiatry Neuropsychol Behav Neurol* 1995;8:38–43.

102. Chan-Palay V, Asan E. Alterations in catecholamine neurons of the locus coeruleus in senile dementia of the Alzheimer type and in Parkinson's disease with and without dementia and depression. *J Comp Neurol* 1989;287:373–92.

103. Forstl H, Burns A, Luthert P *et al.* Clinical and neuropathological correlates of depression in Alzheimer's disease. *Psychol Med* 1992;22:877–84.

104. Zubenko GS, Moossy J. Major depression in primary dementia. *Arch Neurol* 1988;45:1182–6.

105. Zubenko GS, Moossy J, Kopp U. Neurochemical correlates of major depression in primary dementia. *Arch Neurol* 1990;47:209–14.

106. Chen CPL-H, Alder JT, Bowen DM *et al.* Presynaptic serotonergic markers in community-acquired cases of Alzheimer's disease: correlations with depression and neuroleptic medication. *J Neurochem* 1996;66:1592–8.

107. McAllister TW, Hays LR. TRH test, DST, and response to desipramine in primary degenerative dementia. *Biol Psychiatry* 1987;22:189–93.

108. Miller AH, Sastry G, Speranza AJ *et al.* Lack of association between cortisol hypersecretion and nonsuppression on the DST in patients with Alzheimer's disease. *Am J Psychiatry* 1994;151:267–70.

109. Shrimankar J, Soni SD, McMurray J. Dexamethasone suppression test in dementia and depression. *Br J Psychiatry* 1989;154:372–7.

110. Jeste DV, Finkel SI. Psychosis of Alzheimer's disease and related dementias. *Am J Geriatr Psychiatry* 2000;8:29–34.

111. Ballard C, Saad K, Patel A *et al*. The prevalence and phenomenology of psychotic symptoms in dementia sufferers. *Int J Geriatr Psychiatry* 1995;10:477–85.

112. Cooper JK, Mungas D, Verma M *et al*. Psychotic symptoms in Alzheimer's disease. *Int J Geriatr Psychiatry* 1991;6:721–6.

113. Gormley N, Rizwan MR. Prevalence and clinical correlates of psychotic symptoms in Alzheimer's disease. *Int J Geriatr Psychiatry* 1998;13:410–14.

114. Mendez MF, Martin RJ, Smyth KA *et al*. Psychiatric symptoms associated with Alzheimer's disease. *J Neuropsychiatry Clin Neurosci* 1990;2:28–33.

115. Binetti G, Bianchetti A, Padovani A *et al*. Delusions in Alzheimer's disease and multi-infarct dementia. *Acta Neurol Scand* 1993;88:5–9.

116. Burns A, Jacoby R, Levy R. Psychiatric phenomena in Alzheimer's disease, I: Disorders of thought content; II: Disorders of perception. *Br J Psychiatry* 1990;157:72–81.

117. Hwang J-P, Yang C-H, Tsai S-J *et al*. Delusions of theft in dementia of the Alzheimer type: a preliminary report. *Alzheimer Dis Assoc Disord* 1997;11: 110–12.

118. Mendez MF. Delusional misidentification of persons in dementia. *Br J Psychiatry* 1992;160:414–16.

119. Migliorelli R, Petracca G, Teson A *et al*. Neuropsychiatric and neuropsychological correlates of delusions in Alzheimer's disease. *Psychol Med* 1995; 25:505–13.

120. Reisberg B, Borenstein J, Salob SP *et al*. Behavioral symptoms in Alzheimer's disease: phenomenology and treatment. *J Clin Psychiatry* 1987;48:9–15.

121. Venneri A, Shanks MF, Staff RT *et al*. Nurturing syndrome: a form of pathological bereavement with delusions in Alzheimer's disease. *Neuropsychologia* 2000; 38:213–24.

122. Renvoize EB, Kent J, Klar HM. Delusional infestation and dementia: a case report. *Br J Psychiatry* 1987;150:403–5.

123. Drevets WC, Rubin EH. Erotomania and senile dementia of Alzheimer type. *Br J Psychiatry* 1987;151:400–2.

124. Molchan SE, Martinez RA, Lawlor BA *et al*. Reflections of the self: atypical misidentification and delusional syndromes in two patients with Alzheimer's disease. *Br J Psychiatry* 1990;157:605–8.

125. Hirono N, Mori E, Yasuda M *et al*. Factors associated with psychotic symptoms in Alzheimer's disease. *J Neurol Neurosurg Psychiatry* 1998;64:648–52.

126. Chui HC, Lyness SA, Sobel E *et al*. Extrapyramidal signs and psychiatric symptoms predict faster cognitive decline in Alzheimer's disease. *Arch Neurol* 1994;51:676–81.

127. Haupt M, Romero B, Kurz A. Delusions and hallucinations in Alzheimer's disease: results from a two-year longitudinal study. *Int J Geriatr Psychiatry* 1996;11:965–72.

128. Mortimer JA, Ebbitt B, Jun S *et al*. Predictors of cognitive and functional progression in patients with probable Alzheimer's disease. *Neurology* 1992;42: 1689–96.

129. Paulsen JS, Salmon DP, Thal LJ *et al*. Incidence of and risk factors for hallucinations and delusions in patients with probable AD. *Neurology* 2000;54:1965–71.

130. Stern Y, Albert M, Brandt J *et al*. Utility of extrapyramidal signs and psychosis as predictors of cognitive and functional decline, nursing home admission,

and death in Alzheimer's disease: prospective analyses from the Predictors Study. *Neurology* 1994;44:2300–7.

131. Wilson RS, Gilley DW, Bennett DA *et al.* Hallucinations, delusions, and cognitive decline in Alzheimer's disease. *J Neurol Neurosurg Psychiatry* 2000;69: 172–7.

132. Lesser IM, Miller BL, Boone K *et al.* Psychosis as the first manifestation of degenerative dementia. *Bull Clin Neurosci* 1989;54:59–63.

133. Webster J, Grossberg GT. Late-life onset of psychotic symptoms. *Am J Geriatr Psychiatry* 1998;6:196–202.

134. Chemerinski E, Petracca G, Teson A *et al.* Prevalence and correlates of aggressive behavior in Alzheimer's disease. *J Neuropsychiatry Clin Neurosci* 1998; 10:421–5.

135. Deutsch LH, Bylsma FW, Rovner BW *et al.* Psychosis and physical aggression in probable Alzheimer's disease. *Am J Psychiatry* 1991;148:1159–63.

136. Flynn FG, Cummings JL, Gornbein J. Delusions in dementia syndromes: investigation of behavioral and neuropsychological correlates. *J Neuropsychiatry Clin Neurosci* 1991;3:364–70.

137. Bylsma FW, Folstein M, Devanand DP *et al.* Delusions and patterns of cognitive impairment in Alzheimer's disease. *Neuropsychiatry Neuropsychol Behav Neurol* 1994;7:98–103.

138. Lopez OL, Becker JT, Brenner RP. Alzheimer's disease with delusions and hallucinations: neuropsychological and electroencephalophic correlates. *Neurology* 1991;41:906–12.

139. Jeste DV, Wragg RE, Salmon DP *et al.* Cognitive deficits of patients with Alzheimer's disease with and without delusions. *Am J Psychiatry* 1992; 149:184–9.

140. Ballard C, Bannister C, Graham C *et al.* Associations of psychotic symptoms in dementia sufferers. *Br J Psychiatry* 1995;167:537–40.

141. Gilley DW, Whalen ME, Wilson RS *et al.* Hallucinations and associated factors in Alzheimer's disease. *J Neuropsychiatry Clin Neurosci* 1991;3:371–6.

142. Lerner AJ, Koss E, Patterson MB *et al.* Concomitants of visual hallucinations in Alzheimer's disease. *Neurology* 1994;44:523–7.

143. Murgatroyd C, Prettyman R. An investigation of visual hallucinosis and visual sensory status in dementia. Int J Geriat Psychiatry 2001;16:709–13.

144. Chapman FM, Dickinson J, McKeith IG *et al.* Association among visual hallucinations, visual acuity, and specific eye pathologies in Alzheimer's disease: treatment implications. *Am J Psychiatry* 1999;156:1983–5.

145. Edwards-Lee T, Cook I, Fairbanks L *et al.* Quantitative electroencephalographic correlates of psychosis in Alzheimer disease. *Neuropsychiatry Neuropsychol Behav Neurol* 2000;13:163–70.

146. Kotrla KJ, Chacko RC, Harper RG *et al.* SPECT findings on psychosis in Alzheimer's disease. *Am J Psychiatry* 1995;152:1470–5.

147. Mega MS, Lee L, Dinov ID, Mishkin F, Toga AW, Cummings JL. Cerebral correlates of psychotic symptoms in Alzheimer's disease. *J Neurol Neurosurg Psychiatry* 2000; 69:167–71.

148. Ponton MO, Darcourt J, Miller BL *et al.* Psychometric and SPECT studies in Alzheimer's disease with and without delusions. *Neuropsychiatry Neuropsychol Behav Neurol* 1995;8:264–70.

149. Staff RT, Shanks MF, Macintosh L *et al.* Delusions in Alzheimer's disease: SPET evidence of right hemispheric dysfunction. *Cortex* 1999;35:549–60.

150. Starkstein SE, Vazquez S, Petracca G. A SPECT study of delusions in Alzheimer's disease. *Neurology* 1994;44:2055–9.
151. Grady CL, Haxby JV, Schapiro MB. Subgroups in dementia of the Alzheimer type identified using positron emission tomography. *J Neuropsychiatry Clin Neurosci* 1990;2:373–84.
152. Mentis MJ, Weinstein EA, Horwitz B *et al.* Abnormal brain glucose metabolism in the delusional misidentification syndromes: a positron emission tomography study in Alzheimer disease. *Biol Psychiatry* 1995;38:438–49.
153. Förstl H, Burns A, Levy R *et al.* Neuropathological correlates of psychotic phenomena in confirmed Alzheimer's disease. *Br J Psychiatry* 1994;165:53–9.
154. Zubenko GS, Moossy J, Martinez AJ *et al.* Neuropathologic and neurochemical correlates of psychosis in primary dementia. *Arch Neurol* 1991;48:619–24.
155. Farber NB, Rubin EH, Newcomer JW *et al.* Increased neocortical neurofibrillary tangle density in subjects with Alzheimer disease and psychosis. *Arch Gen Psychiatry* 2000;57:1165–73.
156. Lai MKP, Lai O-F, Keene J *et al.* Psychosis of Alzheimer's disease is associated with elevated muscarinic M2 binding in the cortex. *Neurology* 2001;57: 805–11.
157. Rubin EH, Morris JC, Berg L. The progression of personality changes in senile dementia of the Alzheimer's type. *J Am Geriatr Soc* 1987;35:721–5.
158. Rubin EH, Morris JC, Storandt M *et al.* Behavioral changes in patients with mild senile dementia of the Alzheimer's type. *Psychiatry Res* 1987;21: 55–62.
159. Aitken L, Simpson S, Burns A. Personality change in dementia. *Int Psychogeriatr* 1999;11:263–71.
160. Petry S, Cummings JL, Hill MA *et al.* Personality alterations in dementia of the Alzheimer type. *Arch Neurol* 1988;45:1187–90.
161. Petry S, Cummings JL, Hill MA *et al.* Personality alterations in dementia of the Alzheimer type: a three-year follow-up study. *J Geriatr Psychiatry Neurol* 1989;2:203–7.
162. Chatterjee A, Strauss ME, Smyth KA *et al.* Personality changes in Alzheimer's disease. *Arch Neurol* 1992;49:486–91.
163. Strauss ME, Pasupathi M. Primary caregivers' descriptions of Alzheimer patients' personality traits: temporal stability and sensitivity to change. *Alzheimer Dis Assoc Disord* 1994;8:166–76.
164. Welleford EA, Harkins SW, Taylor JR. Personality change in dementia of the Alzheimer's type: relations to caregiver personality and burden. *Exp Aging Res* 1995;21:295–314.
165. Strauss ME, Lee MM, DiFilippo JM. Premorbid personality and behavioral symptoms in Alzheimer disease. *Arch Neurol* 1997;54:257–9.
166. Lyketsos CG, Corazzini K, Steele C. Mania in Alzheimer's disease. *J Neuropsychiatry Clin Neurosci* 1995;7:350–2.
167. Lebert F, Pasquier F, Danel T *et al.* Psychiatric, neuropsychologic, and SPECT evidence of elated mood in dementia of Alzheimer's type. *Neuropsychiatry Neuropsychol Behav Neurol* 1994;7:299–302.
168. Tiberti C, Sabe L, Kuzis G *et al.* Prevalence and correlates of the catastrophic reaction in Alzheimer's disease. *Neurology* 1998;50:546–8.
169. Porter V, Buxton WG, Fairbanks L *et al.* Frequency and characteristics of

anxiety among patients with Alzheimer's disease and related dementias. *J Neuropsychiatry Clin Neurosci* (in press).

170. Derouesne C, Guigot J, Chermat V *et al.* Sexual behavioral changes in Alzheimer disease. *Alzheimer Dis Assoc Disord* 1996;10:86–92.

171. Lilly R, Cummings JL, Benson DF *et al.* Clinical features of the human Kluver-Bucy syndrome. *Neurology* 1983;33:1141-5.

172. Bliwise DL, Watts RL, Watts N *et al.* Disruptive nocturnal behavior in Parkinson's disease and Alzheimer's disease. *J Geriatr Psychiatry Neurol* 1995;8:107–10.

173. Hwang J-P, Tsai S-J, Yang C-H *et al.* Hoarding behavior in dementia. *Am J Geriatr Psychiatry* 1998;6:285–9.

174. Berger A-K, Fratiglioni L, Forsell Y *et al.* The occurrence of depressive symptoms in the preclinical phase of AD: a population-based study. *Neurology* 1999;53:1998–2002.

175. Shimokawa A, Yakomi N, Anamizu S *et al.* Influence of deteriorating ability of emotional comprehension on interpersonal behavior in Alzheimer-type dementia. *Brain Cogn* 2001;47:423–33.

176. Albert MS, Cohen C, Koff E. Perception of affect in patients with dementia of the Alzheimer type. *Arch Neurol* 1991;48:791–5.

177. Cadieux NL, Greve KW. Emotion processing in Alzheimer's disease. *J Int Neuropsychol Soc* 1997;3:411–19.

178. Ogrocki PK, Hills AC, Strauss ME. Visual exploration of facial emotion by healthy older adults and patients with Alzheimer disease. *Neuropsychiatry Neuropsychol Behav Neurol* 2000;13:271–8.

179. Hargrave R, Maddock RJ, Stone V. Impaired recognition of facial expressions of emotion in Alzheimer's disease. *J Neuropsychiatry Clin Neurosci* 2002;14: 64–71.

180. Roberts VJ, Ingram SM, Lamar M *et al.* Prosody impairment and associated affective and behavioral disturbances in Alzheimer's disease. *Neurology* 1996;47:1482–8.

181. Testa JA, Beatty WW, Gleason AC *et al.* Impaired affective prosody in AD. *Neurology* 2001;57:1474–81.

182. Sweet RA, Nimgaonkar VL, Devlin B *et al.* Increased familial risk of the psychotic phenotype of Alzheimer disease. *Neurology* 2002;58:907–11.

183. Holmes C, Smith H, Ganderton R *et al.* Psychosis and aggression in Alzheimer's disease: the effect of dopamine receptor gene variation. *J Neurol Neurosurg Psychiatry* 2001;71:777–9.

184. Sweet R, Nimgaonkar VL, Kamboh MI *et al.* Dopamine receptor genetic variation, psychosis, and aggression in Alzheimer disease. *Arch Neurol* 1998;55:1335–40.

185. Holmes CJ, Arranz MJ, Powell JF *et al.* 5-HT2A and 5-HT2C receptor polymorphisms and psychopathology in late onset Alzheimer's disease. *Hum Mol Genet* 1998;7:1507–9.

186. Nacmias B, Tedde A, Forleo P *et al.* Association between 5-HT2A receptor polymorphism and psychotic symptoms in Alzheimer's disease. *Biol Psychiatry* 2001;50:472–5.

187. Sukonick DL, Pollock BG, Sweet R *et al.* The 5-HTTPR*S/*L polymorphism and aggressive behavior in Alzheimer disease. *Arch Neurol* 2001;58:1425–8.

188. Sweet RA, Pollock BG, Sukonick DL *et al.* The 5-HTTPR polymorphism confers

liability to a combined phenotype of psychotic and aggressive behavior in Alzheimer disease. *Int Psychogeriatr* 2001;13:401–9.

189. Hirono N, Mori E, Yasuda M *et al.* Lack of effect of apolipoprotein E E4 allele on neuropsychiatric manifestations in Alzheimer's disease. *J Neuropsychiatry Clin Neurosci* 1999;11:66–70.

190. Levy ML, Cummings JL, Fairbanks LA *et al.* Apolipoprotein E genotype and non-cognitive symptoms in Alzheimer's disease. *Biol Psychiatry* 1999;45:422–5.

191. Weiner MF, Vega G, Risser RC *et al.* Apolipoprotein Eε4, other risk factors, and course of Alzheimer's disease. *Biol Psychiatry* 1999;45:633–8.

192. Harwood DG, Barker WW, Ownby RL *et al.* Apolipoprotein-E (APO-E) genotype and symptoms of psychosis in Alzheimer's disease. *Am J Geriatr Psychiatry* 1999;7:119–23.

193. Scarmeas N, Brandt J, Albert M *et al.* Association between the *APOE* genotype and psychopathologic symptoms in Alzheimer's disease. *Neurology* 2002;58:1182–8.

194. Sano M, Ernesto C, Thomas RG *et al.* A controlled trial of selegiline, alpha-tocopherol, or both as treatment for Alzheimer's disease. *N Engl J Med* 1997;336:1216–22.

195. Tariot PN, Mack JL, Patterson MB *et al.* The Behavior Rating Scale for Dementia of the consortium to establish a registry for Alzheimer's disease. *Am J Psychiatry* 1995;152:1349–57.

196. Doody RS, Stevens JC, Beck C *et al.* Practice parameter: management of dementia (an evidence-based review). Report of the Quality Standards Subcommittee of the American Academy of Neurology. *Neurology* 2001;56: 1154–66.

197. Giacobini E (ed). Cholinesterase inhibitors: from the Calabar bean to Alzheimer therapy. In: *Cholinesterases and Cholinesterase Inhibitors.* London: Martin Dunitz, 2000: 181–226.

198. Mohs RC, Doody RS, Morris JC *et al.* A 1-year, placebo-controlled preservation of function survival study of donepezil in AD patients. *Neurology* 2001; 57:481–8.

199. Knopman D, Schneider L, Davis K *et al.* Long-term tacrine (Cognex) treatment: effects on nursing home placement and mortality. *Neurology* 1996;47:166–77.

200. Rogers SL, Friedhoff LT. The efficacy and safety of donepezil in patients with Alzheimer's disease: results of a US multicentre, randomized, double-blind, placebo-controlled trial: The Donepezil Study Group. *Dementia* 1996;7: 293–303.

201. Rogers SL, Farlow MR, Doody RS *et al.* A 24-week, double-blind, placebo-controlled trial of donepezil in patients with Alzheimer's disease: Donepezil Study Group. *Neurology* 1998;52:218–19.

202. Feldman H, Gauthier S, Hecker J *et al.* A 24-week, randomized, double-blind study of donepezil in moderate to severe Alzheimer's disease. *Neurology* 2001;57:613–20.

203. Tariot PN, Cummings J, Katz IR *et al.* A randomized, double-blind, placebo-controlled study of the efficacy and safety of donepezil in patients with Alzheimer's disease in the nursing home setting. *J Am Geriatr Soc* 2001;49: 1590–9.

204. Raskind MA, Peskind ER, Wessel T *et al.* Galantamine in AD: a 6-month randomized, placebo-controlled trial with a 6-month extension. *Neurology* 2000;54:2261–8.

205. Tariot PN, Solomon PR, Morris JC *et al.* A 5-month, randomized, placebo-controlled trial of galantamine in AD: The Galantamine USA-10 Study Group. *Neurology* 2000;54:2269–76.

206. Wilcock GK, Lilienfeld S, Gaens E *et al.* Efficacy and safety of galantamine in patients with mild to moderate Alzheimer's disease: multicentre randomised controlled trial. *BMJ* 2000;32:1–7.

207. Cummings J, Mega M. *Neuropsychiatry and Clinical Neuroscience.* New York: Oxford University Press (in press).

208. Corey-Bloom J, Anand R, Veach J. A randomized trial evaluating the efficacy and safety of ENA 713 (rivastigmine tartrate), a new acetylcholinesterase inhibitor, in patients with mild to moderately severe Alzheimer's disease: The ENA 713 B352 Study Group. *Int J Geriatr Psychopharmacol* 1998;1:55–65.

209. Rosler M, Anand R, Cicin-Sain A *et al.* Efficacy and safety of rivastigmine in patients with Alzheimer's disease: international randomized controlled trial. *BMJ* 1999;318:633–40.

210. Rosler M, Retz W, Retz-Junginger P *et al.* Effects of two-year treatment with the cholinesterase inhibitor rivastigmine on behavioural symptoms in Alzheimer's disease. *Behav Neurol* 1998/1999;11:211–16.

211. Cummings JL. Cholinesterase inhibitors: a new class of psychotropic compounds. *Am J Psychiatry* 2000;157:4–15.

212. Mega M, Masterman DM, O'Connor SM *et al.* The spectrum of behavioral responses in cholinesterase inhibitor therapy in Alzheimer's disease. *Arch Neurol* 1999;56:1388–93.

213. Mega MS, Dinov ID, Lee L *et al,* Orbital and dorsolateral frontal perfusion defect associated with behavioral response to cholinesterase inhibitor therapy in Alzheimer's disease. *J Neuropsychiatry Clin Neurosc* 2000;12:209–18.

214. Galynker I, Ieronimo C, Miner C *et al.* Methylphenidate treatment of negative symptoms in patients with dementia. *J Neuropsychiatry Clin Neurosci* 1997;9:231–9.

215. Jeste DV, Rockwell E, Harris MJ *et al.* Conventional vs. newer antipsychotics in elderly patients. *Am J Geriatr Psychiatry* 1999;7:70–6.

216. Jeste DV, Okamoto A, Napolitano J *et al.* Low incidence of persistent tardive dyskinesia in elderly patients with dementia treated with risperidone. *Am J Psychiatry* 2000a;157:1150–5.

217. Katz IR, Jeste DV, Mintzer JE *et al.* Comparison of risperidone and placebo for psychosis and behavioral disturbances associated with dementia: a randomized, double-blind trial: Risperidone Study Group. *J Clin Psychiatry* 1999;60:107–15.

218. De Deyn PP, Rabheru K, Rasmussen A *et al.* A randomized trial of risperidone, placebo, and haloperidol for behavioral symptoms of dementia. *Neurology* 1999;53:946–55.

219. Street J, Clark WS, Gannon KS *et al.* Olanzapine treatment of psychotic and behavioral symptoms in patients with Alzheimer's disease in nursing care

facilities. A double-blind, randomized, placebo-controlled trial. *Arch Gen Psychiatry* 2000;57:968–76.

220. Wood S, Cummings JL, Hsu M-A *et al*. The use of the Neuropsychiatric Inventory in nursing home residents: characterization and measurement. *Am J Geriatr Psychiatry* 2000;8:75–83.

221. Schneider L, Pollock VE, Lyness SA. A meta-analysis of controlled trials of neuroleptic treatment in dementia. *J Am Geriatr Soc* 1990;38:553–63.

222. Devanand DP, Marder K, Michaels KS *et al*. A randomized, placebo-controlled dose-comparison trial of haloperidol for psychosis and disruptive behaviors in Alzheimer's disease. *Am J Psychiatry* 1998;155:1512–20.

223. Tariot PN, Erb R, Leibovici A *et al*. Carbamazepine treatment of agitation in nursing home patients with dementia: a preliminary study. *J Am Geriatr Soc* 1994;42:1160–6.

224. Tariot PN, Erb R, Podgorski CA *et al*. Efficacy and tolerability of carbamazepine for agitation and aggression in dementia. *Am J Psychiatry* 1998;155:54–61.

225. Porsteinsson AP, Tariot PN, Erb R *et al*. Placebo-controlled study of divalproex sodium for agitation in dementia. *Am J Geriatr Psychiatry* 2001;9:58–66.

226. Devarajan S, Dursun SM. Aggression in dementia with lamotrigine treatment. *Am J Psychiatry* 2000;157:1178.

227. Hawkins JW, Tinkleberg JR, Sheikh JI *et al*. A retrospective chart review of gabapentin for the treatment of aggressive and agitated behavior in patients with dementias. *Am J Geriatr Psychiatry* 2000;8:221–5.

228. Roane DM, Feinberg TE, Meckler L *et al*. Treatment of dementia-associated agitation with gabapentin. *J Neuropsychiatry Clin Neurosci* 2000;12:40–3.

229. Pollock BG, Mulsant BH, Rosen J *et al*. Comparison of citalopram, perphenazine, and placebo for the acute treatment of psychosis and behavioral disturbances in hospitalized, demented patients. *Am J Psychiatry* 2002; 159:460–5.

230. Sultzer DL, Gray KF, Gunay I *et al*. A double-blind comparison of trazodone and haloperidol for treatment of agitation in patients with dementia. *Am J Geriatr Psychiatry* 1996;5:60–9.

231. Kyomen HH, Satlin A, Hennen J *et al*. Estrogen therapy and aggressive behavior in elderly patients with moderate-to-severe dementia: results from a short-term, randomized, double-blind trial. *Am J Geriatr Psychiatry* 1999;7:339–48.

232. Lebert F, Pasquier F, Petit H. Behavioral effects of trazodone in Alzheimer's disease. *J Clin Psychiatry* 1994;55:536–8.

233. Pollock BG, Mulsant BH, Sweet R *et al*. An open pilot study of citalopram for behavioral disturbances of dementia. *Am J Geriatr Psychiatry* 1997;5:70–8.

234. Shankle WR, Nielson KA, Cotman CW. Low-dose propranolol reduces aggression and agitation resembling that associated with orbitofrontal dysfunction in elderly demented patients. *Alzheimer Dis Assoc Disord* 1995;9:233–7.

235. Clark WS, Street JS, Feldman PD, Breier A. The effects of olanzapine in reducing the emergence of psychosis among nursing home patients with Alzheimer's disease. *J Clin Psychiatry* 2001;62:34–40.

236. Street JS, Clark WS, Kadam DL *et al*. Long-term efficacy of olanzapine in the control of psychotic and behavioral symptoms in nursing home patients with Alzheimer's dementia. *Int J Geriatr Psychiatry* 2001;16:S62–70.

237. Burke KL, Folks DG, Roccaforte WH *et al.* Serotonin reuptake inhibitors for the treatment of coexisting depression and psychosis in dementia of the Alzheimer type. *Am J Geriatr Psychiatry* 1994;2:352–4.
238. Burke WJ, Dewan V, Wengel SP *et al.* The use of selective serotonin reuptake inhibitors for depression and psychosis complicating dementia. *Int J Geriatr Psychiatry* 1997;12:519–25.
239. Li Y-S, Meyer JS, Thornby J. Longitudinal follow-up of depressive symptoms among normal versus cognitively impaired elderly. *Int J Geriatr Psychiatry* 2001;16:718–27.
240. Petracca G, Teson A, Chemerinski E *et al.* A double-blind placebo-controlled study of clomipramine in depressed patients with Alzheimer's disease. *J Neuropsychiatry Clin Neurosci* 1996;8:270–5.
241. Lyketsos CG, Sheppard J-ME, Steele CD *et al.* Randomized, placebo-controlled, double-blind clinical trial of sertraline in the treatment of depression complicating Alzheimer's disease: initial results from the depression in Alzheimer's disease study. *Am J Psychiatry* 2000;157:1686–9.
242. Tariot PN, Cohen RM, Sunderland T. L-Deprenyl in Alzheimer's disease: preliminary evidence for behavioral change with monoamine oxidase B inhibition. *Arch Gen Psychiatry* 1987;44:427–33.
243. Taragano FE, Lyketsos CG, Mangone CA *et al.* A Double-blind, randomized, fixed-dose trial of fluoxetine vs. amitriptyline in the treatment of major depression complicating Alzheimer's disease. *Psychosomatics* 1997;38:246–52.
244. Katona CL, Hunter BN, Bray J. A double-blind comparison of the efficacy and safety of paroxetine and imipramine in the treatment of depression with dementia. *Int J Geriatr Psychiatry* 1998;13:100–8.
245. Mintzer J, Faison W, Street J *et al.* Olanzapine in the treatment of anxiety symptoms due to Alzheimer's disease: a post hoc analysis. *Int J Geriatr Psychiatry* 2001;16:S71–S77.
246. Cooper AJ. Medroxyprogesterone acetate (MPA) treatment of sexual acting out in men suffering from dementia. *J Clin Psychiatry* 1987;48:368–70.
247. Amadeo M. Antiandrogen treatment of aggressivity in men suffering from dementia. *J Geriatr Psychiatry Neurol* 1996;9:142–5.
248. Levitsky AM, Owens NJ. Pharmacologic treatment of hypersexuality and paraphilias in nursing home residents. *J Am Geriatr Soc* 1999;47:231–4.
249. Ballard C, O'Brien J, James I *et al. Dementia: Management of Behavioural and Psychological Symptoms.* New York: Oxford University Press, 2001.
250. Mittleman M, Ferris S, Shulman E *et al.* A family intervention to delay nursing home placement of patients with Alzheimer's disease. *JAMA* 1996;276: 1725–31.

chapter 4

Dementia with Lewy bodies

Dementia with Lewy bodies (DLB) is a complex neuropsychiatric syndrome including dementia, prominent neuropsychiatric symptoms, and parkinsonism. The disorder shares clinical and pathological features with Alzheimer's disease; a similar syndrome occurs in patients with Parkinson's disease and dementia (Chapter 5). The pathologic hallmark of DLB is the presence of Lewy bodies in the cerebral cortex.

Diagnostic features for DLB are presented in Box 4.1.[1] Patients have a progressive dementia syndrome with prominent attentional deficits, fluctuating cognition, marked visual hallucinations, and parkinsonism (two of these three latter features must be present for diagnosis of probable DLB). Other neuropsychiatric features including delusions, misidentification symptoms, rapid eye movement (REM) sleep behavior disorder, and depression are common. Neuroleptic sensitivity may be marked and use of conventional neuroleptic medications is contraindicated in the treatment of neuropsychiatric symptoms in this disorder. Most studies have shown the criteria for DLB to have high specificity (80–100%), but more limited sensitivity (35–80%).[2–6]

Clinical features

Dementia with Lewy bodies accounts for approximately 20–30% of autopsy series of dementing disorders.[1,7] Onset of the disease varies

Box 4.1 Consensus criteria for the clinical diagnosis of probable and possible DLB[1,62]

- Progressive cognitive decline of sufficient magnitude to interfere with normal social or occupational function. Prominent or persistent memory impairment may not necessarily occur in the early stages but is usually evident with progression. Deficits on tests of attention and of frontal-subcortical skills and visuospatial ability may be especially prominent
- Two of the following core features are essential for a diagnosis of probable DLB, and one is essential for possible DLB:
  - Fluctuating cognition with pronounced variations in attention and alertness
  - Recurrent visual hallucinations that are typically well formed and detailed
  - Spontaneous motor features of parkinsonism
- Features supportive of the diagnosis are:
  - Repeated falls
  - Syncope
  - Transient loss of consciousness
  - Neuroleptic sensitivity
  - Systematized delusions
  - Hallucinations in other modalities
  - REM sleep behavior disorder
  - Depression
- DLB is less likely in the presence of:
  - Stroke disease, evident as focal neurologic signs or on brain imaging
  - Evidence on physical examination and investigation of any physical illness or other brain disorder sufficient to account for the clinical picture

between 50 and 90 years of age and the duration of the illness varies between 6 and 10 years (similar or slightly shorter than the duration of Alzheimer's disease).[7,8] The disease is increasingly common among aged individuals. Men are more likely than women to manifest DLB and the apolipoproteinE-4 genotype has been found to be a risk factor for DLB by most investigators.[9]

The parkinsonian syndrome of DLB consists primarily of bradykinesia and rigidity. Half of the patients manifest a rest tremor and approximately

20% have myoclonus. Seventy percent of patients with DLB have at least a transient beneficial response to treatment with levodopa.[10]

Dementia syndrome

Patients with the common form of DLB present with dementia as the primary manifestation. Patients with Parkinson's disease and DLB present with parkinsonism and progress to a dementia syndrome over the course of several years. Patients with diffuse Lewy body disease (a rare form of DLB, discussed below) present in midlife with an extrapyramidal syndrome and progress to parkinsonism with dementia.

The typical dementia syndrome of DLB includes pronounced attentional fluctuations; in some cases distinguishing the dementia of DLB from a delirium can be difficult. Attentional disturbances are evident when patients are assessed by clinical inquiry or by neuropsychological or electroencephalographic measures. Caregivers report that patients have spontaneous periods of impaired alertness and concentration where they appear drowsy but awake and are not aware of their environment. These periods may vary in duration from several minutes to a day or more.[11] Neuropsychological measures of vigilance and complex reaction time similarly reveal attentional deficits,[12] and electroencephalographic measures demonstrate excessive fluctuation of EEG frequency on a second-to-second basis.[11]

Patients with DLB have prominent visuospatial deficits and perform poorly on tests of visuoperceptual function, such as object size discrimination, form discrimination, overlapping figure identification, and visual counting tasks. They also perform more poorly than patients with Alzheimer's disease on picture arrangement, block design, and object assembly tasks from the Wechsler Adult Intelligence Scale-Revised.[13,14] Memory and naming abilities are less severely impaired in DLB than in Alzheimer's disease.[14,15] Cognitive skills mediated by the frontal lobes or frontal-subcortical circuits including verbal fluency tasks, tests requiring alternation of sets and assessments of response inhibition are more compromised in patients with DLB than patients with Alzheimer's disease.[16]

Neuropsychiatric features

Neuropsychiatric symptoms are among the defining features of DLB. Although the behavioral alterations that occur in DLB are not unique to the disorder and occur in other dementing illnesses, they are present at a much higher frequency in DLB than in other dementias. Visual hallucinations are one of the key diagnostic features of DLB, but hallucinations in other domains, delusions, delusional misidentification, mood changes, and REM sleep behavior disorder are also prominent neuropsychiatric manifestations. The visual hallucinations characteristic of DLB are fully formed and usually involve animals, people, or scenes being acted out near the patient.

Neuropsychiatric change is more common at the time of presentation in patients with DLB than in those with Alzheimer's disease. These differences become less marked in patients in more advanced phases of the two conditions.[17,18] Misidentification delusions such as the Capgras syndrome represent a specific type of delusional disorder that is more common in DLB than in Alzheimer's disease.[17] Figure 4.1 shows the frequency of neuropsychiatric symptoms observed during the course of

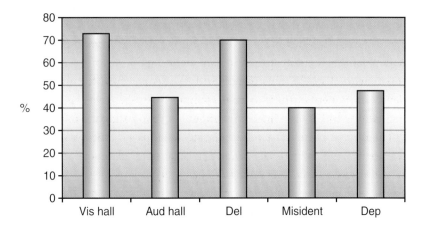

Figure 4.1 Neuropsychiatric symptoms in patients with pathologically confirmed DLB.[17] Vis hall, visual hallucinations; Aud hall, auditory hallucinations; Del, delusions; Misident, misidentification symptoms; Dep, depression.

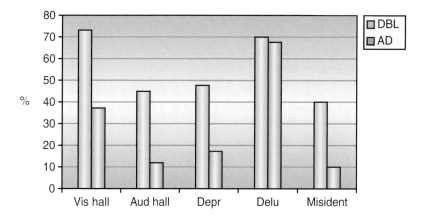

Figure 4.2 *Comparison of neuropsychiatric symptoms in patients with dementia with Lewy bodies (DLB) and in patients with Alzheimer's disease (AD).[17] There were 98 patients in the DLB sample and 92 patients in the AD sample. The proportions of symptoms in this clinically diagnosed cohort were similar to the percent reported in patients with pathologic confirmation. All differences are statistically significant except delusions. Vis hall, visual hallucinations; Aud hall, auditory hallucinations; Depr, depression; Delu, delusions; Misident, misidentification.*

DLB in a group of patients with pathologically confirmed disease.[17] Figure 4.2 contrasts neuropsychiatric symptoms in patients with DLB with those of Alzheimer's disease.[17] Compared to patients with Parkinson's disease following treatment with levodopa, hallucinations and depression are equally common, but delusions are more common in those with DLB.[19,20] Compared with patients with frontotemporal dementia, patients with DLB more commonly exhibit delusions and hallucinations and are less likely to manifest euphoria and disinhibition.[21]

There have been few studies relating neuropsychiatric symptoms to the cognitive deficits of DLB. In general, patients with more severe cognitive disturbances exhibit more marked behavioral changes.[22] Relationships between cognition and neuropsychiatric symptoms are weak in DLB where behavioral disturbances are often present in patients with only mild cognitive changes.

REM sleep behavior disorder is characterized by limb or truncal jerking and complex and sometimes violent behavior associated with dream recall. There is polysomnographic evidence during REM sleep of elevated tonic or phasic limb tone on electromyography. There is an absence of epileptic activity during REM sleep on electroencephalography. Patients with dementia and REM sleep behavior disorder most commonly have DLB as the underlying cause of the dementia syndrome.[23,24] Patients with DLB have a variety of other types of sleep disturbances including excessive daytime sleepiness, nocturnal periodic limb movements, confusion on awakening, and bad dreams.[25]

The Neuropsychiatric Inventory (NPI)[26] has been used to characterize the profile of behavioral changes in neuropsychiatric symptoms in patients with DLB[21] (Figure 4.3). The NPI reveals high rates of apathy, delusions, hallucinations, and aberrant motor behavior. Depression, anxiety, irritability, aggression, and disinhibition were less common and euphoria was not present in any of the patients studied.

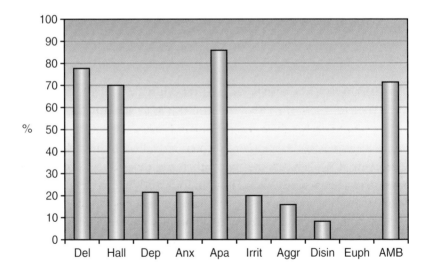

Figure 4.3 Percent of patients with scoreable symptoms on the Neuropsychiatric Inventory (data from Hirono et al. 1999).[21] The sample was based on 23 patients with DLB with Mini-Mental State Scores of 17.7. Depression was less common in this sample than in most studies of patients with DLB. Del, delusions; Hall, hallucinations; Dep, depression; Anx, anxiety; Apa, apathy; Irrit, irritability; Aggr, aggression; Disin, disinhibition; Euph, euphoria; AMB, aberrant motor behavior.

Neuroimaging

Studies with magnetic resonance imaging (MRI) reveal that medial temporal and hippocampal atrophy is significantly greater in DLB than in normal control patients, but less severe than in patients with Alzheimer's disease.[27,28] Studies with single photon emission tomography (SPECT) or fluorodeoxyglucose (FDG) positron emission tomography (PET) reveal diminished cortical perfusion or metabolism sparing the primary somatomotor cortex. Unlike patients with Alzheimer's disease, those with DLB have marked hypoperfusion or hypometabolism of the primary occipital cortex.[29–32]

Neuroimaging studies also reveal diminished dopaminergic activity in the basal ganglia of patients with DLB. F^{18}-fluorodopa PET shows diminished dopamine uptake in the basal ganglia[33] and SPECT studies using a marker for the striatal dopamine transporter reveal diminished transporter activity in the basal ganglia.[34]

Lewy body disorders

Lewy bodies occur in several neurological disorders (Box 4.2). As noted, there are two forms of DLB (one presenting with dementia and parkinsonism and the other presenting with Parkinson's disease and progressing to include a dementia (Chapter 5)). Parkinson's disease is characterized by Lewy bodies and other pathological changes in the brain stem (Chapter 5). Similarly, a syndrome of isolated dysphagia has been related to brain stem Lewy bodies in the region of the vagal nucleus, and patients with clinical syndromes manifesting progressive supranuclear palsy, dystonia, and motor neuron disease have all been found to exhibit Lewy bodies at autopsy.[35]

Patients with DLB typically have concomitant histopathological evidence of neuritic plaques (described below). There is also a syndrome of diffuse (or cortical) Lewy body disease without co-occurring Alzheimer's type pathology. This disorder tends to present in the presenile or even juvenile age group with a parkinsonian syndrome and progressive

---

Box 4.2 Disorders associated with Lewy bodies (modified from Lowe and Dickson[35])

Dementia with Lewy bodies
   Form with dementia preceding parkinsonism
   Form with Parkinson's disease preceding dementia
Diffuse Lewy body disease
   Sporadic
   Familial
Parkinson's disease
   Sporadic
   A-synuclein mutations
   MPTP-parkinsonism
Miscellaneous conditions
   Isolated dysphagia
   Progressive supranuclear palsy-like disorder
   Dystonia-type disorder
   Motor neuron disorder-type disorder
   Pure autonomic failure

---

dementia. Psychotic features including hallucinations are commonly present.[36,37] A familial form of diffuse Lewy body disease has been described.[38]

Neuropathology

The hallmark of DLB is the presence of the Lewy body in brain stem and cortical structures. In the brain stem, Lewy bodies are found in the substantia nigra and the locus ceruleus. They also are common in the nucleus basalis of Meynert. Subcortical Lewy bodies consist of a dense amorphous core surrounded by a filamentous halo. They are typically round and one or more may occur in the cytoplasm of the neuron. Cortical Lewy bodies are smaller, less well-defined, and rarely have a definite core[39] (Figure 4.4). Lewy bodies contain neurofilament subunits, ubiqui-

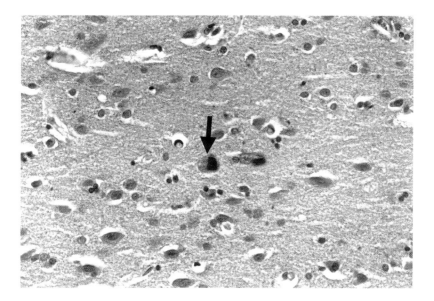

Figure 4.4 *Cortical Lewy body from the neocortex of a patient with DLB (magnification 350×; alpha-synuclein antibody stain) (courtesy of H Vinters, MD, Division of Neuropathology, UCLA School of Medicine).*

tin, and alpha-synuclein.[39,40] In Parkinson's disease, Lewy bodies are prominent in the brain stem structures and rare in the cortex, whereas in DLB they are common in the limbic system (transitional form of DLB) or the limbic system and the neocortex (neocortical form of DLB).[1] Patients with typical DLB (onset over age 60) have beta-amyloid plaques in addition to cortical Lewy bodies. Approximately half of the cases of DLB have neurofibrillary tangles; the abundance of tangle formation is less severe in DLB than in Alzheimer's disease.[39] Amyloid deposits in blood vessels are common in DLB.[41] Clinicopathological correlations reveal that the severity of dementia in DLB is associated significantly with the abundance of cortical Lewy bodies.[42,43]

Neurochemical studies reveal that patients with DLB have reductions in basal ganglia dopamine similar to that observed in Parkinson's disease. Markers of cholinergic functions are reduced in DLB, and cholinergic deficits are more severe in DLB than in Alzheimer's disease.[44,45]

Cholinergic activity is more markedly reduced in DLB patients with visual hallucinations compared with those without[46] (Figure 4.5). In contrast, serotonergic receptor binding and both dopamine and serotonin metabolites are significantly more reduced in cases without hallucinations.[47] Thus, a ratio of reduced cholinergic activity compared with relatively preserved dopaminergic and serotonergic activity is characteristic of DLB patients with hallucinations. Increased muscarinic receptor binding (M1 receptor) and increased D3 receptor density have both been correlated with the occurrence of psychosis in patients with DLB.[48,49]

Pharmacotherapy

Pharmacologic treatment of DLB includes treatment of the parkinsonian syndrome with dopaminergic agents, therapy for the cognitive deficit with cholinesterase inhibitors, and treatment of the behavioral disturbances with cholinesterase inhibitors or psychotropic medications.

Treatment of the parkinsonian syndrome with dopaminergic agents provides at least partial relief of the motor disability in 70% of patients with DLB.[10] Potential exacerbation of visual hallucinations and delu-

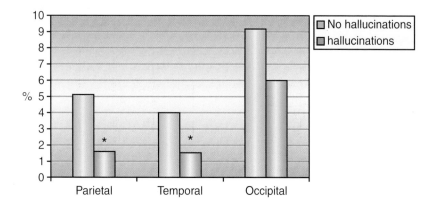

Figure 4.5 *Choline acetyltransferase activity (nmol/H/mg protein) in patients with DLB. Patients with hallucinations had lower choline acetyltranferase activity in parietal and temporal cortex than DLB patients without hallucinations.[46]*

sions must be monitored; these symptoms occur at a high rate before treatment in patients with DLB.

Cholinesterase inhibitors may improve both the cognitive deficits and some behavioral disturbances in patients with DLB. The marked cholinergic deficit of DLB, prominence of attentional deficits, and fluctuating cognition suggest that cholinergic therapy may ameliorate attentional deficits and related cognitive disturbances. Open-label observations with tacrine, donepezil, and rivastigmine support the utility of cholinesterase inhibitors in improving cognition in patients with DLB.[50-52] Side effects with cholinesterase inhibitors involve cholinergic activation of the gastrointestinal system and include nausea, vomiting, diarrhea, and anorexia.

A double-blind placebo-controlled trial of rivastigmine in patients with DLB showed a significant reduction in the four-item cluster of delusions, hallucinations, apathy, and depression as rated by the NPI. The percentage of patients exhibiting at least a 30% reduction in the total of these four items was significantly different in the rivastigmine and placebo groups. Individual symptoms that improved with rivastigmine therapy included apathy, indifference, anxiety, delusions, hallucinations, and aberrant motor behavior.[53] The total NPI score was also reduced (Figure 4.6).

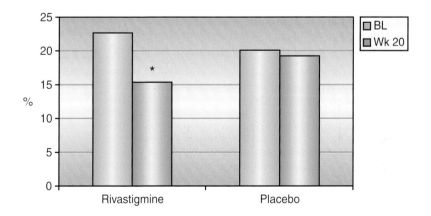

Figure 4.6 *Rivastigmine significantly reduced the Neuropsychiatric Inventory total score (10 items) in the observed case analysis (patients who completed the clinical trial).*[53]

The high frequency of neuropsychiatric symptoms in patients with DLB leads clinicians to use psychotropic agents in many cases. These patients are vulnerable to severe and sometimes fatal neuroleptic sensitivity when treated with conventional neuroleptic agents.[54] Atypical antipsychotic agents are therefore preferred for treatment of delusions, hallucinations, misidentifications, and agitation in patients with DLB if patients do not improve following treatment with a cholinesterase inhibitor. Clozapine, risperidone, olanzapine, and quetiapine are atypical antipsychotic agents that are potentially useful in the treatment of DLB.[55–57] One post-hoc analysis of patients meeting criteria for DLB and included in a double-blind placebo-controlled trial of olanzapine for treatment of psychosis and agitation in patients with Alzheimer's disease revealed a significant antipsychotic effect without concomitant worsening of cognition or motor function.[58] However, even atypical agents may produce parkinsonism in this vulnerable patient population and individuals treated with atypical antipsychotics must be monitored carefully for exacerbation of their parkinsonism.[57,59,60]

Treatment with mood-stabilizing anticonvulsant drugs such as carbamazepine or serotonergic antidepressant agents such as trazodone may ameliorate agitation in some patients with DLB.[61,62]

Depression is common in DLB[63] and treatment with antidepressant agents (usually selective serotonin reuptake inhibitors) is warranted.

References

1. McKeith IG, Galaski D, Kosaka K *et al.* Consensus guidelines for the clinical and pathologic diagnosis of dementia with Lewy bodies (DLB): report of the consortium on DLB international workshop. *Neurology* 1996;47:1113–24.
2. Lopez OL, Litvan I, Catt KE *et al.* Accuracy of four clinical diagnostic criteria for the diagnosis of neurodegenerative dementias. *Neurology* 1999;53:1292–9.
3. McKeith IG, Fairbairn AF, Bothwell RA *et al.* An evaluation of the predictive validity and inter-rater reliability of clinical diagnostic criteria for senile dementia of the Lewy body type. *Neurology* 1994;44:872–7.
4. Mega MS, Masterman DL, Benson DF *et al.* Dementia with Lewy bodies: reliability and validity of clinical and pathologic criteria. *Neurology* 1996; 47:1403–9.
5. Verghese J, Crystal HA, Dickson DW *et al.* Validity of clinical criteria for the diagnosis of dementia with Lewy bodies. *Neurology* 1999;53:1974–82.

6. Lopez OL, Becker JT, Kaufer DI *et al*. Research evaluation and prospective diagnosis of dementia with Lewy bodies. *Arch Neurol* 2002;59:43–6.
7. Papka M, Rubio A, Schiffer RB. A review of Lewy body disease, an emerging concept of cortical dementia. *J Neuropsychiatry Clin Neurosci* 1998;10:267–79.
8. Olichney JM, Galasko D, Salmon DP *et al*. Cognitive decline is faster in Lewy body variant than in Alzheimer's disease. *Neurology* 1998;51:351–7.
9. Galasko D, Saitoh T, Xia Y *et al*. The apolipoprotein E allele e4 is overrepresented in patients with the Lewy body variant of Alzheimer's disease. *Neurology* 1994;44:1950–1.
10. Louis ED, Klatka LA, Liu Y *et al*. Comparison of extrapyramidal features in 31 pathologically confirmed cases of diffuse Lewy body disease and 34 pathologically confirmed cases of Parkinson's disease. *Neurology* 1997;48:376–80.
11. Walker MP, Ayre GA, Cummings JL *et al*. Quantifying fluctuation in dementia with Lewy bodies, Alzheimer's disease, and vascular dementia. *Neurology* 2000;54:1616–24.
12. Ballard C, O'Brien J, Gray A *et al*. Attention and fluctuating attention in patients with dementia with Lewy bodies and Alzheimer disease. *Arch Neurol* 2001;58:977–82.
13. Mori E, Shimomura T, Fujimori M *et al*. Visuoperceptual impairment in dementia with Lewy bodies. *Arch Neurol* 2000;57:489–93.
14. Shimomura T, Mori E, Yamashita H *et al*. Cognitive loss in dementia with Lewy bodies and Alzheimer disease. *Arch Neurol* 1998;55:1547–52.
15. Heyman A, Fillenbaum GG, Gearing M *et al*. Comparison of Lewy body variant of Alzheimer's disease with pure Alzheimer's disease: Consortium to Establish a Registry for Alzheimer's Disease, part XIX. *Neurology* 1999; 52:1839–44.
16. Downes JJ, Priestley NM, Doran M *et al*. Intellectual, mnemonic, and frontal functions in dementia with Lewy bodies: a comparison with early and advanced Parkinson's disease. *Behav Neurol* 1998/1999;11:173–83.
17. Ballard C, Holmes C, McKeith I *et al*. Psychiatric morbidity in dementia with Lewy bodies: a prospective clinical and neuropathological comparative study with Alzheimer's disease. *Am J Psychiatry* 1999;156:1039–45.
18. Weiner MF, Risser RC, Cullum CM *et al*. Alzheimer's disease and its Lewy body variant: a clinical analysis of postmortem verified cases. *Am J Psychiatry* 1996;153:1269–73.
19. Klatka LA, Louis ED, Schiffer RB. Psychiatric features in diffuse Lewy body disease: a clinicopathologic study using Alzheimer's disease and Parkinson's disease comparison groups. *Neurology* 1996;47:1148–52.
20. Aarsland D, Ballard C, Larsen JP, McKeith I. A comparative study of psychiatric symptoms in dementia with Lewy bodies and Parkinson's disease with and without dementia. *Int J Geriatr Psychiatry* 2001;16:528–36.
21. Hirono N, Mori E, Tanimukai S *et al*. Distinctive neurobehavioral features among neurodegenerative dementias. *J Neuropsychiatry Clin Neurosci* 1999; 11:498–503.
22. Del Ser T, McKeith I, Anand R *et al*. Dementia with Lewy bodies: findings from an international multicentre study. *Int J Geriatr Psychiatry* 2000; 15:1034–45.
23. Boeve BF, Silber MH, Ferman TJ *et al*. REM sleep behavior disorder and

degenerative dementia: an association likely reflecting Lewy body disease. *Neurology* 1998;51:363–70.

24. Ferman TJ, Boeve BF, Smith GE *et al*. REM sleep behavior disorder and dementia: cognitive differences when compared with AD. *Neurology* 1999; 52:951–7.

25. Grace JB, Walker MP, McKeith IG. A comparison of sleep profiles in patients with dementia with Lewy bodies and Alzheimer's disease. *Int J Geriatr Psychiatry* 2000;15:1028–33.

26. Cummings JL, Mega M, Gray K *et al*. The Neuropsychiatric Inventory: comprehensive assessment of psychopathology in dementia. *Neurology* 1994; 44:2308–14.

27. Barber R, Gholkar A, Scheltens P *et al*. Medial temporal lobe atrophy in MRI in dementia with Lewy bodies. *Neurology* 1999;52:1153–8.

28. Hashimoto M, Kitagaki H, Imamura T *et al*. Medial temporal and whole-brain atrophy in dementia with Lewy bodies: a volumetric MRI study. *Neurology* 1998;51:357–62.

29. Albin RL, Minoshima S, D'Amato CJ *et al*. Fluoro-deoxyglucose positron emission tomography in diffuse Lewy body disease. *Neurology* 1996;47:462–6.

30. Ishii K, Yamaji S, Kitagaki H *et al*. Regional cerebral blood flow difference between dementia with Lewy bodies and AD. *Neurology* 1999;53:413–16.

31. Lobotesis K, Fenwick JD, Phipps A *et al*. Occipital hypoperfusion on SPECT in dementia with Lewy bodies but not AD. *Neurology* 2001;56:643–9.

32. Minoshima S, Foster NL, Sima AAF *et al*. Alzheimer's disease versus dementia with Lewy bodies: cerebral metabolic distinction with autopsy confirmation. *Ann Neurol* 2001;50:358–65.

33. Hu XS, Okamura N, Arai H *et al*. ^{18}F-fluorodopa PET study of striatal dopamine uptake in the diagnosis of dementia with Lewy bodies. *Neurology* 2000;55:1575–6.

34. Donnemiller E, Heilmann J, Wenning GK *et al*. Brain perfusion scintigraphy with 99m Tc-HMPAO or 99m Tc-ECD and 123I-β-CIT single-photon emission tomography in dementia of the Alzheimer-type and diffuse Lewy body disease. *Eur J Nucl Med* 1997;24:320–5.

35. Lowe J, Dickson DW. Pathological diagnostic criteria for dementia associated with cortical Lewy bodies: review and proposal for a descriptive approach. *J Neural Transm* 1997;51:111–20.

36. Kosaka K. Diffuse Lewy body disease in Japan. *J Neurol* 1990;237:197–204.

37. Hely MA, Reid WGJ, Halliday GM *et al*. Diffuse Lewy body disease: clinical features in nine cases without coexistent Alzheimer's disease. *J Neurol Neurosurg Psychiatry* 1996;60:531–8.

38. Brett FM, Henson C, Staunton H. Familial diffuse Lewy body disease, eye movement abnormalities, and distribution of pathology. *Arch Neurol* 2002; 59:464–7.

39. Lennox G, Lowe J. Dementia with Lewy bodies. In: Markesbery WR (ed) *Neuropathology of Dementing Disorders*. New York: Arnold, 1998: 181–92.

40. Baba M, Nakajo S, Tu P-H *et al*. Aggregation of alpha-synuclein in Lewy bodies of sporadic Parkinson's disease and dementia with Lewy bodies. *Am J Pathology* 1998;152:879.

41. Wu E, Lipton RB, Dickson DW. Amyloid angiopathy in diffuse Lewy body disease. *Neurology* 1992;42:2131–5.

42. Haroutunian V, Serby M, Purohit DP *et al.* Contribution of Lewy body inclusions to dementia in patients with and without Alzheimer disease neuropathological conditions. *Arch Neurol* 2000;57:1145–50.

43. Samuel W, Galasko D, Masliah E *et al.* Neocortical Lewy body counts correlate with dementia in the Lewy body variant of Alzheimer's disease. *J Neuropathol Exp Neurol* 1996;55:44–52.

44. Langlais PJ, Thal L, Hansen L *et al.* Neurotransmitters in basal ganglia and cortex of Alzheimer's disease with and without Lewy bodies. *Neurology* 1993;43:1927–34.

45. Tiraboschi P, Hansen LA, Alford M *et al.* Cholinergic dysfunction in diseases with Lewy bodies. *Neurology* 2000;54:407–11.

46. Perry EK, Kerwin J, Perry RH *et al.* Cerebral cholinergic activity is related to the incidence of visual hallucinations in senile dementia of Lewy body type. *Dementia* 1990;1:2–4.

47. Perry EK, Marshall E, Kerwin J *et al.* Evidence of a monoaminergic-cholinergic imbalance related to visual hallucinations in Lewy body dementia. *J Neurochem* 1990;55:1454–6.

48. Ballard C, Piggott M, Johnson M *et al.* Delusions associated with elevated muscarinic binding in dementia with Lewy bodies. *Ann Neurol* 2000; 48:868–76.

49. Sweet RA, Hamilton RL, Healy MT *et al.* Alterations of striatal dopamine receptor binding in Alzheimer disease are associated with Lewy body pathology and antemortem psychosis. *Arch Neurol* 2001;58:466–72.

50. Levy R, Eagger S, Griffiths M *et al.* Lewy bodies and response to tacrine in Alzheimer's disease. *Lancet* 1994;343:176.

51. Kaufer DI, Catt KE, Lopez OL *et al.* Dementia with Lewy bodies: response of delirium-like features to donepezil. *Neurology* 1998;51:1512.

52. Grace J, Daniel S, Stevens T *et al.* Long-term use of rivastigmine in patients with dementia with Lewy bodies: an open-label trial. *Int Psychogeriatr* 2001; 13:199–205.

53. McKeith I, Del Ser T, Spano PF *et al.* Efficacy of rivastigmine in dementia with Lewy bodies: a randomised, double-blind, placebo-controlled international study. *Lancet* 2000;356:2031–6.

54. McKeith I, Fairbairn A, Perry R *et al.* Neuroleptic sensitivity in patients with senile dementia of Lewy body type. *BMJ* 1992;305:673–8.

55. Allen RL, Walker Z, D'Ath PJ *et al.* Risperidone for psychotic and behavioural symptoms in Lewy body dementia. *Lancet* 1995;346:185.

56. Chacko RC, Hurley RA, Jankovic J. Clozapine use in diffuse Lewy body disease. *J Neuropsychiatry Clin Neurosci* 1993;5:206–8.

57. Walker Z, Grace J, Overshot R *et al.* Olanzapine in dementia with Lewy bodies: a clinical study. *Int J Geriatr Psychiatry* 1999;14:459–66.

58. Cummings JL, Street J, Masterman DL *et al.* Efficacy of olanzapine in the treatment of psychosis in dementia with Lewy bodies. *Dement Geriatr Cogn Disord* 2002;13:67–73.

59. Burke WJ. Neuroleptic sensitivity to clozapine in dementia with Lewy bodies. *J Neuropsychiatry Clin Neurosci* 1998;10:227–9.

60. McKeith I, Ballard C, Harrison RWS. Neuroleptic sensitivity to risperidone in Lewy body dementia. *Lancet* 1995;346:699.

61. Geroldi C, Frisoni GB, Bianchetti A *et al.* Drug treatment in Lewy body dementia. *Dement Geriatr Cogn Disord* 1997;8:188–97.
62. Stewart JT, Yelton JA. Treatment of organic hallucinosis with carbamazepine. *Am J Psychiatry* 1995;152:150.
63. McKeith IG, Perry EK, Perry RH. Report of the second dementia with Lewy body international workshop: diagnosis and treatment. *Neurology* 1999; 53:902–5.

chapter 5

Parkinson's disease and related parkinsonian syndromes

The diagnosis of Parkinson's disease (PD) is based on clinical criteria and there are no confirmatory laboratory studies. An alternative diagnosis is found at autopsy in 10–30% of patients and is most commonly an extrapyramidal disorder with overlapping clinical signs such as progressive supranuclear palsy or corticobasal degeneration. Dementia is present in approximately 40% of patients with PD and another 30–40% have intellectual impairment, predominantly deficits in executive function, that impair cognition but do not meet full criteria for a dementia syndrome. Patients with dementia are more vulnerable than those without to the development of neuropsychiatric symptoms.

Box 5.1 presents clinical criteria for diagnosis of idiopathic PD. Requirements are a beneficial response to levodopa and at least two of the symptoms of rest tremor, bradykinesia, cogwheel rigidity, or postural reflex impairment.[1] Other causes of parkinsonism such as trauma, brain tumor, infection, vascular disease, other known neurological diseases, or drugs, chemicals, or toxins exclude the diagnosis of PD. Similarly, signs that are prominent in other non-PD parkinsonian syndromes exclude the diagnosis of PD – including prominent oculomotor palsy, cerebellar signs, vocal cord paresis, orthostatic hypotension, pyramidal tract signs, or amyotrophy. Finally, hypointensity of the striatum on magnetic resonance imaging (MRI) is also more indicative of atypical parkinsonism than PD and is an exclusionary criterion for the diagnosis of PD.

Box 5.1 Criteria for the diagnosis of Parkinson's disease[1]

- Beneficial response to levodopa ($\geq$33% improvement on at least one timed test)
- Two of:
  - Rest tremor*
  - Bradykinesia*
  - Cogwheel rigidity
  - Postural reflex impairment
  (*Must include one of these two items)

Exclusionary criteria:
- Parkinsonism due to trauma, brain tumor, infection, cerebrovascular disease, other known neurological disease, or known drugs, chemicals, toxins
- Prominent oculomotor palsy, cerebellar signs, vocal cord paresis, orthostatic hypotension (blood pressure drop of >20 mmHg on standing), pyramidal signs, amyotrophy
- Hypointensity of the striatum on MRI

Demography and clinical features

Parkinson's disease is a common disorder of the elderly, affecting 1.5–2.5% of individuals over the age of 70. The reported prevalence of the illness varies from 100 to 250 per 100,000 population and is more common among white subjects than black and Asian individuals.[2] The disease is rare before the age of 30 and most patients develop the first symptoms of their disease between the ages of 50 and 79. Men are more often affected than women. The duration of the disease without levodopa therapy varies from 9 to 10 years and with optimal therapy longevity is 13–14 years.[2] Rural living, possibly associated with pesticide exposure, has been identified in several studies as a risk factor for PD, while cigarette smoking has emerged as a protective factor.[2] The role of genetics in the etiology of PD is controversial, but the concordance rate among identical twins is low,[3] suggesting that in most cases hereditary factors play a limited role in the disease. Autosomal dominant varieties of the disease have been associated with mutations of the alpha-synuclein gene on chromosome 4 and the parkin gene on chromosome 6.[4]

The clinical manifestations of PD include rest tremor, bradykinesia, cogwheel rigidity, postural reflex impairment, and response to levodopa.[1] Not all patients have all signs. The typical tremor of PD is a six cycle-per-second rest tremor present when the patient is in alert repose; it disappears with sleep and with action of the affected limb. The hands are most commonly affected; the tongue is involved in some patients. Cogwheel rigidity occurs when the examiner is able to palpate the occurrence of the tremor during passive flexion and extension of the limbs. It is most commonly identified in the upper extremities, whereas a plastic or 'lead-pipe' rigidity without a ratchet or cogwheel quality is typically present in the lower extremities.[5] Patients with mild or incipient rigidity will have a marked increase in limb tone when they perform active movements with the contralateral limb (Froment's sign). To elicit this sign, the clinician performs passive limb movements and then asks the patient to perform an active movement such as drawing a square in the air with the contralateral upper extremity. Bradykinesia in PD is manifested by slowness of movements. There is often a start hesitation when asked to rise from a chair or initiate other movements. Walking, writing, and talking also may be slowed. There may be festination with an uncontrollable increase in speed as the patient continues the activity. Paradoxically, patients may occasionally be able to respond rapidly to an unexpected event such as a thrown ball even though such rapid movements would be impossible under other circumstances.[6] Bradykinesia has a variety of associated manifestations including changes in gait, typically reduced step height and reduced stride length on a narrow base producing a shuffling type of walk; reduced arm swing while walking; micrographia with progressively reduced height of usual writing and decreased space between letters leading to small and sometimes illegible written productions. A variety of postural reflex impairments also occur in PD. Patients lose their postural writing reflexes, which contributes both to festination with uncontrollable forward movement while walking and to difficulty adjusting to a sudden backward pull conducted in the course of the examination. Patients also exhibit a progressive tendency towards a flexion posture with increasing flexion of the head on the neck, forward flexion of the trunk on the pelvis, and flexion of the knees. Asymmetrical onset of parkinsonism with tremor or rigidity in one limb is more common than symmetrical onset and asymmetry typically persists throughout the disease course.

A variety of other signs has also been observed in patients with PD. Examination of the eyes and eye movements reveal that they often have a reduction in spontaneous blink rate and may have an abnormal persistence of blinking with recurrent tapping of the glabellar region between and above the eyes (Myerson's sign). Convergence movements and upgaze may be mildly reduced in patients with PD, but they lack the marked eye movement abnormalities characteristic of progressive supranuclear palsy.[7] Speech changes are common in patients with PD. Hypophonia with reduced speech volume is the most frequently observed abnormality. Patients may exhibit festination of speech with increasingly rapid output as they count or perform other serial tasks. Articulatory precision may be compromised with an ensuing dysarthria. Patients with PD often have reduced voice inflexion with a monotonic vocal output.[8,9]

Dementia syndrome

The reported frequency of dementia with Parkinson's disease varies between 18 and 40%.[10-13] Dementia is associated with increased mortality and crude prevalence figures underestimate the frequency with which dementia complicates PD.[14] Risk factors for the occurrence of dementia in PD include reduced verbal fluency (number of words beginning with a specified letter named in 1 minute or number of items belonging to a specific category named in 1 minute), more advanced Parkinson's disease, depression, and any evidence of cognitive impairment.[15-17] Patients who develop tremor are less likely to develop a dementia syndrome in the course of their illness while those with a more prominent akinetic rigid state are more likely to evidence a dementia syndrome.[18,19] Dementia is also more common in patients who are older at the time of onset of PD and who have had PD for a longer period of time.[10,12,13]

Multiple types of dementias have been linked to PD.[20] Patients with dementia typically exhibit cortical Lewy bodies and it is this histopathologic finding that correlates most strongly with the occurrence of dementia.[21,22] In addition, some patients exhibit cortical changes typical of those of Alzheimer's disease.[23] At least two syndromes are recognizable clinically, a subcortical dementia syndrome associated primarily with executive dysfunction[24,25] and a dementia syndrome consistent with dementia with Lewy bodies (DLB) with fluctuating cognition and more severe involvement with language and visuospatial skills as well as executive deficits.[11,26-30]

Neuroimaging

Magnetic resonance imaging is typically normal in patients with PD with and without dementia. Imaging can be useful to exclude other types of parkinsonism: mixed low and high signal intensity may be evident in the putamen in patients with striatonigral degeneration; pontine and cerebellar changes may be evident in olivopontocerebellar atrophy; midbrain atrophy is typical of progressive supranuclear palsy; asymmetrical cortical atrophy may be seen in patients with corticobasal degeneration; and a mixture of lacunar infarcts and periventricular and deep white matter hyperintensities may be evident in patients with vascular parkinsonism.[31]

Functional imaging may be useful in distinguishing PD from other parkinsonian syndromes. Striatal glucose metabolism is normal or increased in patients with PD studied with fluorodeoxyglucose (FDG) positron emission tomography (PET).[32,33] Studies with fluoro-dopa PET and studies of dopamine transporters using PET reveal diminished striatal dopaminergic activity affecting putamen more than caudate.[34,35] In contrast, dopamine receptors are upregulated in the early phases of the illness and decline as the disease progresses in severity.[32,36] Fluoro-dopa scans aid in distinguishing between PD and progressive supranuclear palsy. The latter exhibits involvement of both anterior and posterior putamen, whereas PD patients have involvement primarily of posterior putaminal regions.[37] Studies using single photon emission computed tomography (SPECT) and FDG PET reveal that PD patients without dementia have generalized hypometabolism or hypoperfusion compared with normal elderly individuals. PD patients with dementia exhibit reductions in frontal, temporal, and parietal regions with sparing of primary motor and sensory cortices.[38,39] These scans have a distribution of metabolic and perfusion changes similar to those seen in patients with Alzheimer's disease. Dorsolateral hypoperfusion of patients with PD correlates most strongly with perseveration and depression.[40] Reductions in dopamine transporter activity in the orbitofrontal cortex correlate with summary cognitive scores on the Unified PD Rating Scale and with depression scale scores. Diminished dopamine transporter activity in the putamen is associated with motor scores on the Unified PD Rating Scale.[1,41] Measurement of presynaptic cholinergic terminal densities using I-iodobenzobesamicol binding reveals reductions in parietal and occipital cortex in patients with PD and no dementia, whereas PD patients with dementia have severe reductions in binding throughout the entire cerebral cortex and hippocampus.[42]

Pathology

A transverse section through the upper midbrain reveals loss of cells and depigmentation of the substantia nigra in patients with PD (Figures 5.1 and 5.2). The two primary histopathologic abnormalities occurring in PD are loss of nerve cells and the occurrence of Lewy bodies in many of the residual neurons or in the neuropil in areas where cells have disappeared. The Lewy body is a cytoplasmic inclusion with a dense hyalin core and clear halo (Figure 5.3). These spherical inclusions have a variety of constituents including neurofilament subunits.[31] Vulnerable cell

a

b

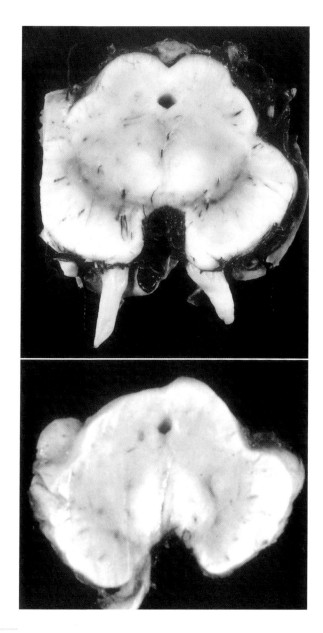

Figure 5.1 Horizontal section of brain stem of patient with Parkinson's disease (b) with reduced pigmentation in the substantia nigra compared with a normal elderly control (a) (courtesy of H Vinters, MD, Neuropathology, UCLA School of Medicine).

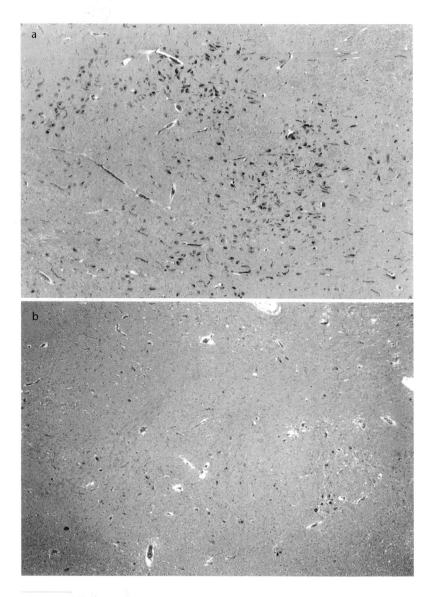

Figure 5.2 *(a) Normally pigmented substantia nigra (low magnification); (b) substantia nigra of patient with Parkinson's disease has dramatic reduction in pigmented cells (courtesy of H Vinters, MD, Neuropathology, UCLA School of Medicine).*

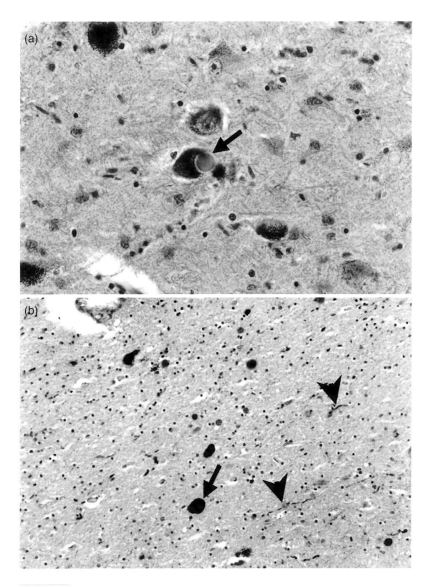

Figure 5.3 *Lewy bodies in the substantia nigra of a patient with Parkinson's disease (435 × 220 magnification): (a) hematoxylin stain; (b) antibody to alpha-synuclein stain) (courtesy of H Vinters, MD, Neuropathology, UCLA School of Medicine).*

populations in PD that exhibit pathological changes include the substantia nigra, locus ceruleus, raphe nuclei, the nucleus basilis of Meynert, hypothalamic neurons, and small cortical neurons – particularly those of the cingulate gyrus or entorhinal cortex.[31]

Dementia in PD has been related to atrophy of the nucleus basilis and loss of cholinergic innervation of the cortex.[20,43] Within the substantia nigra, the lateral area of the pars compacta is more affected than the medial region and medial involvement correlates with the presence of cognitive impairment.[44] Degenerating neuronal processes or neurites (Lewy neurites) are found in all affected brain regions; their occurrence correlates with the dementia of PD.[45] The presence of cortical Lewy bodies is highly specific and sensitive for the presence of dementia in PD.[21,46,47] As in dementia with Lewy bodies (Chapter 4), there is a stronger relationship between neuritic plaques and Lewy bodies than between neurofibrillary tangles.[22,46]

These observations suggest that the prominent dementia syndrome observed in patients with PD is one form of DLB. As noted in Chapter 4, there appear to be two pathways to DLB. One begins with dementia and is evidenced pathologically by neuritic plaques, cortical Lewy bodies, a cholinergic deficit, and a dopaminergic deficit. Clinically, the patients exhibit parkinsonism, fluctuating cognition, and visual hallucinations (Figure 5.4). Another trajectory to DLB begins with PD. In a subset of PD patients, Lewy bodies are abundant in the cortex and there is a concomitant marked cholinergic deficiency. Dementia and increased vulnerability to neuropsychiatric symptoms and fluctuating cognition are characteristic of this disorder.

Studies contrasting patients with Alzheimer's disease and PD with dementia demonstrate that even when matched for dementia severity there are identifiable clinical differences. Patients with Alzheimer's disease have more impaired verbal memory and logical memory, more impaired language with aphasic type abnormalities, less severe executive dysfunction, and less marked cognitive slowing as measured by complex reaction times.[11,24,48-50]

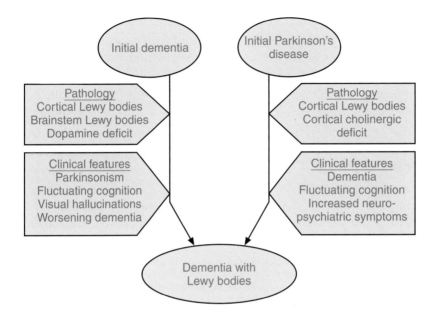

Figure 5.4 *Diagrammatic representation of two principal pathways to dementia with Lewy bodies. One pathway begins with dementia and progresses with addition of the clinical features of parkinsonism, fluctuating cognition, visual hallucinations, and worsening dementia in concert with the occurrence of cortical Lewy bodies, brain stem Lewy bodies, and a dopamine deficit. Alternatively, patients may begin with Parkinson's disease and progress to include dementia, fluctuating cognition, and increased neuropsychiatric symptoms as cortical Lewy bodies accrue and cortical cholinergic deficits emerge.*

Neuropsychiatric features

Neuropsychiatric symptoms are common among patients with PD. In a comprehensive community sample of PD patients, 61% had at least one behavior when interviewed using the Neuropsychiatric Inventory (NPI)[51] (Figures 5.5 and 5.6). The most common behaviors observed were dysphoric mood (38%) and hallucinations (27%). Psychiatric symptoms were more common among PD patients residing in nursing homes and correlated with the severity of disease and severity of cognitive impairment.[52] Twenty-five percent of patients had three or more neuropsychiatric

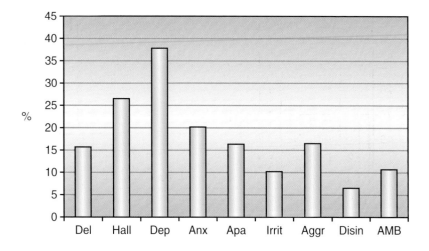

Figure 5.5 *Percent of patients with Parkinson's disease exhibiting neuropsychiatric symptoms (patients were assessed in an epidemiologic study).[52] (See legend to Figure 5.12 for explanation of abbreviations.)*

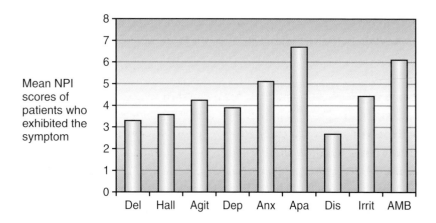

Figure 5.6 *Neuropsychiatric Inventory scores of Parkinson's disease patients exhibiting behavioral and neuropsychiatric symptoms.[52] Agit, agitation. (See legend to Figure 5.12 for rest of abbreviations.)*

symptoms simultaneously. Of those symptoms that were present, the highest mean scores were for anxiety, apathy, depression, agitation, and irritability (Figure 5.6). Neuropsychiatric symptoms are more common

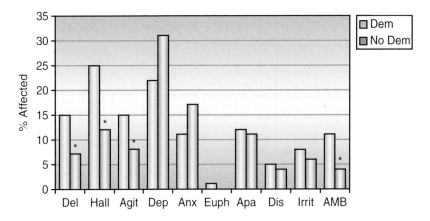

Figure 5.7 *Neuropsychiatric Inventory scores of Parkinson's disease patients with and without dementia. Neuropsychiatric symptoms are more common in those with cognitive impairment. (Data courtesy of D Aarsland.) Dem, dementia; Agit, agitation; *, p = 0.05. (See legend to Figure 5.12 for rest of abbreviations.)*

in PD patients with dementia compared with those without cognitive impairment (Figure 5.7).[53] A summary of neuropsychiatric symptoms and syndromes observed in patients with PD is presented in Box 5.2.

Depression

Some degree of depression has been identified in approximately 40% of patients with PD.[54,55] Relatively few patients (approximately 10%) meet criteria for a major depressive episode in cross-sectional studies and up to a third have major depression when followed longitudinally.[56] The incidence of depression is approximately 2% per year.[57] A variety of risk factors have been associated with the occurrence of depression in PD including greater cognitive impairment. Among patients with Mini-Mental State Examination (MMSE) scores above 20, approximately 5% have major depression, whereas of those with scores below 20, the prevalence of depression is approximately 25%.[55,58] Early onset of PD, the presence of hallucinations or delusions, and the akinetic-rigid clinical syndrome (as opposed to the tremor-dominant syndrome) also have been identified as risk factors for major depression.[59–61] Some studies have found that those with right-sided parkinsonism (greater left brain involvement)

Box 5.2 Neuropsychiatric disorders reported in Parkinson's disease

Depression
• Major depression
• Minor depression
Anxiety
• Without depression
• With depression
Obsessive-compulsive disorder
Personality traits
• Shy, cautious, not novelty-seeking
• Apathy
• Irritability
Sleep disturbance
• Sleep fragmentation
• REM sleep behavior disorder
• Daytime drowsiness
Treatment-associated neuropsychiatric symptoms
• Hallucinations
• Delusions
• Hedonistic homeostatic dysregulation
• Euphoria/mania
• Hypersexuality/paraphilia
• Sleep attacks

---

are more likely to exhibit depressive symptoms.[56] Several investigations have revealed that depression scores predict disability in PD.[56,61]

The clinical features of PD-related depression vary somewhat from those of late-onset idiopathic depression. Patients tend to exhibit pessimism, hopelessness, diminished motivation and drive, and increased concern for health with relatively low levels of guilt, self-blame, and feelings of worthlessness.[62] The profile of symptoms of depression may evolve over the course of the illness. Self-reproach has been found to be present in the earliest phases of PD, giving way to more somatic features with increased disease progression and the predominance of vegetative symptoms in the later phases of the disease.[63] Autonomic symptoms are prominent in patients with PD and depression.[64,65] Parkinson's disease patients with major depression show greater cognitive decline, faster progression of disease, and more deterioration of activities of daily living when followed longitudinally than patients with minor depression or no mood abnormalities.[66] Depression is associated with worse cognitive function in patients with PD compared with PD patients without depression and elderly controls. Those with major mood changes exhibit greater abnormalities on tests of executive function and memory.[59,67–70]

Mood fluctuations are common in patients with the 'on-off' phenomenon. These represent abrupt fluctuations in motor ability varying from 'off' periods with nearly complete immobility to 'on' periods with nearly normal ambulation and motoric abilities. On-off phenomena may occur at regular periods as 'end of dose deterioration' or irregularly and unpredictably. Increased depression and anxiety are common in patients with PD who experience the on-off phenomenon. Approximately 70% of patients have some degree of mood change and nearly 40% describe themselves as moderately more or very much more depressed when in the 'off' state[67,71–73] (Figure 5.8). Infusion with levodopa reduces the degree of depression and agitation in patients with motor fluctuations,

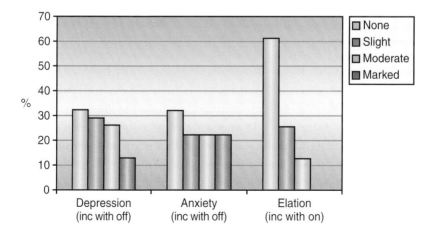

Figure 5.8 *Graph demonstrating the percent of patients who experience no change in mood, anxiety or elation during on-off fluctuations or slight, moderate, or marked changes.[72] Inc, increased.*

suggesting that the mood and anxiety alterations are related in part to levodopa deficiency.[74]

Several biologic measures have been linked to depression in PD. Studies of cerebrospinal fluid levels of 5-hydroxyindoleacetic acid (the major metabolite of serotonin) reveal decreased levels in patients with major depression compared with PD patients without depression or to normal elderly controls.[75–77] Fluorodeoxyglucose PET studies reveal diminished metabolic activity in the caudate, inferior frontal and medial frontal regions in patients with PD and depression.[78,79] Infusion of methylphenidate is usually followed by a euphoric response. In PD patients with depression such infusions cause no mood changes, suggesting that the responsiveness of limbic terminals of dopamine neurons is reduced.[80] Most post-mortem examinations reveal greater loss of neurons in the locus ceruleus in PD patients with depression compared with those without mood changes.[81]

Neuroendocrine tests such as the dexamethasone suppression test have proven to be of limited utility in patients with PD since there is a relatively high rate of nonsuppression among patients without mood changes.[82,83]

Anxiety

Anxiety disorders are common in PD and usually co-occur with depression. Most studies find that of patients attending clinics approximately 30–40% meet criteria for an anxiety disorder.[84–88] Using the NPI in a community survey of neuropsychiatric symptoms in patients with PD, anxiety was identified in approximately 20% of patients and the severity of the anxiety was relatively high in those patients exhibiting symptoms.[52] The anxiety is commonly associated with a depressive disorder. In a community questionnaire survey of PD patients, 7% reported having anxiety symptoms without depression while 38% reported a combination of anxiety and depression (23% reported depression without anxiety).[84] Anxiety has not been found to correlate with severity of parkinsonian symptoms,[89] treatment with levodopa, or other disease variables. Approximately 70% of patients experience anxiety during their 'off' periods, with approximately equal numbers experiencing slight, moderate, or marked anxiety symptoms (Figure 5.8).

Apathy

Apathy is common in patients with PD. Community-based studies reveal a frequency of approximately 15%.[52] Clinical samples have shown a frequency of 12% in the absence of depression and 30% of patients exhibit a combination of apathy and depression.[66] When present, apathy is one of the most severe symptoms exhibited by patients with PD.[52]

Obsessive-compulsive disorder

Severe obsessive-compulsive disorder is an uncommon finding in patients with PD, but obsessive and compulsive characteristics are frequent. Using inventories to measure obsessional and compulsive features, patients with PD have been found to have elevated levels of checking, doubting, cleaning, and ordering.[90,91] These symptoms appear to be related to left-sided parkinsonism suggesting a relationship to right basal ganglia dysfunction.[92]

Sleep disorders

Sleep disorders are a common and often overlooked complication of PD. Use of a sleep questionnaire to identify sleep disturbances led to identification of significant sleep abnormalities in 50% of patients with PD.[93,94] Compared with normal controls, PD patients have worse sleep quality, longer sleep latency (time to fall asleep after going to bed), more night-time awakenings, more daytime sleepiness, and more night-time jerks and restless leg symptoms.[95] Studies of sleep architecture reveal numerous nocturnal movement arousals and awakenings. Sleep spindle density is significantly reduced.[96] Some patients (15–40%) have sudden narcolepsy-like sleep attacks.[97,98] Sleep attacks are independent of cognitive impairment or type of treatment. Depression and anxiety may contribute to abnormal sleep, but do not appear to account for a major amount of the variance[95] of sleep changes observed in PD.

Patients with treatment-associated hallucinations have a reduced total rapid eye movement (REM) sleep time and a reduced percentage of time spent in REM sleep compared with those without hallucinations.[99] Nearly all patients with drug-associated neuropsychiatric symptoms have concomitant sleep complaints.[100] Sleep attacks and excessive daytime sleepiness have been associated with dopaminergic therapy particularly use of dopamine receptor agonists.[93]

REM sleep behavior disorder is a dramatic condition in which dreams appear to be 'acted out'. Between 15 and 40% of PD patients report evidence of REM sleep behavior disorder.[93,101] At least a third of those with REM sleep behavior disorder report causing injury to themselves or to caregivers.

Personality

The existence of a characteristic premorbid personality in patients with PD has been a focus of debate. An emerging consensus using several different types of personality inventories and measures suggests that before the onset of illness, PD patients feature a predominant behavioral style characterized variously as shy, quiet, cautious, less extroverted, less exploratory and curious, and less motivated by novelty-seeking.[102–106] Some studies have found a link between this personality style and the presence of depression and anxiety.[102,103] In normal individuals, higher scores on scales assessing novelty-seeking are correlated with decreased fluoro-dopa uptake in the caudate nuclei, suggesting that the reduced novelty-seeking in PD may be a reflection of the reduced striatal dopamine possibly present for many years before the emergence of more overt parkinsonism.[107]

Treatment-associated neuropsychiatric symptoms

A variety of symptoms have been associated with treatment of PD including sleep disturbances, hallucinations, delusions, mania/euphoria, and hypersexuality/sexual paraphilias. While these syndromes evolve after the introduction of treatment, the dosage of dopaminergic agents in patients with and without these psychiatric symptoms is not usually significantly different.[108–111] Host factors determine which individuals develop psychiatric phenomena following initiation of therapy. Among these factors the presence of cognitive impairment is the most influential. Dementia patients exhibit significantly more psychiatric symptoms than those without dementia (Figure 5.7). Thus, the term 'treatment-associated' is superior to 'treatment-induced,' since it is the critical interaction between treatment and host factors that determines the behavioral manifestations.

Hallucinations

Hallucinations occur in 25–40% of PD patients treated with dopaminergic agents.[110,111] The most common hallucination reported is a fully formed visual image that is silent, in full color, and well-defined. There may be movement such as walking or gesturing by the images. They may be recognized as false visual images by the patient or they may comprise part of a psychosis with delusional endorsement of the reality of the vision. Typically, the hallucinated images are not aggressive and neither threaten the patient nor are involved with other violent activities. The patient with paranoid or persecutory delusions may experience them as aggressive or threatening. Once hallucinations have begun, they are highly likely to persist and be present on subsequent assessments.[109,112,113] Risk factors for visual hallucinations include the presence of dementia and the occurrence of reduced REM sleep.[99,110,111] Deficits in color and contrast discrimination may be more common among those with hallucinations, and these visual changes may make patients more vulnerable to the occurrence of this phenomenon.[114] Hallucinations represent a risk factor for nursing home placement.[108,112] Genetic investigations suggest that the apolipoprotein e4 genotype increases the risk of drug-associated hallucinations and preliminary studies suggest that the allele 2 form of the dopamine D3 gene may also be over-represented among patients with visual hallucinations.[109] Patients who develop visual hallucinations soon after the introduction of dopaminergic therapy may represent a distinct subgroup of patients more likely to progress to DLB with more severe cognitive impairment, greater likelihood of placement in nursing home, and greater mortality. They also experience more nonvisual hallucinations than those whose visual hallucinations begin after more chronic therapy.[115] Patients with visual hallucinations that emerge after chronic levodopa therapy experience their onset in concert with the appearance of cognitive impairment and increasing postural instability.[116,117]

Delusions

Delusions are less common in PD than hallucinations, occurring in 6–10% of patients.[52,118] Delusions are typically of a paranoid or persecutory type and are often combined with visual or other types of hallucinations. Patients may feel that neighbors are threatening them, that they are watched, or that they are the victim of a plot. They may arm themselves or otherwise seek to protect themselves from those who intend harm. Delusional misidentification syndromes such as the Capgras syndrome also have been reported in the context of PD with delusions.[119,120] Patients may believe that a family member has been replaced by an identical appearing stranger (Capgras syndrome) or that there are multiple versions of the same individual performing different roles in the patient's life. Compared with patients without delusions, PD patients with psychosis have greater cognitive impairment, more depression, and more advanced PD.[52,121] Sleep disturbances are also more common among those with delusions compared with those without. It has been hypothesized that delusions and hallucinations in PD represent a REM-like sleep disorder resulting from chronically inadequate night-time REM sleep.[121,122] The relationship between declining cognitive ability and increasing psychiatric phenomena is shown in Figure 5.9.

Mania, hypomania, and euphoria

Anti-parkinsonian therapy with dopaminergic agents produces mood elevation in some patients. This can vary from increased feelings of well being, to euphoria, hypomanic feelings, or occasionally full blown manic episodes with grandiosity, pressured speech, racing thoughts, and hyperactivity.[118] Euphoria and hypomania are rare phenomena, recorded in approximately 2% of patients. Elation has occasionally been reported in association with the on-off phenomenon, where approximately 25% of patients feel slight elation and 12% of patients feel moderate elation during 'on' periods[72] (Figure 5.8).

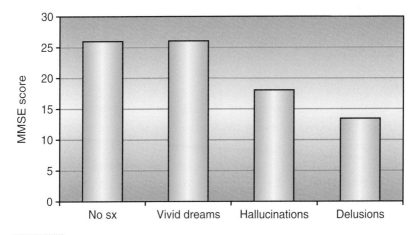

Figure 5.9 Mini-Mental State Examination (MMSE) scores are lower in patients with increasing psychiatric symptomatology.[52] No sx, no symptoms.

Hypersexuality and sexual paraphilias

The typical change in sexual behavior in patients with PD is a reduction in the frequency of sexual contact with their spouse.[123] Eighty percent of both male and female patients report reduced frequency of sexual activity. Approximately 60% of men with PD report impotence while a third of women report vaginismus or anorgasmia. Treatment with levodopa may allow resumption of sexual activity and occasionally results in hypersexuality or sexual deviations.

Hypersexuality may occur independent of other symptoms of mania or hypomania and is not related to known premorbid or disease variables. It is more common in men than women. Hypersexuality typically includes increased sexual desire, increased sexual activity, and approaching prostitutes or other surrogate sexual partners.[124,125] Paraphilic behavior is ameliorated by reducing treatment doses. Increased sexual behavior also may be seen as part of manic or hypomanic episode or in conjunction with the hedonistic homeostatic dysregulation syndrome (discussed below).

Exhibitionism, masochistic behavior, and zoophilia have also been reported in patients with PD following treatment with levodopa or increase in dopaminergic drug dosage.[126,127]

Hedonistic homeostatic dysregulation

Some patients develop an addiction syndrome to levodopa. It is characterized by excessive use of dopamine replacement therapy beyond that required to alleviate motor impairment. There is impairment in social and occupational functioning as a result of levodopa misuse; dose requirements increase over time as drug tolerance develops; and withdrawal reactions with dysphoria, irritability, and anxiety occur when levodopa replacement therapy is not available. Patients engage in classic substance abuse behaviors including drug hoarding and denying their behaviors. Frequently associated with the syndrome are repetitive, purposeless motor acts (called punding), hypersexuality, the urge to walk, pathological gambling and shopping, and anorexia. The syndrome is most common in men with early-onset PD who exhibit drug-induced dyskinesias.[128,129]

Treatment of Parkinson's disease and associated neuropsychiatric symptoms

The treatment of patients with PD begins with therapy of the parkinsonian motor disorder. Therapy also must address the neuropsychiatric symptoms that commonly accompany this condition. In addition, there is increasing evidence that the dementia syndrome of PD may be responsive to treatment with cholinesterase inhibitors. Drug interactions between the powerful agents used to treat PD and psychotropic agents are common.

Treatment of the motor disorder

Table 5.1 lists the treatments commonly used for PD. Anticholinergic agents should be avoided in PD patients with dementia as they may increase confusion, delusions or hallucinations. It is controversial whether selegiline is a disease-modifying treatment. Some evidence suggests that this agent, which has antioxidant properties, may reduce the rate of cell loss in PD and delay required initiation of therapy with dopaminergic compounds.[130–132]

Table 5.1 Drugs used to treat Parkinson's disease

Class	Drug (trade name)	Initial dose	Final dose
Monoamine oxidase B inhibitor	Selegiline (Deprenyl, Eldepryl)	5 mg q.d. (a.m.)	5 mg 2 times/day
Dopamine release facilitation and reuptake blockade	Amantadine (Symmetrel)	100 mg q.d.	100 mg 2 or 3 times/day
Dopamine precursor	Levodopa Given with peripheral dopa decarboxylase inhibitor (carbidopa (in 4:1 and 10:1 ratios)) (Sinemet)	25/100 t.i.d.	Variable; late in disease patients may require multiple doses/day (up to 2 g levodopa/day)
	Controlled-release formulations (with carbidopa (4:1)) (Sinemet-CR)	50/200 b.i.d.	50/200 q.i.d.
Dopamine agonist; ergot-derived	Bromocriptine (Parlodel)	1.25 mg b.i.d.	30–40 mg/day
	Pergolide (Permax)	0.05 mg q.d.	3–5 mg/day
Dopamine agonist; non-ergot derived	Ropinerole (Requip)	0.25 mg t.i.d.	Up to 24 mg/day in 3 divided doses
	Pramipexole (Mirapex)	0.125 mg t.i.d.	Up to 4.5 mg/day in 3 divided doses
Catechol-o-methyltransferase inhibitor	Entacapone (Comtan)	200 mg administered with each levodopa dose	200 mg 4–10 times/day (given with levodopa)

Treatment with dopaminergic agents is initiated when patients consider that their motor symptoms cause disability in occupational, social, or personal function. Initial treatment with dopaminergic receptor agonists (bromocriptine, pergolide, ropinerole, pramipexole) may reduce the rate of occurrence of long-term complications such as dyskinesias and the on-off phenomenon.[134] Alternatively, treatment may be initiated with levodopa administered in conjunction with carbidopa, a peripheral dopa decarboxylase inhibitor (Sinemet, Madopar). After several years, combination therapy is typically required. If treatment was begun with levodopa then a dopaminergic agonist is added. If treatment was begun with a dopaminergic agonist, then a levodopa compound is added to the regimen. Catechol-o-methyltransferase inhibitors reduce the rate of peripheral metabolism of levodopa and raise brain levels associated with each administered dose. Thus, these agents may be administered in conjunction with levodopa to optimize the response with each levodopa dose. Patients intolerant of one compound in the drug class may benefit from treatment with another compound within the same class. Amantadine is a useful adjunctive agent that may provide benefit in patients who lose response to other medications.[134]

Patients who are intolerant or unresponsive to medical therapies – typically those late in their disease course – may benefit from surgical intervention. Thalamotomy may be useful for treatment of tremor, particularly when the tremor is asymmetric, and reduction on one side with contralateral thalamotomy will produce substantial functional benefit. Deep brain stimulation or pallidotomy can provide substantial relief to patients with levodopa-induced dyskinesias and marked on-off fluctuations. Transplantation of fetal nigral cells to the striatum remains an experimental procedure whose utility is under study. The presence of dementia has generally been considered a contraindication to surgical therapy in patients with PD.

Treatment of depression

Several pharmacologic options are available for the treatment of depression in PD.[135] Only a few randomized placebo-controlled trials have been done in PD and thus treatment decisions are guided largely by experience with open-label trials and information derived from elderly patients without PD.

Dopaminergic agents may have antidepressant properties. Deprenyl is a monoamine oxidase B inhibitor and has been reported to have anti-depressant effects in PD.[136,137] Bromocriptine also has been reported to have antidepressant qualities.[138] The non-ergot dopamine receptor ago-nists with preferential D2-D3 dopamine receptor effects may suppress the emergence of depression in patients with PD and may reduce depres-sive symptoms in patients manifesting mood disorders.[139,140]

Treatment with a selective serotonin reuptake inhibitor (SSRI) is the initial step in the treatment of depression in PD in view of the limited side effects of these agents in elderly persons. Selegiline must be stopped before an SSRI is initiated since this combination of treatment may produce a toxic serotonergic syndrome. Selective serotonin reuptake inhibitors have been reported to increase parkinsonism in some patients, but this is a relatively rare phenomenon and this should not dissuade clinicians from using this class of agents in patients with PD. SSRIs are the most commonly used agents for the treatment of depres-sion in PD.[141] Sertraline and paroxetine have been reported to reduce symptoms of depression in patients with PD and a mood disorder.[142,143] Selective noradrenergic reuptake inhibitors are also effective in relieving mood symptoms in patients with PD.[144] If the patient does not benefit from treatment with the first agent chosen then this should be dis-continued and treatment with a tricyclic antidepressant initiated. A tri-cyclic agent with few anticholinergic side effects such as nortriptyline or desipramine should be chosen.[135] Lack of response should be followed by changing the patient to a combined reuptake inhibitor such as ven-lafaxin which has reuptake inhibition effects on both norepinephrine and serotonin. Both these transmitters are reduced in PD and mood changes may benefit from the combined reuptake effect. Combined reuptake inhibitors are used as the agents of choice for treatment of depression by some clinicians. Continued resistance to treatment should lead to referral for electroconvulsive therapy. Therapeutic agents and choices used to treat depression in PD are provided in Chapter 10 (Table 10.1).

Electroconvulsive therapy (ECT) is consistently effective in improving both the motor syndrome and the mood disorder in patients with PD and depression.[145,146] Patients with PD and depression have essentially the same efficacy when treated with ECT as patients with depression not associated with PD.[147] Prolonged delirium may follow ECT in PD patients, and families of patients should be warned that post-ECT delirium is expected.[148] In most cases the delirium resolves within 1 week of therapy but occasionally patients may have persistent confusion for up to 3 weeks. Dyskinesias may also occur following ECT.[145] Parkinsonism typically improves in concert following the second or third treatment episode and tends to relapse to pretreatment levels within a few weeks of discontinuing therapy. Mood changes typically require six or seven treatments with ECT before benefit is evident and the therapeutic response may persist for months or years.

Treatment of psychosis

Delusions are difficult to treat in patients with PD because dopamine blocking agents typically used to treat psychosis exacerbate parkinsonism. Conversely, attempts to reduce dopaminergic agents largely responsible for precipitating these psychotic events also result in worsening parkinsonism. This clinical conundrum has been alleviated somewhat by the introduction of atypical antipsychotic agents. Of these, clozapine is the most efficacious and has the fewest side effects. Low doses are usually adequate to control symptoms (6.25–75 mg per day), and the response is typically evident within a few days of introducing therapy.[149,150] In addition to improvement in psychosis, patients also may experience reduced anxiety, depression, and sleep disturbances following treatment with clozapine. Tremor, torticollis, limb dystonia, and akathisia also may be improved.[151] No worsening of parkinsonism has been reported in conjunction with treatment with clozapine.[149,152] Clozapine causes a potentially fatal agranulocytosis in 1–2% of patients exposed to this agent and the US Food and Drug Administration requires weekly blood counts for patients taking this agent. Figure 5.10 shows the response of the Brief Psychiatric Rating Scale, a clinical global depression scale, and a scale for positive symptoms including delusions and halluci-

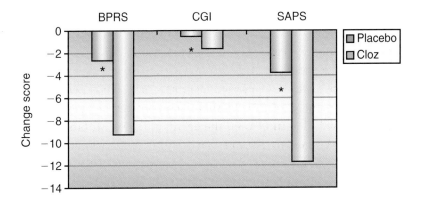

Figure 5.10 Reductions in Brief Psychiatric Rating Scale (BPRS), Clinical Global Impression Scale (CGIS), and Scale for the Assessment of Positive Symptoms (SAPS) scores induced by clozapine (cloz) compared with placebo (n = 60; mean dose of clozapine was 24.7 mg per day).[149] All differences were statistically significant.

nations in patients treated with placebo compared with those treated with clozapine in a controlled clinical trial.[149]

Alternative antipsychotic agents that may be useful in treating psychosis in PD include risperidone, olanzapine and quetiapine. Both risperidone and olanzapine have been reported to be efficacious in reducing psychosis in some patients with PD and delusions; these agents have also been reported to increase parkinsonism in some patients receiving therapy.[153–156] Quetiapine has been reported to improve psychosis without worsening of parkinsonism.[157–159] Quetiapine doses range from 50 to 300 mg daily.

Ondansatron, a serotonergic receptor antagonist, has been shown to reduce hallucinations and delusions in PD patients with psychosis in open-label trials.[160] ECT may be useful in patients with PD and psychosis who cannot tolerate treatment with an antipsychotic agent or adjunctive therapy combining an atypical antipsychotic agent, and ECT may prove to be of benefit.[161,162]

Treatment of other neuropsychiatric symptoms

Treatment of other neuropsychiatric symptoms in PD has not been subject to rigorous study. Mania/hypomania is typically approached by reducing the dosage of levodopa. Carbamazepine or valproate represent treatment alternatives. Lithium and clozapine also have benefited manic symptoms in patients with PD.[163] Anxiety is treated with anxiolytics that are well-tolerated in the elderly such as lorazepam or oxazepam (Table 10.1). Hypersexuality and paraphilic behaviors are diminished by reducing the dosage of levodopa and clozepine has been noted to reduce these symptoms. Hedonistic homeostatic dysregulation is treatment-resistant and is approached with therapeutic modalities used in substance abuse disorders.

Cholinesterase inhibitors

Patients with PD, dementia, and neuropsychiatric symptoms may benefit from therapy with cholinesterase inhibitors (see Chapter 3, Table 3.1). An open-label trial of tacrine in patients with PD and dementia revealed improvement in cognition, reduction in hallucinations, and no exacerbation of parkinsonism.[164] A structured open-label trial of rivastigmine to treat patients with parkinsonism and hallucinations revealed significant improvement in cognition, hallucinations, and sleep disturbance[165] (Figure 5.11). Caregiver stress was significantly improved compared with baseline. There are many similarities between patients with Parkinson's disease with dementia and DLB (Figure 5.3), including the presence of a cholinergic deficit, and there may be a substantial role for the use of cholinesterase inhibitors in patients with PD, dementia, and neuropsychiatric symptoms.

Other parkinsonian syndromes

The basal ganglia are critical to human cognition and emotional function (Chapter 9) and basal ganglia disorders are frequently manifested by cognitive and neuropsychiatric abnormalities in addition to motor system disturbances. Choreiform disorders (e.g. Huntington's disease, Sydenham's chorea) present in early life or in midlife and are not considered in this discussion of late-onset dementias with neuropsychi-

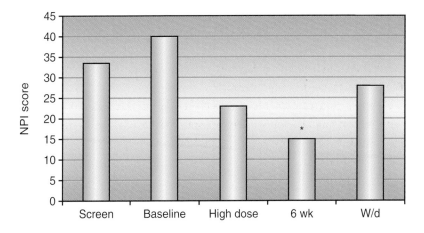

Figure 5.11 Total NPI scores from patients with Parkinson's disease and hallucinations at screen and baseline after high dose rivastigmine, following 6 weeks of therapy with rivastigmine and after withdrawal (w/d) of rivastigmine. There was a significant reduction in total NPI score after 6 weeks of therapy with the cholinesterase inhibitor.[165]

atric symptoms. Box 5.3 provides a list of the principal causes of parkinsonism in the elderly.

Progressive supranuclear palsy

Progressive supranuclear palsy (PSP) is the degenerative disorder most commonly confused with PD. Clinical criteria for its diagnosis are presented in Box 5.4.[166] Key components of PSP are a paralysis of vertical gaze, parkinsonism with predominant extensor posturing and axial rigidity, a prominent disarthria often leading to unintelligibility of speech, and a subcortical type of dementia.[167–169] The typical oculomotor abnormalities of PSP begin with limitations of volitional vertical downgaze followed by decreased volitional upgaze. Vertical pursuit movements and lateral movements are affected next. Oculocephalic reflexes remain intact through most of the disease course.

The cognitive disturbance associated with PSP is primarily one of executive dysfunction. Abnormalities of set shifting on card sorting tests and reductions in verbal fluency are typical.[170,171] The type of memory

Box 5.3 Principal causes of parkinsonism in the elderly

Idiopathic (Lewy body) Parkinson's disease
Familial Parkinson's disease
Parkinsonism in other degenerative diseases
- Progressive supranuclear palsy
- Dementia with Lewy bodies
- Creutzfeldt-Jakob disease
- Corticobasal degeneration
- Frontotemporal lobar degeneration
- Multiple-system atrophies
  - Olivopontocerebellar degeneration
  - Shy-Drager syndrome
  - Striatonigral degeneration
- Calcification of the basal ganglia (idiopathic and symptomatic)
- Hallervorden-Spatz disease
Vascular dementia with parkinsonism
Post-encephalitic parkinsonism
- Encephalitis lethargica
- Other encephalitides, including syphilis
Secondary parkinsonism
- Drug- or toxin-induced parkinsonism (especially neuroleptic agents and other dopamine blocking drugs); carbon monoxide intoxication, cyanide poisoning, carbon disulfide, methanol, ethanol
- Post-anoxic, parkinsonism
- 'Punch drunk' syndrome (dementia pugilistica)
- Hydrocephalus (normal pressure)
- Space-occupying lesions: tumors, etc.

abnormality observed in PSP is also consistent with an executive disorder with involvement of frontal-subcortical circuits. Learning of new information and retrieval of learned information are impaired while recognition of consolidated information is preserved.[171–173] Reaction time procedures reveal cognitive slowing in patients with PSP, in excess of that observed in PD or normal elderly controls.[174]

Investigation of neuropsychiatric symptoms in patients with PSP are also consistent with frontal lobe dysfunction. Patients experience a high

Box 5.4 National Institute of Neurological Diseases and Stroke-Society for Progressive Supranuclear Palsy (NINDS-SPSP) criteria for diagnosis of PSP[166]

- Definite
  - Clinically probable or possible PSP and histopathologic evidence of typical PSP
- Probable
  - Gradually progressive disorder
  - Onset at age 40 or later
  - Vertical (upward or downward gaze) supranuclear palsy and prominent postural instability with falls in the first year of disease onset
  - No evidence of other diseases that could explain the foregoing features, as indicated by mandatory exclusion criteria
- Possible
  - Gradually progressive disorder
  - Onset at age 40 or later
  - Either vertical (upward or downward gaze) supranuclear palsy or both slowing of vertical saccades and prominent postural instability with falls in the first year of disease onset
  - No evidence of other diseases that could explain the foregoing features, as indicated by mandatory exclusion criteria
- Supportive criteria
  - Symmetric akinesia or rigidity, proximal more than distal
  - Abnormal neck posture, especially retrocollis
  - Poor or absent response of parkinsonism to levodopa therapy
  - Early dysphagia and dysarthria
  - Early onset of cognitive impairment including at least two of the following: apathy, impairment in abstract thought, decreased verbal fluency, utilization or imitation behavior, or frontal release signs
- Exclusion criteria
  - Recent history of encephalitis
  - Alien limb syndrome, cortical sensory deficits, focal frontal or temporoparietal atrophy
  - Hallucinations or delusions unrelated to dopaminergic therapy
  - Cortical dementia of Alzheimer's type (severe amnesia and aphasia or agnosia, according to NINCDS-ADRDA criteria)

continued

Box 5.4 *continued*

– Prominent, early cerebellar symptoms or prominent, early unexplained dysautonomia (marked hypotension and urinary disturbances)
– Severe, asymmetric parkinsonian signs (i.e. bradykinesia)
– Neuroradiologic evidence of relevant structural abnormality (i.e. basal ganglia or brain stem infarcts, lobar atrophy)
– Whipple's disease, confirmed by polymerase chain reaction, if indicated

rate of apathy (present in 91%) and disinhibition (present in one third of patients)[175] (Figure 5.12). Depression and anxiety are also observed in PSP although at lower levels. Other neuropsychiatric phenomena are relatively uncommon.[175,176] Compared with patients with PD, those with PSP have significantly more apathy and disinhibition while those with PD evidence more delusions, hallucinations, and depression.[15] Sleep abnormalities occur

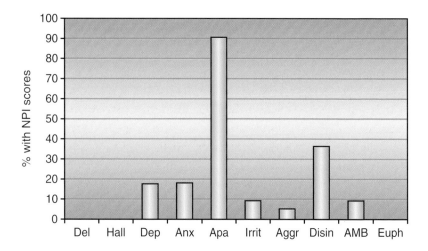

Figure 5.12 *Neuropsychiatric Inventory profile for progressive supranuclear palsy (*n *= 22; mean Mini-Mental State Examination score = 25.1).*[175] *Del, delusions; Hal, hallucinations; Dep, depression/dysphoria; Anx, anxiety; Apa, apathy; Irrit, irritability; Aggr, aggression/agitation; Disin, disinhibition; AMB, aberrant motor behavior; Euph, euphoria. No patient had delusions, hallucinations, or euphoria in this study.*

in PSP and may be severe. There is a shortened sleep time and a lower percentage of time spent in REM sleep. Awakenings are common.[177,178]

Electroencephalographic studies reveal theta range slowing over the frontal lobes of patients with PSP. Magnetic resonance imaging (MRI) demonstrates marked midbrain and tectal atrophy in moderate to advanced phases of the disease.[179] Studies with FDG PET show globally diminished cortical metabolism with more pronounced reductions in the frontal lobes including motor and premotor structures. Subcortical regions including the caudate, putamen, thalamus, and pons are also hypometabolic.[180,181] Studies of the presynaptic dopaminergic system with fluoro-dopa, dopamine receptors, and dopamine transporters all reveal abnormalities in dopaminergic function in patients with PSP.[182–184]

At autopsy, patients with PSP have marked atrophy of the midbrain and microscopically they have numerous neurofibrillary tangles or neuropil threads, or both, in the basal ganglia or brain stem. These are most abundant in the pallidum, subthalamic nucleus, substantia nigra, and pons. Abnormalities are also evident in the striatum, oculomotor complex, medulla, and dentate nucleus of the cerebellum. Tau-positive astrocytes in these areas are common[185] and PSP is regarded as a tauopathy (Chapter 9). Dopamine is reduced in the subcortical regions of PSP and markers of the cholinergic system are reduced in the frontal cortex as well as subcortical structures.[186]

Progressive supranuclear palsy is a treatment-resistant condition.[187] Some patients show improved functional status when treated with tricyclic antidepressants even if mood symptoms are not prominent.[188,189] Parkinsonism may respond to dopaminergic agents, particularly dopamine receptor agonists in some cases.[190] Patients are intolerant of anticholinergic compounds, which should be avoided.[191] Local treatment with botulinum toxin injections may relieve blepharospasm or painful spasms in affected limbs.[192]

Corticobasal degeneration

The clinical features of corticobasal degeneration are listed in Box 5.5.[193] Patients have a parkinsonian syndrome manifested by rigidity which is often asymmetric with dystonia and focal reflex myoclonus. Cognitive

---

Box 5.5 Diagnostic criteria for corticobasal degeneration[193]

- Inclusion criteria
  - Rigidity plus one cortical sign (apraxia, cortical sensory loss, or alien limb phenomenon); or
  - Asymmetric rigidity, dystonia, and focal reflex myoclonus
- Qualification of inclusion factors
  - Rigidity: easily detectable without reinforcement
  - Apraxia: more than simple use of limb as object; clear absence of cognitive or motor deficit sufficient to explain disturbance
  - Cortical sensory loss: preserved primary sensation; asymmetric
  - Alien limb phenomenon: more than simple levitation
  - Dystonia: focal in limb; present at rest at onset
  - Myoclonus: reflex myoclonus spreads beyond stimulated digits
- Exclusion criteria
  - Early dementia (this will exclude some patients who have CBD, but whose illness cannot clinically be distinguished from other primary dementing diseases)
  - Early vertical gaze palsy
  - Rest tremor
  - Severe autonomic disturbances
  - Sustained responsiveness to levodopa
  - Lesions on imaging studies indicating another responsible pathologic process

---

features include apraxia, cortical sensory loss, or alien hand phenomenon. The sensitivity of the diagnosis of corticobasal degeneration is low, but the specificity is high. Thus, most patients who are diagnosed with the illness have the diagnosis confirmed at autopsy while many patients in whom the illness is not suspected have autopsy features consistent with the disorder. The most common misdiagnosis is to mistake cases of corticobasal degeneration for PSP.[194] Although most patients present with both motor and cognitive changes, in some cases the earliest detectable abnormalities involve a dementia syndrome.[195,196] Myoclonus of corticobasal degeneration is typically focal, confined to one limb (typically the arm) and most prominent during voluntary action.[197] The apraxia of corticobasal degeneration is of the ideomotor type with the inability to perform movements on command and is not explained by motor and sensory abnormalities. The ideomotor apraxia affects the limbs and rarely involves bucculofacial structures.[198] The apraxia is typically most severe in the limb affected by dystonia or myoclonus.[199] The alien limb phenomenon, an extreme manifestation of apraxia, is not limited to a simple involuntary grasp reflex, but includes actions performed by the affected limb that are not consciously intended by the patient.

The cognitive deficits of corticobasal degeneration include a unique combination of cortical and frontal-subcortical-type disturbances. Executive disturbances are prominent, including difficulty with card sorting tests and verbal fluency. Visuospatial disturbances also are marked. The typical memory disturbance is one of a retrieval deficit disorder without the marked amnesia typical of Alzheimer's disease.[200,201] Half of the patients manifest an aphasic syndrome with characteristics of anomic, Broca's, or transcortical motor aphasia.[202] Occasional patients with corticobasal degeneration exhibit Balint's syndrome manifested by simultanagnosia, optic ataxia, and reduced volitional eye movements.[203]

The profile of neuropsychiatric symptoms in corticobasal degeneration is unique. Depression is frequent and is often severe. In addition, apathy is prominent while most other symptoms are less common[204] (Figure 5.13).

Neuroimaging studies with MRI reveal asymmetric frontal-parietal atrophy.[205] Single photon emission computerized tomography (SPECT) demonstrates reduced perfusion of the frontal and parietal cortex as well as the striatum and thalamus.[206] Similarly, studies with FDG PET show diminished dorsolateral frontal, medial frontal, parietal, lateral temporal, striatal and thalamic metabolism. Changes are most severe contralateral to the affected limbs.[207,208] Studies with fluoro-dopa PET reveal reduced dopamine uptake in the caudate, putamen, and medial frontal cortical regions. The uptake is asymmetric and reflects the asymmetry of the clinical disorder.[209]

At autopsy there is cortical degeneration involving primarily the frontal and parietal regions and disproportionately affecting the frontal poles and parasagittal regions. Ballooned achromatic cells are observed

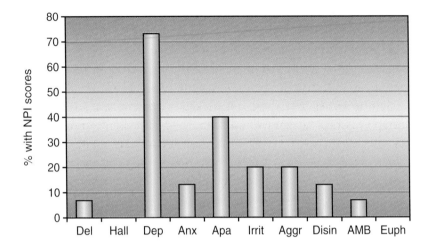

Figure 5.13 *Neuropsychiatric Inventory profile for patients with corticobasal degeneration (*n *= 15; mean Mini-Mental State Examination score = 26.1).[203] Depression is particularly common in this patient group (see legend to Figure 5.12 for abbreviations).*

in the involved cortex as well as subcortical regions. There is typically severe degeneration with loss of nerve cells in the substantia nigra with less but variable involvement of the globus pallidus, striatum, and subthalamic nucleus. Corticobasal degeneration is a tauopathy and tau-positive neurofibrillary tangles are observed in the cortex, subcortical nuclei, and brain stem. Tau immunohistochemistry reveals prominent neuropil threads and grains with glial and neuronal inclusions in the degenerated cortex, underlying white matter, basal ganglia, and pons.[210] There is substantial overlap between the syndromes of frontotemporal lobar degeneration and corticobasal degeneration. The shared aspects include both clinical and pathologic features.[211]

Multiple system atrophy

Multiple system atrophy includes striatonigral degeneration (when parkinsonian features predominate), sporadic olivopontocerebellar atrophy (when cerebellar features predominate), and Shy-Drager syndrome (when autonomic failure is predominant).[212] Diagnostic features currently used to identify multiple system atrophy have high specificity but low sensitivity and many patients go unrecognized (Box 5.6).[213] Multiple system atrophy is most commonly diagnosed as PD or PSP. The highest accuracy is present when six of the following eight features are present: sporadic, adult onset, autonomic dysfunction, parkinsonism, pyramidal tract signs, cerebellar signs, absence of a response to levodopa therapy, normal cognitive function, and absent downward gaze supranuclear palsy.[214] The features that discriminate multiple system atrophy from PD are rapid progression and the presence of autonomic dysfunction.[215] Patients with multiple system atrophy tend to have an earlier age at onset (50–55 years of age) than patients with PD.[216] Progression is more rapid than in idiopathic PD, with 40% of patients markedly disabled or wheelchair-bound within 5 years of onset.[216]

Cognitive changes are typically mild in patients with multiple system atrophy, but an executive disorder with reduced verbal fluency, reduced free recall, and abnormalities on trail making tests are identified in many patients.[217,218] Patients with multiple system atrophy may manifest

---

Box 5.6 Diagnostic features of multiple system atrophy (MSA)[212]

MSA is a sporadic, progressive, adult-onset disorder characterized by autonomic dysfunction, parkinsonism, and ataxia in any combination. The features of this disorder include:
- Parkinsonism (bradykinesia with rigidity or tremor or both), usually with a poor or unsustained motor response to chronic levodopa therapy
- Cerebellar or corticospinal signs
- Orthostatic hypotension, impotence, urinary incontinence or retention, usually preceding or within 2 years of the onset of the motor symptoms

Exclusion criterion:
- These features cannot be explained by medications or other disorder

Note: When parkinsonian features predominate, the term striatonigral degeneration is often used; when cerebellar features predominate, the term sporadic olivopontocerebellar atrophy is often used; when autonomic failure predominates, the term Shy-Drager syndrome is used[212]

depression, and scores on depression rating scales are similar to those with PD.[219,220] REM sleep behavior disorder also has been observed in patients with multiple system atrophy.[221]

A majority of patients with multiple system atrophy have hyperintense lateral and putaminal rims and a region of hypointense signal attenuation on T2-weighted images in the dorsolateral putaminal region.[222] Fluorodeoxyglucose PET shows reduced metabolism in the putamen and cerebellum with significant hypometabolism in the motor, premotor, and prefrontal cortex of some patients.[223,224] Studies with fluoro-dopa PET reveal reduced dopamine uptake capacity of both caudate and putamen.[37]

Pathological examination reveals gliosis and cell loss in the putamen, caudate nucleus, external pallidum, substantia nigra, locus ceruleus, inferior olives, pontine nuclei, cerebellum, and intermediolateral columns of the spinal cord.[225] Histologically, all the clinical subtypes of multiple system atrophy have glial cytoplasmic inclusions in oligodendrocytes of the cerebral white matter. These cytoplasmic inclusions contain alphasynuclein and multiple system atrophies are synucleinopathies (Chapter 9). Neuronal cytoplasmic inclusions similar to those observed in glial cells are less abundant but occur in involved structures.[226]

Treatment is aimed at symptomatic relief of symptoms. Fluoroenef or midodrene may be used to help orthostatic hypotension when it is symptomatic.

Other extrapyramidal syndromes

Parkinsonism is associated with DLB as discussed in Chapter 4; parkinsonism in the context of vascular dementia is described in Chapter 6; parkinsonism is one manifestation of frontotemporal lobar degeneration as described in Chapter 7; and parkinsonism in conjunction with Creutzfeldt-Jakob disease is discussed in Chapter 8. Box 5.3 presents the principal causes of parkinsonism in the elderly.

References

1. Langston JW, Widner H, Goetz CG *et al.* Core assessment program for intracerebral transplantations (CAPIT). *Mov Disord* 1992;7:2–13.
2. Marttila RJ. Epidemiology. In: Koller WC (ed) *Handbook of Parkinson's Disease*, 2nd edn. New York: Marcel Dekker, 1992: 35–57.
3. Tanner CM, Ottman R, Goldman SM *et al.* Parkinson disease in twins: an etiologic study. *JAMA* 1999;281:341–6.
4. Farrer M, Chan P, Chen R *et al.* Lewy bodies and parkinsonism in families with Parkin mutations. *Ann Neurol* 2001;50:293–300.
5. DeJong RN. *The Neurologic Examination*, 4th edn. New York: Harper and Row, 1979.
6. Glickstein M, Stein J. Paradoxical movement in Parkinson's disease. *Trends Neurosci* 1991;14:480–2.
7. Vidailhet M, Rivaud S, Gouider-Khouja N *et al.* Eye movements in parkinsonian syndromes. *Ann Neurol* 1994;35:420–6.
8. Stewart C, Winfield L, Hunt A *et al.* Speech dysfunction in early Parkinson's disease. *Mov Disord* 1995;10:562–5.
9. Caekebeke JFV, Jennekens-Schinkel A, van der Linden ME *et al.* The interpretation of dysprosody in patients with Parkinson's disease. *J Neurol Neurosurg Psychiatry* 1991;54:145–8.
10. Aarsland D, Tandberg E, Larsen JP *et al.* Frequency of dementia in Parkinson disease. *Arch Neurol* 1996;53:538–42.
11. Cummings JL, Darkins A, Mendez M *et al.* Alzheimer's disease and Parkinson's disease: comparison of speech and language alterations. *Neurology* 1988; 38:680–4.
12. Mayeux R, Denaro J, Hemenegildo N *et al.* A population-based investigation of Parkinson's disease with and without dementia. *Arch Neurol* 1992;49:492–7.
13. Tison F, Dartigues JF, Auriacombe S *et al.* Dementia in Parkinson's disease: a population-based study in ambulatory and institutionalized individuals. *Neurology* 1995;45:705–8.
14. Marder K, Leung D, Tang M *et al.* Are demented patients with Parkinson's disease accurately reflected in prevalence surveys? A survival analysis. *Neurology* 1991;41:1240–3.
15. Aarsland D, Litvan I, Larsen JP. Neuropsychiatric symptoms of patients with progressive supranuclear palsy and Parkinson's disease. *J Neuropsychiatry Clin Neurosci* 2001;13:42–9.
16. Jacobs DM, Marder K, Cote L *et al.* Neuropsychological characteristics of preclinical dementia in Parkinson's disease. *Neurology* 1995;45:1691–6.
17. Marder K, Tang M-X, Cote L *et al.* The frequency and associated risk factors for dementia in patients with Parkinson's disease. *Arch Neurol* 1995; 52:695–701.
18. Hershey LA, Feldman BJ, Kim KY *et al.* Tremor at onset: predictor of cognitive and motor outcome in Parkinson's disease. *Arch Neurol* 1991;48: 1049–51.
19. Huber SJ, Christy JA, Paulson GW. Cognitive heterogeneity associated with clinical subtypes of Parkinson's disease. *Neuropsychiatry Neuropsychol Behav Neurol* 1991;4:147–57.

20. Whitehouse PJ, Hedreen JC, White CL III et al. Basal forebrain neurons in the dementia of Parkinson disease. Ann Neurol 1983;13:243–8.
21. Hurtig H, Trojanowski JQ, Galvin J et al. Alpha-synuclein cortical Lewy bodies correlate with dementia in Parkinson's disease. Neurology 2000; 54:1916–21.
22. Mattila PM, Rinne JO, Helenius H et al. Alpha-synuclein-immunoreactive cortical Lewy bodies are associated with cognitive impairment in Parkinson's disease. Acta Neuropathol 2000;100:285–90.
23. Gaspar P, Gray F. Dementia in idiopathic Parkinson's disease. Acta Neuropathol 1984;64:43–52.
24. Freedman AM, Oscar-Berman M. Selective delayed response deficits in Parkinson's and Alzheimer's disease. Arch Neurol 1986;43:886–90.
25. Huber SJ, Shuttleworth EC, Paulson GW et al. Cortical vs subcortical dementia: neuropsychological differences. Arch Neurol 1986;43:392–4.
26. Appollonio I, Grafman J, Clark K et al. Implicit and explicit memory in patients with Parkinson's disease with and without dementia. Arch Neurol 1994;51:359–67.
27. Levin BE, Llabre MM, Reisman S et al. Visuospatial impairment in Parkinson's disease. Neurology 1991;41:365–9.
28. Gabrieli JDE, Singh J, Stebbins GT et al. Reduced working memory span in Parkinson's disease: evidence for the role of a frontostriatal system in working and strategic memory. Neuropsychology 1996;10:322–32.
29. Owen AM, James M, Leigh PN et al. Fronto-striatal cognitive deficits at different stages of Parkinson's disease. Brain 1992;115:1727–51.
30. Taylor AE, Saint-Cyr JA, Lang AE. Subcognitive processing in the frontocaudate 'complex loop': the role of the striatum. Alzheimer Dis Assoc Disord 1990;4:150–60.
31. Lang AE, Lozano AM. Parkinson's disease. N Engl J Med 1998;339:1044–53, 1130–43.
32. Antonini A, Vontobel P, Psylla M et al. Complementary positron emission tomographic studies of the striatal dopaminergic system in Parkinson's disease. Arch Neurol 1995;52:1183–90.
33. Eidelberg D, Takikawa S, Moeller JR et al. Striatal hypometabolism distinguishes striatonigral degeneration from Parkinson's disease. Ann Neurol 1993;33:518–27.
34. Brooks DJ, Salmon EP, Mathias CJ et al. The relationship between locomotor disability, autonomic dysfunction, and the integrity of the striatal dopaminergic system in patients with multiple system atrophy, pure autonomic failure, and Parkinson's disease, studied with PET. Brain 1990;113:1539–52.
35. Seibyl JP, Marek KL, Quinlan D et al. Decreased single-photon emission computed tomographic {123 I} β-CIT striatal uptake correlates with symptom severity in Parkinson's disease. Ann Neurol 1995;38:589–98.
36. Laulumaa V, Kuikka JT, Soininen H et al. Imaging of D2 dopamine receptors of patients with Parkinson's disease using single photon emission computed tomography and iodobenzamide I-123. Arch Neurol 1993;50:509–12.
37. Brooks DJ, Ibanez V, Sawle GV et al. Differing patterns of striatal [18]f-dopa uptake in Parkinson's disease, multiple system atrophy, and progressive supranuclear palsy. Ann Neurol 1990;28:547–55.

38. Peppard R, Martin RW, Carr GD *et al.* Cerebral glucose metabolism in Parkinson's disease with and without dementia. *Arch Neurol* 1992;49:1262–8.
39. Starkstein SE, Chemerinski E, Sabe L *et al.* A prospective longitudinal study of depression and anosognosia in Alzheimer's disease. *Br J Psychiatry* 1997; 171:47–52.
40. Jagust WJ, Reed B, Martin EM *et al.* Cognitive function and regional cerebral blood flow in Parkinson's disease. *Brain* 1992;115:521–37.
41. Ouchi Y, Yoshikawa E, Okada H *et al.* Alterations in binding site density of dopamine transporter in the striatum, orbitofrontal cortex, and amygdala in early Parkinson's disease: compartment analysis for β-CFT binding with positron emission tomography. *Ann Neurol* 1999;45:601–10.
42. Kuhl DE, Minoshima S, Fessler JA *et al.* In vivo mapping of cholinergic terminals in normal aging, Alzheimer's disease, and Parkinson's disease. *Ann Neurol* 1996;40:399–410.
43. Arendt T, Bigl V, Arendt A. Loss of neurons in the nucleus basalis of Meynert in Alzheimer's disease, paralysis agitans and Korsakoff's disease. *Acta Neuropathol* 1983;61:101–8.
44. Rinne JO, Rummukainen J, Paljarvi L *et al.* Dementia in Parkinson's disease is related to neuronal loss in the medial substantia nigra. *Ann Neurol* 1989;26:47–50.
45. Churchyard A, Lees AJ. The relationship between dementia and direct involvement of the hippocampus and amygdala in Parkinson's disease. *Neurology* 1997;49:1570–6.
46. Zweig RM, Cardillo JE, Cohen M *et al.* The locus ceruleus and dementia in Parkinson's disease. *Neurology* 1993;43:986–91.
47. Apaydin H, Ahlskog E, Parisi J *et al.* Parkinson disease neuropathology. *Arch Neurol* 2002;59:102–12.
48. Litvan I, Mohr E, Williams J *et al.* Differential memory and executive functions in demented patients with Parkinson's and Alzheimer's disease. *J Neurol Neurosurg Psychiatry* 1991;54:25–9.
49. Pate DS, Margolin DI. Cognitive slowing in Parkinson's and Alzheimer's patients: distinguishing bradyphrenia from dementia. *Neurology* 1994;44: 669–74.
50. Pillon B, Dubois B, Lhermitte F *et al.* Heterogeneity of cognitive impairment in progressive supranuclear palsy, Parkinson's disease, and Alzheimer's disease. *Neurology* 1986;36:1179–85.
51. Cummings JL, Mega M, Gray K *et al.* The Neuropsychiatric Inventory: comprehensive assessment of psychopathology in dementia. *Neurology* 1994;44:2308–14.
52. Aarsland D, Larsen JP, Lim NH *et al.* Range of neuropsychiatric disturbances in patients with Parkinson's disease. *J Neurol Neurosurg Psychiatry* 1999;67:492–6.
53. Aarsland D, Ballard C, Larsen JP *et al.* A comparative study of psychiatric symptoms in dementia with Lewy bodies and Parkinson's disease with and without dementia. *Int J Geriatr Psychiatry* 2001;16:528–36.
54. Cummings JL. Depression and Parkinson's disease: a review. *Am J Psychiatry* 1992;149:443–54.
55. Tandberg E, Larsen JP, Aarsland D *et al.* The occurrence of depression in Parkinson's disease: a community-based study. *Arch Neurol* 1996;53:175–9.

56. Cole SA, Woodard JL, Juncos JL *et al.* Depression and disability in Parkinson's disease. *J Neuropsychiatry Clin Neurosci* 1996;8:20–5.

57. Dooneief G, Mirabello E, Bell K *et al.* An estimate of the incidence of depression in idiopathic Parkinson's disease. *Arch Neurol* 1992;49:305–7.

58. Holroyd S, Currie L, Wooten GF. Prospective study of hallucinations and delusions in Parkinson's disease. *J Neurol Neurosurg Psychiatry* 2001;70:734–8.

59. Starkstein SE, Berthier ML, Bolduc PL *et al.* Depression in patients with early versus late onset of Parkinson's disease. *Neurology* 1989;39:1441–5.

60. Starkstein SE, Petracca G, Chemerinski E *et al.* Depression in classic versus akinetic-rigid Parkinson's disease. *Mov Disord* 1998;13:29–33.

61. Tandberg E, Larsen JP, Aarsland D *et al.* Risk factors for depression in Parkinson disease. *Arch Neurol* 1997;54:625–30.

62. Gotham A-M, Brown RG, Marsden CD. Depression in Parkinson's disease: a quantitative and qualitative analysis. *J Neurol Neurosurg Psychiatry* 1986;49:381–9.

63. Huber SJ, Freidenberg DL, Paulson GW *et al.* The pattern of depressive symptoms varies with progression of Parkinson's disease. *J Neurol Neurosurg Psychiatry* 1990;53:275–8.

64. Starkstein SE, Preziosi TJ, Forrester AW *et al.* Specificity of affective and autonomic symptoms of depression in Parkinson's disease. *J Neurol Neurosurg Psychiatry* 1990;53:869–73.

65. Berrios GE, Campbell C, Politynska BE. Autonomic failure, depression and anxiety in Parkinson's disease. *Br J Psychiatry* 1995;166:789–92.

66. Starkstein SE, Mayberg JS, Preziosi TJ *et al.* Reliability, validity, and clinical correlates of apathy in Parkinson's disease. *J Neuropsychiatry Clin Neurosci* 1992;4:134–9.

67. Kuzis G, Sabe L, Tiberti C *et al.* Cognitive functions in major depression and Parkinson disease. *Arch Neurol* 1997;54:982–6.

68. Troster AI, Paolo AM, Lyons KE *et al.* The influence of depression on cognition in Parkinson's disease: a pattern of impairment distinguishable from Alzheimer's disease. *Neurology* 1995;45:672–6.

69. Troster AI, Stalp LD, Paolo AM *et al.* Neuropsychological impairment in Parkinson's disease with and without depression. *Arch Neurol* 1995;52:1164–9.

70. Norman S, Tröster AI, Fields JA, Brooks R. Effects of depression and Parkinson's disease on cognitive functioning. *J Neuropsychiatry Clin Neurosc* 2002;14:31–6.

71. Menza M, Sage J, Marshall E *et al.* Mood changes and 'on-off' phenomena in Parkinson's disease. *Mov Disord* 1990;5:148–51.

72. Nissenbaum H, Quinn NP, Brown RG *et al.* Mood swings associated with the 'on-off' phenomenon in Parkinson's disease. *Psychol Med* 1987;17:899–904.

73. Richard IH, Justus AW, Kurlan R. Relationship between mood and motor fluctuations in Parkinson's disease. *J Neuropsychiatry Clin Neurosci* 2001; 13:35–41.

74. Maricle RA, Nutt JG, Valentine RJ *et al.* Dose-response relationship of levodopa with mood and anxiety in fluctuating Parkinson's disease: a double-blind, placebo-controlled study. *Neurology* 1995;45:1757–60.

75. Kostic VS, Djuricic BM, Covichovic-Sternic N *et al.* Depression and Parkin-

son's disease: possible role of serotonergic mechanisms. *J Neurol* 1987; 234:94–6.

76. Mayeux R, Stern Y, Cote L *et al.* Altered serotonin metabolism in depressed patients with Parkinson's disease. *Neurology* 1984;34:642–6.

77. Mayeux R, Stern Y, Williams JBW *et al.* Clinical and biochemical features of depression in Parkinson's disease. *Am J Psychiatry* 1986;143:756–9.

78. Mayberg HS, Starkstein SE, Sadzot B *et al.* Selective hypometabolism in inferior frontal lobe in depressed patients with Parkinson's disease. *Ann Neurol* 1990;28:57–64.

79. Ring JA, Bench CJ, Trimble MR *et al.* Depression in Parkinson's disease: a positron emission study. *Br J Psychiatry* 1994;165:333–9.

80. Cantello R, Aguggia M, Gilli M *et al.* Major depression in Parkinson's disease and the mood response to intravenous methylphenidate: possible roles of the 'hedonic' dopamine synapse. *J Neurol Neurosurg Psychiatry* 1989;52: 724–31.

81. Chan-Palay V, Asan E. Alterations in catecholamine neurons of the locus coeruleus in senile dementia of the Alzheimer type and in Parkinson's disease with and without dementia and depression. *J Comp Neurol* 1989;287:373–92.

82. Kostic VS, Covichovic-Sternic N, Beslac-Bumbasirevic L *et al.* Dexamethasone suppression test in patients with Parkinson's disease. *Mov Disord* 1990; 5:23–6.

83. Frochtengarten ML, Villares JCB, Maluf E *et al.* Depressive symptoms and the dexamethasone suppression test in parkinsonian patients. *Biol Psychiatry* 1987;22:386–9.

84. Henderson R, Kurlan R, Kersun JM *et al.* Preliminary examination of the comorbidity of anxiety and depression in Parkinson's disease. *J Neuropsychiatry Clin Neurosci* 1992;4:257–64.

85. Menza MA, Robertson-Hoffman DE, Bonapace AS. Parkinson's disease and anxiety: comorbidity with depression. *Biol Psychiatry* 1993;34:465–70.

86. Richard IH, Schiffer RB, Kurlan R. Anxiety and Parkinson's disease. *J Neuropsychiatry Clin Neurosci* 1996;8:383–92.

87. Starkstein SE, Robinson RG, Leiguarda R *et al.* Anxiety and depression in Parkinson's disease. *Behav Neurol* 1993;6:151–4.

88. Stein MB, Heuser IJ, Juncos JL *et al.* Anxiety disorders in patients with Parkinson's disease. *Am J Psychiatry* 1990;147:217–20.

89. Fernandez HH, Friedman JH. Punding on L-Dopa. *Mov Disord* 1999;14: 836–8.

90. Alegret M, Junque C, Valldeoriola F *et al.* Obsessive-compulsive symptoms in Parkinson's disease. *J Neurol Neurosurg Psychiatry* 2001;70:394–6.

91. Müller N, Putz A, Kathmann N *et al.* Characteristics of obsessive-compulsive symptoms in Tourette's syndrome, obsessive-compulsive disorder, and Parkinson's disease. *Psychiatry Res* 1997;70:105–14.

92. Tomer R, Levin BE, Weiner WJ. Obsessive-compulsive symptoms and motor asymmetries in Parkinson's disease. *Neuropsychiatry Neuropsychol Behav Neurol* 1993;6:26–30.

93. Ondo WG, Vuong KD, Khan H *et al.* Daytime sleepiness and other sleep disorders in Parkinson's disease. *Neurology* 2001;57:1392–6.

94. Hobson DE, Lang AE, Martin WR et al. Excessive daytime sleepiness and sudden-onset sleep in Parkinson disease. *JAMA* 2002;287:455–63.
95. Menza M, Rosen RC. Sleep in Parkinson's disease: the role of depression and anxiety. *Psychosomatics* 1995;36:262–6.
96. Emser W, Brenner M, Stober T et al. Changes in nocturnal sleep in Huntington's and Parkinson's disease. *J Neurol* 1988;235:177–9.
97. Tan EK, Lum RN, Fook-Chong SM et al. Evaluation of somnolence in Parkinson disease: comparison with age- and sex-matched controls. *Neurology* 2002;58:465–8.
98. Arnulf I, Konofal E, Merino-Andreu M et al. Parkinson's disease and sleepiness: an integral part of PD. *Neurology* 2002;58:1019–24.
99. Comella CL, Tanner CM, Ristanovic RK. Polysomnographic sleep measures in Parkinson's disease patients with treatment-induced hallucination. *Ann Neurol* 1993;34:710–14.
100. Nausieda PA, Weiner WJ, Kaplan LR et al. Sleep disruption in the course of chronic levodopa therapy: an early feature of the levodopa psychosis. *Clin Neuropharmacol* 1982;5:183–94.
101. Comella C, Nardine T, Diedrich N et al. Sleep-related violence, injury, and REM sleep behavior disorder in Parkinson's disease. *Neurology* 1998;51:526–9.
102. Bell IR, Amend D, Kaszniak AW et al. Trait shyness in the elderly: evidence for an association with Parkinson's disease in family members and biochemical correlates. *J Geriatr Psychiatry Neurol* 1995;8:16–22.
103. Glosser G, Clark C, Freundlich B et al. A controlled investigation of current and premorbid personality: characteristics of Parkinson's disease patients. *Mov Disord* 1995;10:201–6.
104. Hubble J, Venkatesh R, Hassanein RES et al. Personality and depression in Parkinson's disease. *J Nerv Ment Dis* 1993;181:657–62.
105. Menza M, Forman NE, Goldstein HS et al. Parkinson's disease, personality, and dopamine. *J Neuropsychiatry Clin Neurosci* 1990;2:282–7.
106. Menza MA, Golbe LI, Cody RA et al. Dopamine-related personality traits in Parkinson's disease. *Neurology* 1993;43:505–8.
107. Menza M, Mark MH, Burn DJ et al. Personality correlates of [18F] Dopa striatal uptake: results of positron-emission tomography in Parkinson's disease. *J Neuropsychiatry Clin Neurosci* 1995;7:176–9.
108. Aarsland D, Larsen JP, Tandberg E et al. Predictors of nursing home placement in Parkinson's disease: a population-based, prospective study. *J Am Geriatr Soc* 2000;48:938–42.
109. Goetz CG, Leurgans S, Pappert EJ et al. Prospective longitudinal assessment of hallucinations in Parkinson's disease. *Neurology* 2001;57:2078–82.
110. Haeske-Dewick HC. Hallucinations in Parkinson's disease: characteristics and associated clinical features. *Int J Geriatr Psychiatry* 1995;10:487–95.
111. Sanchez-Ramos J, Ortoll R, Paulson G. Visual hallucinations associated with Parkinson disease. *Arch Neurol* 1996;53:1265–8.
112. Goetz CG, Stebbins GT. Mortality and hallucinations in nursing home patients with advanced Parkinson's disease. *Neurology* 1995;45:669–71.
113. Fernandez W, Stern G, Lees AJ. Hallucinations and parkinsonian motor fluctuations. *Behav Neurol* 1992;5:83–6.

114. Diederich NJ, Goetz CG, Raman R et al. Poor visual discrimination and visual hallucinations in Parkinson's disease. *Clin Neuropharmacol* 1998; 21:289–95.
115. Goetz CG, Vogel C, Tanner CM et al. Early dopaminergic drug-induced hallucinations in parkinsonian patients. *Neurology* 1998;51:811–14.
116. Graham JM, Grunewald RA, Sagar HJ. Hallucinosis in idiopathic Parkinson's disease. *J Neurol Neurosurg Psychiatry* 1997;63:434–40.
117. Barnes J, David AS. Visual hallucinations in Parkinson's disease: a review and phenomenological survey. *J Neurol Neurosurg Psychiatry* 2001;70:727–33.
118. Cummings JL. Behavioral complications of drug treatment of Parkinson's disease. *J Am Geriatr Soc* 1991;39:708–16.
119. Edelstyn NMJ, Oyebode F, Barrett K. Delusional misidentification: a neuropsychological case study in dementia associated with Parkinson's disease. *Neurocase* 1998;4:181–8.
120. Roane DM, Rogers J, Robinson JH et al. Delusional misidentification in association with parkinsonism. *J Neuropsychiatry Clin Neurosci* 1998;10: 194–8.
121. Naimark D, Jackson E, Rockwell E et al. Psychotic symptoms in Parkinson's disease patients with dementia. *J Am Geriatr Soc* 1996;44:296–9.
122. Arnulf I, Bonnet A-M, Damier P et al. Hallucinations, REM sleep, and Parkinson's disease. *Neurology* 2000;55:281–8.
123. Brown RG, Jahanshahi M, Quinn N et al. Sexual function in patients with Parkinson's disease and their partners. *J Neurol Neurosurg Psychiatry* 1990; 53:480–6.
124. Uitti RJ, Tanner CM, Rajput AH et al. Hypersexuality with antiparkinsonian therapy. *Clin Neuropharmacol* 1989;12:375–83.
125. Harvey NS. Serial cognitive profiles in levodopa-induced hypersexuality. *Br J Psychiatry* 1988;153:833–6.
126. Quinn NP, Toone B, Lang AE et al. Dopa dose-dependent sexual deviation. *Br J Psychiatry* 1983;142:296–8.
127. Fernandez HH, Durso R. Clozapine for dopaminergic-induced paraphilias in Parkinson's disease. *Mov Disord* 1998;13:597–621.
128. Giovannoni G, O'Sullivan JD, Turner K et al. Hedonistic homeostatic dysregulation in patients with Parkinson's disease on dopamine replacement therapies. *J Neurol Neurosurg Psychiatry* 2000;68:423–8.
129. Nausieda PA. Sinemet 'abusers'. *Clin Neuropharmacol* 1985;8:318–27.
130. Olanow CW, Hauser RA, Gauger L et al. The effect of deprenyl and levodopa on the progression of Parkinson's disease. *Ann Neurol* 1995;38:771–7.
131. Palhagen S, Heinonen EH, Hagglund J et al. Selegiline delays the onset of disability in de novo parkinsonian patients. *Neurology* 1998;51:520–5.
132. Tetrud JW, Langston JW. The effect of deprenyl (selegiline) on the natural history of Parkinson's disease. *Science* 1989;245:519–22.
133. Miyasaki JM, Martin W, Suchowersky O et al. Practice parameter: initiation of treatment for Parkinson's disease: an evidence-based review. *Neurology* 2002;58:11–17.
134. Olanow CW, Watts RL, Koller WC. An algorithm (decision tree) for the management of Parkinson's disease (2001): treatment guidelines. *Neurology* 2001;56:S1–S88.

135. Tom T, Cummings JL. Depression in Parkinson's disease: pharmacological characteristics and treatment. *Drugs Aging* 1998; 12;55–74.
136. Allain H, Pollak P, Neukirch HC *et al.* Symptomatic effect of selegiline in De Novo parkinsonian patients. *Mov Disord* 1993;8:S36–S40.
137. Baronti F, Davis TL, Boldry RC *et al.* Deprenyl effects on levodopa pharmacodynamics, mood, and free radical scavenging. *Neurology* 1992;42:541–4.
138. Jouvent R, Abensour P, Bonnet AM *et al.* Antiparkinsonian and antidepressant effects of high doses of bromocriptine: an independent comparison. *J Affect Disord* 1983;5:141–5.
139. Cummings JL. D-3 receptor agonists: combined action neurologic and neuropsychiatric agents. *J Neurol Sci* 1999;163:2–3.
140. Pogarell O, Kunig G, Oertel WH. A non-ergot dopamine agonist, pramipexole, in the therapy of advanced Parkinson's disease: improvement of parkinsonian symptoms and treatment-associated complications: a review of three studies. *Clin Neuropharmacol* 1997;20:S28–S35.
141. Richard IH, Kurlan R, Parkinson Study Group. A survey of antidepressant drug use in Parkinson's disease. *Neurology* 1997;49:1168–70.
142. Ceravolo R, Nuti A, Piccinni A *et al.* Paroxetine in Parkinson's disease: effects on motor and depressive symptoms. *Neurology* 2000;55:1216–18.
143. Hauser R, Zesiewicz TA. Sertraline for the treatment of depression in Parkinson's disease. *Mov Disord* 1997;12:756–9.
144. Lemke MR. Effect of reboxetine on depression in Parkinson's disease patient. *J Clin Psychiatry* 2002;63:300–4.
145. Douyon R, Serby M, Klutchko B *et al.* ECT and Parkinson's disease revisited: a 'naturalistic' study. *Am J Psychiatry* 1989;146:1451–5.
146. Faber R, Trimble MR. Electroconvulsive therapy in Parkinson's disease and other movement disorders. *Mov Disord* 1991;6:293–303.
147. Moellentine C, Rummans T, Ahlskog JE *et al.* Effectiveness of ECT in patients with parkinsonism. *J Neuropsychiatry Clin Neurosci* 1998; 10:187–93.
148. Figiel GS, Hassen MA, Zorumski C *et al.* ECT-induced delirium in depressed patients with Parkinson's disease. *J Neuropsychiatry Clin Neurosci* 1991; 3:405–11.
149. Parkinson Study Group T. Low-dose clozapine for the treatment of drug-induced psychosis in Parkinson's disease. *N Engl J Med* 1999;340:757–63.
150. Rabey JM, Treves TA, Neufeld MY *et al.* Low-dose clozapine in the treatment of levodopa-induced mental disturbances in Parkinson's disease. *Neurology* 1995;45:432–4.
151. Trosch RM, Friedman JH, Lannon MC *et al.* Clozapine use in Parkinson's disease: a retrospective analysis of a large multicentered clinical experience. *Mov Disord* 1998;13:377–82.
152. Ruggieri S, De Pandis MF, Bonamartini A *et al.* Low dose of clozapine in the treatment of dopaminergic psychosis in Parkinson's disease. *Clin Neuropharmacol* 1997;20:204–9.
153. Aarsland D, Larsen JP, Lim NG *et al.* Olanzapine for psychosis in patients with Parkinson's disease with and without dementia. *J Neuropsychiatry Clin Neurosci* 1999;11:392–4.
154. Goetz CG, Blasucci LM, Leurgans S *et al.* Olanzapine and clozapine: compar-

ative effects on motor function in hallucinating PD patients. *Neurology* 2000;55:789.

155. Wolters EC, Jansen ENH, Tuynman-Qua HG *et al.* Olanzapine in the treatment of dopaminomimetic psychosis in patients with Parkinson's disease. *Neurology* 1996;47:1085–7.

156. Workman RH Jr, Orengo CA, Bakey AA *et al.* The use of risperidone for psychosis and agitation in demented patients with Parkinson's disease. *J Neuropsychiatry Clin Neurosci* 1997;9:594–7.

157. Fernandez HH, Friedman JH, Jacques C *et al.* Quetiapine for the treatment of drug-induced psychosis in Parkinson's disease. *Mov Disord* 1999;14:484–7.

158. Targum SD, Abbott JL. Efficacy of quetiapine in Parkinson's patients with psychosis. *J Clin Psychopharmacol* 2000;20:54–60.

159. Brandstadter D, Oertel WH. Treatment of drug-induced psychosis with quetiapine and clozapine in Parkinson's disease. *Neurology* 2000;58:156–62.

160. Zoldan J, Friedberg G, Livneh M *et al.* Psychosis in advanced Parkinson's disease: treatment with ondansetron, a 5-HT3 receptor antagonist. *Neurology* 1995;45:1305–8.

161. Hurwitz TA, Calne DB, Waterman K. Treatment of dopaminomimetic psychosis in Parkinson's disease with electroconvulsive therapy. *Can J Neurol Sci* 1988;15:32–4.

162. Factor SA, Molho ES, Brown DL. Combined clozapine and electroconvulsive therapy for the treatment of drug-induced psychosis in Parkinson's disease. *J Neuropsychiatry Clin Neurosci* 1995;7:304–7.

163. Kim E, Zwil AS, McAllister TW *et al.* Treatment of organic bipolar mood disorders in Parkinson's disease. *J Neuropsychiatry Clin Neurosci* 1994;6: 181–4.

164. Hutchinson M, Fazzini E. Cholinesterase inhibition in Parkinson's disease. *J Neurol Neurosurg Psychiatry* 1996;61:324–5.

165. Reading PJ, Luce AK, McKeith IG. Rivastigmine in the treatment of parkinsonian psychosis and cognitive impairment: preliminary findings from an open trial. *Mov Disord* 2001;16:1171–95.

166. Litvan I, Agid Y, Calne D *et al.* Clinical research criteria for the diagnosis of progressive supranuclear palsy (Steele-Richardson-Olszewski syndrome): report of the NINDS-SPSP international workshop. *Neurology* 1996;47:1–9.

167. Steele JC, Richardson JC, Olszewski J. Progressive supranuclear palsy: a heterogeneous degeneration involving the brain stem, basal ganglia, and cerebellum with vertical gaze and pseudobulbar palsy, nuchal dystonia and dementia. *Arch Neurol* 1964;10:333–59.

168. de Bruin VMS, Lees AJ. The clinical features of 67 patients with clinically definite Steele-Richardson-Olszewski syndrome. *Behav Neurol* 1992;5:229–32.

169. Santacruz P, Uttl B, Litvan I *et al.* Progressive supranuclear palsy. *Neurology* 1998;50:1637–47.

170. Bak TH, Hodges JR. The neuropsychology of progressive supranuclear palsy. *Neurocase* 1998;4:89–94.

171. Grafman J, Litvan I, Gomez C *et al.* Frontal lobe function in progressive supranuclear palsy. *Arch Neurol* 1990;47:553–8.

172. Litvan I, Grafman J, Gomez C *et al.* Memory impairment in patients with progressive supranuclear palsy. *Arch Neurol* 1989;46:765–7.

173. Pillon B, Deweer B, Michon A *et al.* Are explicit memory disorders of progressive supranuclear palsy related to damage to striatofrontal circuits? *Neurology* 1994;44:1264–70.

174. Dubois B, Pillon B, Legaut-Demare F *et al.* Slowing of cognitive processing in progressive supranuclear palsy. *Arch Neurol* 1988;45:1194–9.

175. Litvan I, Mega MS, Cummings JL *et al.* Neuropsychiatric aspects of progressive supranuclear palsy. *Neurology* 1996;47:1184–9.

176. Menza MA, Cocchiola J, Golbe LI. Psychiatric symptoms in progressive supranuclear palsy. *Psychosomatics* 1995;36:550–4.

177. Aldrich MS, Foster NL, White RF *et al.* Sleep abnormalities in progressive supranuclear palsy. *Ann Neurol* 1989;25:577–81.

178. Montplaisir J, Petit D, Decary A *et al.* Sleep and quantitative EEG in patients with progressive supranuclear palsy. *Neurology* 1997;49:999–1003.

179. Osborn AG. *Diagnostic Neuroradiology.* St Louis, MO: Mosby, 1994.

180. Foster NL, Gilman S, Berent S *et al.* Cerebral hypometabolism in progressive supranuclear palsy studied with positron emission tomography. *Ann Neurol* 1988;24:399–406.

181. Goffinet AM, DeVolder AG, Gillain C *et al.* Positron tomography demonstrates frontal lobe hypometabolism in progressive supranuclear palsy. *Ann Neurol* 1989;25:131–9.

182. Bhatt MH, Snow BJ, Martin WRW *et al.* Positron emission tomography in progressive supranuclear palsy. *Arch Neurol* 1991;48:389–91.

183. Ilgin N, Zubieta J, Reich SG *et al.* PET imaging of the dopamine transporter in progressive supranuclear palsy and Parkinson's disease. *Neurology* 1999;52:1221–6.

184. van Royan E, Verhoeff NFLG, Speelman JD *et al.* Multiple system atrophy and progressive supranuclear palsy. *Arch Neurol* 1993;50:513–16.

185. Hauw JJ, Daniel SE, Dickson D *et al.* Preliminary NINDS neuropathologic criteria for Steele-Richardson-Olszewski syndrome (progressive supranuclear palsy). *Neurology* 1994;44:2015–19.

186. Ruberg M, Javoy-Agid F, Hirsch E *et al.* Dopaminergic and cholinergic lesions in progressive supranuclear palsy. *Ann Neurol* 1985;18:523–9.

187. Kompoliti K, Goetz CG, Litvan I *et al.* Pharmacological therapy in progressive supranuclear palsy. *Arch Neurol* 1998;55:1099–102.

188. Engel PA. Treatment of progressive supranuclear palsy with amitriptyline: therapeutic and toxic effects. *J Am Geriatr Soc* 1996;44:1072–4.

189. Newman GC. Treatment of progressive supranuclear palsy with tricyclic antidepressants. *Neurology* 1985;35:1189–93.

190. Jackson JA, Jankovic J, Ford J. Progressive supranuclear palsy: clinical features and response to treatment in 16 patients. *Ann Neurol* 1983;13:273–8.

191. Litvan I, Blesa R, Clark K *et al.* Pharmacological evaluation of the cholinergic system in progressive supranuclear palsy. *Ann Neurol* 1994;36:55–61.

192. Polo KB, Jabbari B. Botulinum Toxin-A improves the rigidity of progressive supranuclear palsy. *Ann Neurol* 1994;35:237–9.

193. Riley DE, Lang AE. Clinical diagnostic criteria. In: Litvan I, Goetz CG, Lang AE (eds) *Corticobasal Degeneration and Related Disorders.* Philadelphia: Lippincott & Williams, 2000: 29–34.

194. Litvan I, Agid Y, Goetz C *et al.* Accuracy of the clinical diagnosis of corticobasal degeneration: a clinicopathologic study. *Neurology* 1997;48:119–25.
195. Bergeron C, Pollanen MS, Weyer L *et al.* Unusual clinical presentations of cortical-basal ganglionic degeneration. *Ann Neurol* 1996;40:893–900.
196. Grimes DA, Lang AE, Bergeron C. Dementia as the most common presentation of cortical-basal ganglionic degeneration. *Neurology* 1999;53:1969–74.
197. Thompson PD, Rothwell JC, Brown P *et al.* The myoclonus in corticobasal degeneration: evidence for two forms of cortical reflex myoclonus. *Brain* 1994;117:1197–207.
198. Leiguarda R, Lees AJ, Merello M *et al.* The nature of apraxia in corticobasal degeneration. *J Neurol Neurosurg Psychiatry* 1994;57:455–9.
199. Moreaud O, Naegele B, Pellat J. The nature of apraxia in corticobasal degeneration. *Neuropsychiatry Neuropsychol Behav Neurol* 1996;9:288–92.
200. Mimura M, White RF, Albert ML. Corticobasal degeneration: neuropsychological and clinical correlates. *J Neuropsychiatry Clin Neurosci* 1997;9:94–8.
201. Pillon B, Blin J, Vidailhet M *et al.* The neuropsychological pattern of corticobasal degeneration: comparison with progressive supranuclear palsy and Alzheimer's disease. *Neurology* 1995;45:1477–83.
202. Frattali CM, Grafman J, Patronas N *et al.* Language disturbances in corticobasal degeneration. *Neurology* 2000;54:990–2.
203. Mendez MF. Corticobasal ganglionic degeneration with Balint's syndrome. *J Neuropsychiatry Clin Neurosci* 2000;12:273–5.
204. Litvan I, Cummings JL, Mega M. Neuropsychiatric features of corticobasal degeneration. *J Neurol Neurosurg Psychiatry* 1998;65:717–21.
205. Soliveri P, Monza D, Paridi D *et al.* Cognitive and magnetic resonance imaging aspects of corticobasal degeneration and progressive supranuclear palsy. *Neurology* 1999;53:502–7.
206. Markus HS, Lees AJ, Lennox G *et al.* Patterns of regional cerebral blood flow in corticobasal degeneration studied using HMPAO SPECT; comparison with Parkinson's disease and normal controls. *Mov Disord* 1995;10:179–87.
207. Hirono N, Ishii K, Sasaki M *et al.* Features of regional cerebral glucose metabolism abnormality in corticobasal degeneration. *Dement Geriatr Cogn Disord* 2000;11:139–46.
208. Nagahama Y, Fukuyama H, Turjanski N *et al.* Cerebral glucose metabolism in corticobasal degeneration: comparison with progressive supranuclear palsy and normal controls. *Mov Disord* 1997;12:691–6.
209. Sawle GV, Brooks DJ, Marsden CD *et al.* Corticobasal degeneration: a unique pattern of regional cortical oxygen hypometabolism and striatal fluorodopa uptake demonstrated by positron emission tomography. *Brain* 1991;114:541–56.
210. Schneider JA, Watts RL, Gearing M *et al.* Corticobasal degeneration: neuropathologic and clinical heterogeneity. *Neurology* 1997;48:959–69.
211. Kertesz A, Martinez-Lage P, Davidson W *et al.* The corticobasal degeneration syndrome overlaps progressive aphasia and frontotemporal dementia. *Neurology* 2000;55:1368–75.
212. Consensus Committee of the American Autonomic Society and the American Academy of Neurology. Consensus statement on the definition of

orthostatic hypotension, pure autonomic failure, and multiple system atrophy. *Neurology* 1996;46:1470.

213. Litvan I, Goetz CG, Jankovic J *et al.* What is the accuracy of the clinical diagnosis of multiple system atrophy? A clinicopathologic study. *Arch Neurol* 1997;54:937–44.

214. Litvan I, Booth V, Wenning GK *et al.* Retrospective application of a set of clinical diagnostic criteria for the diagnosis of multiple system atrophy. *J Neural Transm* 1998;105:217–27.

215. Colosimo C, Albanese A, Hughes AJ *et al.* Some specific clinical features differentiate multiple system atrophy (striatonigral variety) from Parkinson's disease. *Arch Neurol* 1995;52:294–8.

216. Wenning GK, Ben Shlomo Y, Magalhaes M *et al.* Clinical features and natural history of multiple system atrophy. An analysis of 100 cases. *Brain* 1994;117:835–45.

217. Pillon B, Gouider-Khouja N, Deweer B *et al.* Neuropsychological pattern of striatonigral degeneration: comparison with Parkinson's disease and progressive supranuclear palsy. *J Neurol Neurosurg Psychiatry* 1995;58:174–9.

218. Robbins TW, James M, Lange KW *et al.* Cognitive performance in multiple system atrophy. *Brain* 1992;115:271–91.

219. Kwentus JA, Auth TL, Foy JL. Shy-Drager syndrome presenting as depression: case report. *J Clin Psychiatry* 1984;45:137–9.

220. Pilo L, Ring H, Quinn N *et al.* Depression in multiple system atrophy and in idiopathic Parkinson's disease: a pilot comparative study. *Biol Psychiatry* 1996;39:803–7.

221. Wright BA, Rosen JR, Buysse DJ *et al.* Shy-Drager syndrome presenting as a REM behavioral disorder. *J Geriatr Psychiatry Neurol* 1990;3:110–13.

222. Kraft E, Schwarz J, Trenkwalder C *et al.* The combination of hypointense and hyperintense signal changes on T_2-weighted magnetic resonance imaging sequences. *Arch Neurol* 1999;56:225–8.

223. De Volder AG, Francart J, Laterre C *et al.* Decreased glucose utilization in the striatum and frontal lobe in probable striatonigral degeneration. *Ann Neurol* 1989;26:239–47.

224. Perani D, Bressi S, Testa D *et al.* Clinical/metabolic correlations in multiple system atrophy. *Arch Neurol* 1995;52:179–85.

225. Wenning GK, Tison F, Shlomo B *et al.* Multiple system atrophy: a review of 203 pathologically proven cases. *Mov Disord* 1997;12:133–47.

226. Lantos P, Papp MI. Cellular pathology of multiple system atrophy: a review. *J Neurol Neurosurg Psychiatry* 1994;57:129–33.

chapter 6

Vascular dementia

Vascular dementia (VaD) is a complex neuropsychiatric disorder with cognitive and behavioral manifestations resulting from multiple infarctions, ischemic brain injury, or occasionally, hemorrhagic intracranial events. The course is typically progressive with a stepwise or fluctuating course. Focal neurological signs are usually present on neurological examination and identification of VaD is greatly aided by structural neuroimaging. Cerebrovascular disease is common in the elderly and syndromes of ischemic brain injury mixed with degenerative disorders including Alzheimer's disease, frontotemporal lobar degeneration, dementia with Lewy bodies, and Parkinson's disease are common.

Box 6.1 presents the consensus diagnostic criteria developed by the National Institute of Neurological Disorders and Stroke and the Association Internationale pour la Recherche et l'Enseignement en Neurosciences (NINDS-AIREN).[1,2] These criteria have been shown to have modest sensitivity (0.58) and fair specificity (0.80).[3,4] Ninety percent of patients with Alzheimer's disease are successfully excluded by the criteria and approximately 25% of patients with mixed Alzheimer's disease and cerebrovascular disease are classified as VaD.[3] The NINDS-AIREN criteria have moderately good inter-rater reliability. The diagnostic accuracy of the available criteria for VaD do not perform as well as the current diagnostic criteria for Alzheimer's disease.[5,6]

Box 6.1 NINDS-AIREN diagnostic criteria for definite, probable, and possible vascular dementia (VaD)[1]

Definite VaD
- Clinical criteria for probable VaD
- Autopsy demonstration of appropriate ischemic or hemorrhagic brain injury and no other cause of dementia

Probable VaD
- *Dementia*
  - Decline from a previous higher level of cognitive functioning
  - Impairment of two or more cognitive domains
  - Deficits severe enough to interfere with activities of daily living and not due to physical effects of stroke alone
  - Absence of delirium; absence of psychosis, aphasia, or sensorimotor impairment that precludes neuropsychologic testing; and absence of any other disorder capable of producing a dementia syndrome
- *Cerebrovascular disease*
  - Focal neurologic signs consistent with stroke, and
  - Neuroimaging evidence of extensive vascular lesions
- *Relationship between dementia and cerebrovascular disease*, as evidenced by one or more of the following:
  - Onset of dementia within 3 months of a recognized stroke
  - Abrupt deterioration or fluctuating or stepwise progression of the cognitive deficit

Supporting features
- Subtle onset and variable course of cognitive deficits
- Early presence of gait disturbance
- History of unsteadiness, frequent and unprovoked falls
- Early urinary frequency, urgency, and other urinary symptoms not explained by urologic disease
- Pseudobulbar palsy
- Personality and mood changes, abulia, depression, emotional incontinence, and subcortical deficits, including psychomotor retardation and abnormal executive function

Possible VaD
- Dementia with focal neurologic signs but without neuroimaging confirmation of definite cerebrovascular disease
- Dementia with focal signs but without a clear temporal relationship between dementia and stroke
- Dementia and focal signs but with subtle onset and variable course of cognitive deficits

Alzheimer's disease with cerebrovascular disease
- Clinical criteria for possible Alzheimer's disease
- Clinical and imaging evidence of cerebrovascular disease

Clinical features and types of vascular dementia

Vascular dementia takes several clinical forms depending on the location of the associated brain injury (Table 6.1). The most common lesions associated with VaD are subcortical ischemic infarctions or areas of ischemic injury occurring in the subcortical white matter. Lacunar state refers to the occurrence of multiple lesions in the basal ganglia, thalami, and subcortical white matter. 'Binswanger's disease' refers to extensive ischemic injury of the subcortical white matter in a patient with dementia. Subcortical lacunar infarction involving the basal ganglia and the white matter account for a majority of cases of VaD.[7-9] Thalamic dementia occurs when there are bilateral infarctions of the paramedian thalamic nuclei. Multiple cortical infarctions involving either hemisphere may occur particularly with emboli arising from the heart or carotid arteries. Infarction of the angular gyrus region of the left hemisphere will produce a strategic dementia with interruption of multiple converging pathways critical to normal cognitive function. Borderzone syndromes arise when hypotension leads to infarction in the borderzone or watershed areas between the territories of the major cerebral vessels.[1,10-12] Multi-infarct dementia (MID) refers to the combination of multiple cortical and subcortical vascular lesions.

Vascular dementia is a common cause of cognitive impairment in the elderly, accounting for between 15 and 30% of cases of dementia in most clinicopathological series. In addition to patients meeting criteria for VaD, there are a larger number of patients who have cognitive impairment on a vascular basis that do not meet all criteria for VaD. 'Vascular cognitive impairment' has been proposed as a more inclusive term, embracing patients with VaD and those with ischemic brain injury producing less severe cognitive impairment.[13]

Risk factors for VaD include coronary artery disease, elevated serum low-density lipoprotein levels, high blood pressure, diabetes, obesity hypercholesterolemia, and habitual cigarette smoking.[7,14-18] Protective factors that reduce the risk of VaD include regular physical exercise and supplementary use of vitamin E.[7,18]

Predictors of the occurrence of dementia in patients who have

Table 6.1 Types of vascular dementia

Clinical type	Region of injury	Vessels affected
Multi-infarct dementia	Cortical and subcortical structures	Large and small vessels
Lacunar state	Basal ganglia, thalamus, subcortical white matter	Small penetrating vessels arising from circle of Willis and stems of ACA, MCA, PCA
Binswanger's disease	Hemispheric white matter	Small vessels penetrating from superficial cortical vessels toward the ventricular margin
Thalamic dementia	Thalamic nuclei (especially bilateral paramedian nuclei)	Penetrating vessels arising from the PCA
Anterior cerebral artery syndrome	Medial frontal regions including the anterior angulate cortex	Anterior cerebral arteries
Cortical dementia	Multiple cortical regions	ACA, MCA, PCA
Angular gyrus syndrome (strategic infarct dementia)	Angular gyrus of left hemisphere	Superior branch of left MCA
Borderzone syndromes	Borderzones between ACA/MCA or MCA/PCA	Hypotension; brain ischemia

ACA, anterior cerebral artery; MCA, middle cerebral artery; PCA, posterior cerebral artery.

experienced a stroke have been assessed. More advanced age, pre-existing cognitive decline, severity of the neurological deficit at admission, the presence of diabetes, the presence of 'silent' infarctions on neuroimaging, occurrence of lesions in the hemispheres rather than in brain stem or cerebellar locations, lesions of the left hemisphere as compared to the right hemisphere, lower levels of education, non-White race, and larger size of the stroke-related lesion were all found to be associated with the occurrence of dementia following stroke.[19-23]

Clinical features of VaD will differ according to the etiology of the syndrome. Some characteristics, however, are common across VaD disorders and the Hachinski Ischemic Score (HIS)[24] (Table 6.2) is a common means of capturing signs and symptoms that distinguish VaD from degenerative dementia syndromes. Features that are most characteristic of cerebrovascular disease receive higher weightings (abrupt onset, fluctuating course, history of stroke, focal neurological symptoms, focal neurological signs), while others that are less specific to cerebrovascular

Table 6.2 Hachinski Ischemic Score items[24]

Feature	Value
Abrupt onset	2
Stepwise deterioration	1
Fluctuating course	2
Nocturnal confusion	1
Preservation of personality	1
Depression	1
Somatic complaints	1
Emotional incontinence	1
History of hypertension	1
History of stroke	2
Associated atherosclerosis	1
Focal neurologic symptoms	2
Focal neurologic signs	2
Total ≤4 – not VaD	
Total ≥7 – VaD	

disease receive less weight in the score (stepwise deterioration, nocturnal confusion, preservation of personality, depression, somatic complaints, emotional incontinence, history of hypertension, and associated atherosclerosis). A score of ≤4 on the HIS is most consistent with the degenerative disorder and a score of ≥7 is consistent with VaD. Based on a pathologically proven sample of patients with VaD, these cut-off scores had a sensitivity of 89% and a specificity of 89%.[25] The HIS is less successful in distinguishing VaD from mixed Alzheimer's disease and cerebrovascular disease. Those features that best distinguished VaD from Alzheimer' disease were stepwise deterioration, fluctuating course, history of stroke, and focal neurological symptoms. Stepwise deterioration and emotional incontinence were the factors that optimally distinguished VaD from mixed degenerative and vascular dementia.

Gait disturbance is a common sign of ischemic injury to the subcortical white matter.[26,27] The gait change has features of 'lower-half parkinsonism' – hesitation, diminished stride length, and diminished step height are characteristic. Movement of the face and upper limbs is much less affected. In some cases, VaD may imitate the clinical syndrome of progressive supranuclear palsy.[28] Lesions affecting the upper motor neuron projections will produce a contralateral pyramidal syndrome including hemiparesis, increased tone, exaggerated muscle stretch reflexes, and an extensor plantar response (Babinski sign). When there is disruption of descending pyramidal tracts bilaterally patients frequently exhibit pseudobulbar palsy manifested by a pseudobulbar affect (exaggerated emotional responses that are disproportionate to or inconsistent with the patient's emotional state), dysarthria, dysphagia, exaggerated facial and jaw muscle stretch reflexes, and increased gag reflex. Focal lesions involving the geniculocalcarine radiations produce a contralateral homonymous visual field defect. Focal interruption of ascending sensory projections causes a contralateral hemisensory disturbance. Incontinence is a common early feature of VaD, and the triad of dementia, incontinence, and gait disturbance is more often produced by VaD than by obstructive hydrocephalus.

Cognitive impairment in vascular dementia

The type of cognitive impairment observed in patients with VaD reflects the size of blood vessel involved, the region of the brain infarcted, the size of the injured area, and the time between the onset of the injury and the assessment. When the cerebral hemispheres are involved there are corresponding regional signature syndromes (Table 6.3). With local injury to the left hemisphere, aphasias, apraxias, and related syndromes such as alexia, agraphia, and acalculia are most frequently observed. With injury to the right hemisphere, the observed signature syndromes include the aprosodias, amusia, neglect, anosognosia syndromes, dressing disturbance, constructional abnormalities, prosopagnosia, and environmental agnosia.[29] The concept of 'patchy' deficits is most applicable to the multi-infarct or multiple cortical infarct syndrome where the relationship among cognitive deficits is less regular than in subcortical VaD or progressive degenerative disorders such as Alzheimer's disease.[30]

Subcortical ischemic vascular injury and lacunar infarctions relevant to VaD tend to preferentially involve the subcortical white matter of the frontal lobes and the anterior aspects of the basal ganglia including the caudate nucleus and globus pallidus.[9,31,32] There is a corresponding disproportionate involvement of executive functions mediated by frontal-subcortical circuits.[33,34] Compared with matched normal controls, patients with subcortical VaD exhibit deficits in shifting mental set, response inhibition (such as the Stroop Color Word Interference test), word list generation, and motor programming tests such as alternating sequences and multiple loops[35,36] (Chapter 2). Patients manifest deficits in attention and psychomotor speed as tested by the digit-symbol substitution test, digit span, and trail making tests.[37] Anomia may be present and articulation abnormalities are common.[38] Patients with subcortical VaD exhibit more severe impairment of executive function and less impairment of memory, particularly recognition memory, than patients with Alzheimer's disease.[39–43]

Some VaD patients have a predominance of white matter ischemic injury and a clinical syndrome which tends to be gradually progressive as opposed to one punctuated by periods of acute decline. These patients

Table 6.3 Principal region-related cognitive syndromes occurring in patients with vascular dementia

Vessel	Clinical syndrome
Left hemisphere	
• Anterior cerebral artery	Akinetic neoplasm (transient)
	Transcortical motor aphasia
	Executive dysfunction
	Disinhibition
	Callosal apraxia
• Middle cerebral artery	Broca's aphasia
	Sympathetic apraxia
	Conduction aphasia
	Parietal apraxia
	Wernicke's aphasia
	Anomic aphasia
	Global aphasia
	Transcortical sensory aphasia
	Gerstmann's syndrome (agraphia, right–left disorientation, acalculia, finger agnosia)
	Angular gyrus syndrome (Gerstmann's syndrome plus alexia, anomia, constructional disturbance)
• Posterior cerebral artery	Alexia without agraphia
	Hemiachromatopia
	Homonymous hemianopsia
Right hemisphere	
• Anterior cerebral artery	Callosal apraxia
• Middle cerebral artery	Executive aprosodia
	Receptive aprosodia
	Amusia
	Unilateral (left neglect)
	Anosognosia
	Dressing disturbance
	Constructional disturbance
• Posterior cerebral artery	Prosopagnosia
	Environmental agnosia
	Hemiachromatopsia

are diagnosed as suffering from Binswanger's disease.[44,45] Clinically, the patients manifest pseudobulbar palsy, gait disturbances, and urinary incontinence. There may be focal neurological deficits. Neuroimaging reveals bilateral leukoariosis on computed tomography (CT) or bilateral, multiple, or diffuse high signal areas on T2-weighted magnetic resonance imaging (MRI). Cognitively and behaviorally, patients manifest prominent frontal executive dysfunction with diminished motivation, loss of insight, apathy, and abulia. A retrieval deficit type of memory abnormality may be present and there may be variable changes in language and visuospatial skills.[44,45] Measures of speed of mental processing and of attention are particularly sensitive to white matter changes.[46] Box 6.2 presents criteria for the clinical diagnosis of Binswanger's disease.[47] Subcortical lacunar infarctions are frequently present in patients

---

Box 6.2 Criteria for the clinical diagnosis of possible Binswanger's disease[47]

- Dementia established by clinical examination and confirmed by neuropsychological tests
- One finding from two of the following three groups:
  - Vascular risk factor or evidence of systemic vascular disease (e.g. hypertension, diabetes, a history of myocardial infarction, cardiac arrhythmia, or congestive heart failure)
  - Focal cerebrovascular disease (e.g. a history of stroke, or demonstration of a focal pyramidal or sensory sign)
  - 'Subcortical' cerebral dysfunction (e.g. a parkinsonian, magnetic, or 'senile' gait, parkinsonian or gegenhalten rigidity, or a history of incontinence secondary to a spastic bladder)
- Bilateral leukoariosis on computed tomography (CT), or bilateral and, multiple or diffuse, subcortical high signal T2-weighted lesions $>2 \times 2$ mm on magnetic resonance imaging (MRI)

The proposed criteria lose their validity in the presence of:
- multiple or bilateral cortical lesions on CT or MR; or
- severe dementia

diagnosed with Binswanger's disease and the distinction between Binswanger's disease and lacunar state is somewhat artificial.

Neuropsychiatric features of vascular dementia

Neuropsychiatric disturbances are common in VaD. Both cortical and subcortical VaD syndromes manifest neuropsychiatric abnormalities, although the characteristic features may differ. Studies with the Neuropsychiatric Inventory (NPI)[48] reveal more severe agitation, depression, anxiety, and apathy in patients with subcortical VaD compared with patients with Alzheimer's disease[49] (Figure 6.1). Several studies have confirmed that depression is more common and more severe in VaD than in Alzheimer's disease, while delusions tend to be less common[50–52] (Figure 6.2).

Delusions may occur in patients with VaD and are more common in

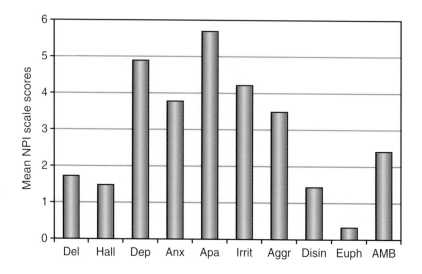

Figure 6.1 Mean scores on the Neuropsychiatric Inventory in patients with subcortical vascular dementia (n = 30).[49] Del, delusions; Hall, hallucinations; Dep, depression; Anx, anxiety; Apa, apathy; Irrit, irritability; Aggr, aggression/agitation; Disin, disinhibition; Euph, euphoria; AMB, aberrant motor behavior.

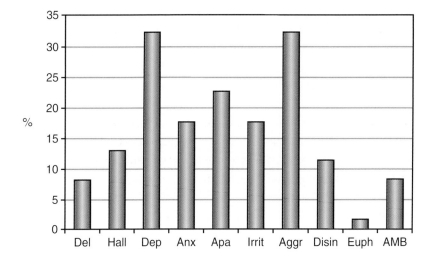

Figure 6.2 *Percent of community-dwelling patients with vascular dementia exhibiting symptoms scoreable on the Neuropsychiatric Inventory (n = 62; community-based study).[51] For explanation of abbreviations see legend to Figure 6.1.*

patients with bilateral subcortical disease. Patients may have mono-symptomatic delusions or complex late-onset paraphrenic disorders.[53,54] VaD patients with delusions tend to be more aggressive and exhibit more activity disturbances than nondelusional patients.[55] Misidentification syndromes occur in about one quarter of VaD patients with delusions; jealousy, persecution, somatic delusions, and delusions of theft represent the other common delusional symptoms of VaD.[56]

Infarction of the anterior thalamic area has been associated with a unique thought disorder called palipsychism manifested by a preservation and superimposition of mental activities normally processed sequentially (e.g. giving biographical information while working on a calculation test).[57]

Personality alterations are frequent in VaD. Studies using personality inventories reveal that VaD patients are more out of touch, more childish, more dependent, more listless, less happy, more labile, and less sensitive than matched elderly subjects without VaD.[58] Compared with patients with Alzheimer's disease they are more apathetic.[59] Disinhibition syndromes also have been observed with both cortical and subcortical lesions in patients with VaD.[60] Patients may become impulsive, disinhibited, and lewd. They may have poor hygiene despite previous fastidiousness. Shoplifting and other legal offenses may be a manifestation of the disinhibition syndrome.[60,61]

With lateralized cortical lesions involving the geniculocalcarine radiations, visual hallucinations may occur and palinopsia with preservation of visual images may be reported by patients, particularly those with lesions of the right posterior hemisphere.[62]

Depression in the acute phases following stroke is associated with left frontal lesions, while depression in more chronic post-stroke patients is more likely to be associated with right posterior lesions.[63] Mania occurring with focal brain lesions typically follows injury to the right hemisphere particularly the frontal regions.[64] Patients with lesions of the caudate nuclei or globus pallidus may exhibit obsessive-compulsive symptoms.[65,66] Table 6.4 presents a list of neuropsychiatric symptoms and commonly associated focal brain lesions.

Neuroimaging

Neuroimaging is essential to the diagnosis of VaD and is required by the NINDS-AIREN criteria (Box 6.1). MRI is the most useful modality for identifying stroke and subcortical ischemic injury. CT is less revealing than MRI but is an adequate means of defining cerebrovascular pathology in most dementia evaluations. Increased lucency is evident on CT at the site of stroke or white matter ischemic injury. Functional imaging such as positron emission tomography (PET) or single photon emission computerized tomography (SPECT) reveal focal lesions at the site of stroke (Figure 6.3), and may show reduced perfusion in functionally related regions. The area of functional disturbance is typically larger than the area of anatomic injury identified by structural imaging.

Dementia is correlated with the total area of infarction and the area of infarction of the left hemisphere as shown by the MRI. Total area of

a   b

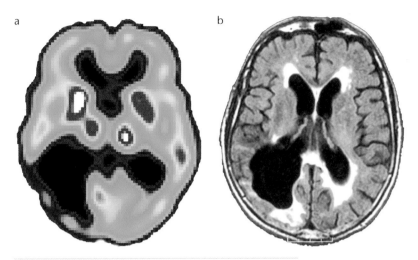

Figure 6.3 MRI with focal lesion and white matter ischemic injury (right), and corresponding area of reduced perfusion on SPECT (left).

white matter ischemic injury and area of white matter ischemic injury in both right and left hemispheres[21] also correlate with degree of cognitive impairment. Severity of abnormalities on CT (infarcts and/or white matter lucency) correlates with the presence of VaD.[67] Diffusion-weighted MRI, a technology that reveals recent infarction, commonly demonstrates the presence of new foci of stroke in patients with VaD even when there has been no corresponding clinical event.[68]

Each of the types of VaD has a corresponding abnormality on neuro-imaging studies (Table 6.1). Patients with multi-infarct dementia will have areas of infarction in both cortical and subcortical regions on CT or MRI. Patients with lacunar state, Binswanger's disease, or the lacunar-Binswanger complex have evidence of small infarctions in the basal ganglia, thalamus, and subcortical white matter in addition to extensive areas of increased signal in the white matter on MRI (Figure 6.4). On CT, there is increased periventricular and deep white matter lucency (Figure 6.5). Patients with strategic infarct dementia such as a stroke involving the left angular gyrus will have a corresponding lesion in the inferior parietal region of the left hemisphere (Figure 6.6). Individuals with

Table 6.4 Neuropsychiatric symptoms commonly associated with focal brain lesions

Neuropsychiatric symptoms	Focal brain lesions
Apathy/abulia	Medial frontal/anterior cingulate
	Nucleus accumbens
	Globus pallidus
	Medial thalamus
Disinhibition	Orbitofrontal
	Ventral caudate
Visual hallucinations	Geniculocalcarine radiations (typically associated with a visual field defect)
	Brain stem (peduncular hallucinosis)
Palinopsia (persistent or recurrent visual images)	Posterior hemisphere (usually right)
Auditory hallucinations	Brain stem
Delusions	Bilateral subcortical (white matter or basal ganglia); right temporo-parietal cortex
Depression	Left frontal (acute period following stroke)
	Right posterior (chronic post-stroke period)
Anxiety	Left frontal
Obsessions/compulsions	Caudate nuclei, globus pallidus (usually bilateral)
Palipsychism (concurrent mental activities usually performed sequentially)	Anterior thalamus
Anosognosia	Right parietal (may be seen with left parietal lesions; it is less severe and less persistent with left-sided injury)

sudden acute hypotension may have areas of infarction in the border-zone or watershed regions between the major cerebrovascular territories of the anterior cerebral, posterior cerebral, and middle cerebral arteries.

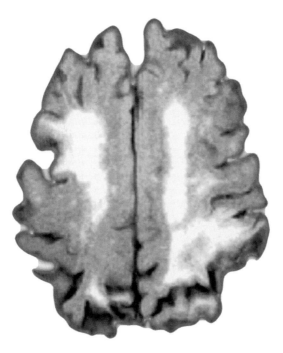

Figure 6.4 *MRI showing extensive changes in the white matter in a patient with Binswanger's disease type of vascular dementia.*

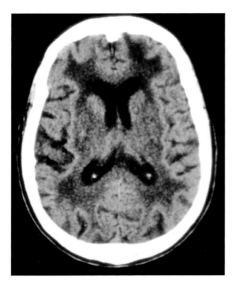

Figure 6.5 *CT showing extensive changes in the white matter in a patient with Binswanger's disease type of vascular dementia.*

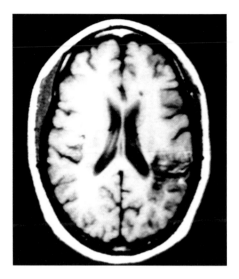

Figure 6.6 MRI showing region of stroke in the left inferior parietal region (angular gyrus) of a patient with strategic infarct type of vascular dementia.

Periventricular white matter changes are common in normal aged individuals without evidence of cognitive impairment. This can be a source of confusion in deciding whether high signal areas observed on an MRI are sufficient to account for cognitive abnormalities observed in individual patients. Depression, gait disturbances, and cognitive impairment without dementia are observed in patients with modest degrees of white matter abnormalities. Neuropsychological studies suggest that a threshold of area of white matter injury must be exceeded before cognitive deficits appear. Patients with white matter lesions exceeding 10 cm^2 in size exhibit cognitive abnormalities while those with smaller lesions do not.[69] Both neuropsychological deficits and impairment of activities of daily living correlate with the degree of subcortical white matter injury.[70–72]

The severity of metabolic abnormalities observed on PET correlates with the severity of cognitive impairment in VaD. These relationships have consistently involved reductions in frontal lobe metabolism bilaterally and occasionally have been involved in reductions in other cortical areas.[73–75] Periventricular hyperintensities and lacunar infarcts of the basal ganglia or thalamus are associated with reduced cortical metabolism.[76]

Differential diagnosis

The common vascular pathologies underlying VaD are atherosclerosis of the large vessels and arteriosclerosis of the small vessels. Atherosclerosis involves the development of fatty streaks that evolve into fibrous plaques and ultimately into complicated plaques that occlude large vessels or send emboli distally into the intracranial vasculature. The principal type of small vessel disease observed in VaD is segmental fibrinoid arterial degeneration with lipohyalinosis involving the deep perforating vessels and vessels of similar size that penetrate from the superficial vessels into the cerebral white matter (Figure 6.7). The principal risk factors for this type of arteriosclerosis are age, arterial hypertension, and diabetes. Hypertension is present in 60% of patients with VaD.[77] Cardiac sources of multiple cerebral emboli account for a smaller

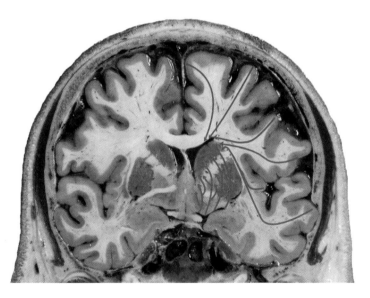

Figure 6.7 *Schematic representation of the distribution of small vessels most commonly involved in vascular dementia. The distribution accounts for the periventricular location of white matter ischemia and the typical location of lacunar infarctions.*

number of cases of VaD. Hemorrhagic disorders and hereditary cerebral vascular conditions such as amyloid angiopathy and cerebral autosomal dominant arteriopathy with subcortical infarcts and leukoencephalopathy (CADASIL) are rare etiologies of VaD. Box 6.3 provides a differential diagnosis of the principal causes of VaD.

The extensive white matter abnormalities associated with Binswanger's disease must be distinguished from the many other causes of white matter hyperintensities (on MRI) or lucencies (on CT).[78] Some of these disorders present with a dementia syndrome and may have prominent neuropsychiatric symptoms. Box 6.4 lists the principal disorders that can present in midlife or later with diffuse white matter changes, cognitive impairment, and behavioral alterations. The differential diagnosis includes several types of vascular dementia (Binswanger's disease, CADASIL, and amyloid angiopathy) as well as adult-onset leukodystrophies, infectious disorders including human immunodeficiency virus (HIV) dementia complex and progressive multi-focal leukoencephalopathy, inflammatory diseases, a variety of toxic leukoencephalopathies (cranial irradiation, anti-neoplastic therapies, 'glue sniffing', carbon monoxide), metabolic disorders including vitamin B12 deficiency, traumatic brain injury with damage to axons, neoplasms such as lymphomas and gliomas, and the periventricular white matter changes that may be associated with hydrocephalus.

Neuropathology

Pure VaD without other concomitant cerebral lesions is relatively rare. Patients diagnosed with VaD clinically, commonly have concomitant Alzheimer's type pathology at autopsy,[79,80] and similarly, patients diagnosed clinically with probable Alzheimer's disease have cerebrovascular pathology of varying severity in up to 25% of cases.[81] However, VaD with no or limited associated degenerative brain changes can be identified accurately using research diagnostic criteria (Box 6.1).[80,81] When VaD is the clinical and pathological diagnosis there are typically extensive and multi-focal vascular lesions. There is an imprecise relationship

Box 6.3 Principal causes of vascular dementia

Atherosclerosis

Arteriosclerosis

Cardiac disease
- Atrial fibrillation
- Myocardial infarction with mural thrombosis
- Cardiac surgery
- Infectious endocarditis
- Cardiomyopathy

Hereditary vascular disorders
- Cerebral autosomal dominant arteriopathy with subcortical infarcts and leukoencephalopathy (CADASIL)
- Hereditary cerebral amyloid angiopathy
- Fibromuscular dysphasia
- Fabry's disease
- Mitochondrial myopathy, encephalopathy, lactic acidosis, and stroke-like episodes (MELAS)

Inflammatory vascular disorders
- Systematic lupus erythematosus (SLE)
- Antiphospholipid antibody syndrome
- Giant cell arteritis (temporal arthritis)
- Sarcoidosis

Chemical and physical causes of vascular disease
- Amphetamines
- Cocaine
- Cerebral radiation

Hematologic disorders
- Leukemia
- Sickle cell disease
- Polycythemia vera

Meningovascular infections
- Syphilis
- Tuberculosis
- Fungal meningitis

Box 6.4 Principal disorders associated with white matter abnormalities

Vascular dementias
- Binswanger's disease
- Cerebral autosomal dominant arteriopathy with subcortical infarcts and leukoencephalopathy (CADASIL)
- Amyloid angiopathy

Multiple sclerosis

Leukodystrophies
- Metachromatic leukodystrophy
- Adrenoleukodystrophy
- Cerebrotendinous xanthomatosis
- Membranous lipodystrophy

Infectious disorders
- Human immunodeficiency virus (HIV) dementia complex
- Progressive multi-focal leukoencephalopathy
- Lyme encephalopathy

Inflammatory diseases
- Systemic lupus erythematosus
- Temporal arteritis
- Sarcoidosis

Toxic leukoencephalopathies
- Cranial irradiations
- Antineoplastic therapies
- Solvents ('glue sniffing')
- Carbon monoxide

Metabolic disorders
- Vitamin B12 deficiency
- Hypertensive encephalopathy
- Marchiafava-Bignami disease

Traumatic brain injury with diffuse axonal injury

Neoplasms
- Gliomatosis cerebri
- Diffuse infiltrating gliomas
- Primary cerebral lymphoma

Hydrocephalus with periventricular white matter changes

between the volume of infarcted tissue and the presence and severity of cognitive deterioration and neuropsychiatric symptoms. The volume of injured tissue has been found to account for 60% of the variance of the clinical symptomatology.[83,84]

The pathological changes reflect the corresponding type of VaD (Table 6.1). Those with multi-infarct dementia, multiple cortical infarctions, borderzone infarctions, and strategic infarct dementia have classical infarctions of the cerebral cortex and underlying white matter (Figure 6.8). Patients with lacunar state have multiple subcortical lacunar infarctions involving the thalamus and basal ganglia (Figure 6.9); those with Binswanger's disease show widespread ischemic injury of the cerebral white matter.

Complete infarctions are characterized pathologically by gliosis, absence of neurons and oligodendroglial cells; less severe anoxic ischemic injury results in laminar necrosis of the neocortex, hippocampal degeneration, and deep white matter demyelination.[85] When areas of increased signal intensity on MRI are analyzed pathologically, the associated regions are areas of pallor with ill-defined margins and sparing the subcortical U-fibers. There is depletion of both myelin and axons, diffuse vacuolization, and significant reduction in the density of glial cells.[86] There is associated pathology of the cerebral arteries and arterioles.[87] Compared with Alzheimer's disease, those with VaD have significantly more white matter involvement including vacuolization and myelin loss.[88] U-fibers immediately beneath the cortical ribbon tend to be least affected and periventricular white matter areas have the greatest abnormalities.

Mixed cerebrovascular disease and Alzheimer-type pathology are common at the time of post-mortem, accounting for approximately 25–35% of cases of late-onset dementia.[89] Diagnostic criteria tend to be insensitive to this mixed state. Combined cerebrovascular disease and Alzheimer's disease exaggerated the cognitive deficits associated with either disorder.[90]

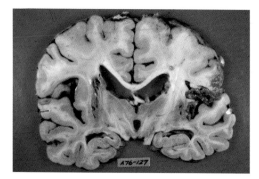

Figure 6.8 *Coronal brain section showing multiple cortical and subcortical infarctions in a patient with multi-infarct type of vascular dementia.*

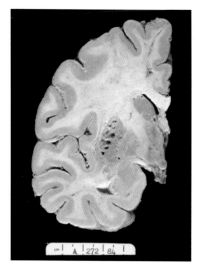

Figure 6.9 *Coronal brain section showing multiple lacunar infarctions in a patient with lacunar type of vascular dementia.*

Treatment

Pharmacologic management of the patient with VaD must address multiple dimensions including prevention of recurrent stroke; management of neuropsychiatric disturbances; use of cognitive enhancing agents, management of stroke-related disabilities such as spasticity, parkinsonism and incontinence; and management risk factors for cerebrovascular disease including hypertension, hypercholesterolemia, diabetes, and cardiac disease (Box 6.5).

Box 6.5 Pharmacologic treatment of vascular dementia

Stroke prevention
- Coumadin (only in disorders with risk of recurrent emboli such as atrial fibrillation)
- Platelet anti-aggregants
  - Aspirin (50–325 mg/day)
  - Aspirin (30–325 mg/day) plus dipyridamole (400 mg) extended-release tablets
  - Clopidogrel (75 mg/day)
  - Ticlopidine (500 mg/day)

Psychotropic agents
- Psychostimulants
- Antidepressants
- Antipsychotics
- Mood-stabilizing agents
- Anxiolytics
- Sedative-hypnotics

Cholinesterase inhibitors

Management of stroke-related physical disturbance
- Anti-spasticity agents
- Anti-incontinence (spastic bladder) agents
- Antiparkinsonian agents
- Treatment of pseudobulbar palsy

Treatment of cerebrovascular disease risk factors
- Antihypertensives
- Cholesterol-lowering agents
- Cardiac agents (anti-arrythmics, digitalis, etc.)

Stroke prevention

VaD is a significant risk factor for recurrent stroke[89] and diffusion-weighted MRI in patients with VaD reveals areas of signal abnormality consistent with new ischemic injury even in patients without recent stepwise decline.[68] Prevention of current stroke is important in minimizing further decline in patients with VaD. Use of anticoagulants such as warfarin is warranted only in patients with risk of recurrent emboli such as those with atrial fibrillation. In patients with evidence of arterial disease including infarctions and subcortical ischemic injury, platelet anti-aggregants are indicated. Aspirin in doses of 50–325 mg daily is the most widely used agent and is appropriate for those without a history of gastrointestinal hemorrhage. There is a synergy between aspirin and extended-release dipyridamole (400 mg per day) in stroke risk reduction. Patients intolerant of aspirin or aspirin/dipyridamole may be treated with clopidogrel or ticlopidine. Biweekly monitoring of the white blood cell and serum count is required during the first 4 months of treatment with ticlopidine because of potential neutropenia and thrombocytopenia.[92] Preliminary evidence suggests that use of platelet anti-aggregants in patients with VaD stabilizes or improves cognitive test performance.[93]

Psychotropic agents

Neuropsychiatric symptoms are common in VaD (Figures 6.1 and 6.2). There have been few randomized clinical trials addressing the utility of psychotropic agents in patients with VaD. The response of these symptoms in other clinical settings combined with the disability produced by neuropsychiatric symptoms suggest that it is reasonable to cautiously approach treatment of neuropsychiatric symptoms in VaD with psychopharmacologic agents.

Apathy is a common manifestation of VaD, particularly those with diffuse white matter ischemic injury, Binswanger's disease, or frontal lobe infarction. Psychostimulants may have a useful role in this condition, including methylphenidate, dextroamphetamine, or modafinil. In some cases, dopamine agonists such as bromocriptine, pergolide, ropinerol, or pramipexole may be valuable in restoring normal motivation. Indirect dopaminergic agents such as amantadine may be beneficial for some patients and others may respond to activating antidepressants such as buproprione, tranylcypramine, desipramine, or fluoxetine.[94]

Depression is a common feature in VaD. It exacerbates disability and limits engagement with rehabilitation. Treatment of depression in VaD follows similar principles to those used in treatment of depression in other elderly individuals. Selective serotonin reuptake inhibitors are preferable to tricyclic agents and monoamine oxidase inhibitors because of the lower risk of side effects. Selective serotonin reuptake inhibitors have been shown to be useful in the treatment of post-stroke depression by most,[95,96] but not all[97] investigators. Tricyclic antidepressants, particularly nortriptyline, have been shown to be effective in post-stroke depressive symptoms.[97,98] Buspirone and psychostimulants also have been shown to be useful in relieving the symptoms of some patients with post-stroke depression.[99,100] Patients with subcortical vascular lesions and frontal lobe syndromes respond more poorly to treatment with antidepressants than patients with idiopathic late life depression.[101] Patients resistant to pharmacotherapy may be treated with electroconvulsive therapy (ECT);[102] post-ECT confusion may be more severe in patients with VaD.

Psychosis and agitation are treated with antipsychotic agents as the first line of therapy. Atypical antipsychotics are preferred over conventional neuroleptics because of the lower rate of adverse events associated with atypical agents. Risperidone has been shown to reduce psychosis and agitation in patients with VaD.[103,104] Olanzapine and quetiapine are atypical antipsychotics that have been shown to reduce similar symptoms in other populations of patients with dementia such as Alzheimer's disease (Chapters 3 and 10). Neuroleptic agents such as haloperidol represent efficacious alternatives in settings where atypical antipsychotics are unavailable or not well tolerated by the patient. The patient must be monitored for the occurrence of parkinsonism and tardive dyskinesia.

Agitation may not respond or may respond incompletely to treatment with antipsychotic agents. In such cases, use of mood-stabilizing agents may be used as an alternative or as co-therapy to antipsychotic compounds (Chapter 10). The largest experience in this setting has been with carbamazepine and valproic acid. Other anticonvulsant agents such as lomatrigine, gabapentin, and tiagabine have mood-stabilizing properties that may be useful in treating agitation. These agents also are used in patients with post-stroke mania.

Anxiety may be controlled with benzodiazepine-type anxiolytics such as lorazepam or oxazepam that are well metabolized in the elderly, or nonbenzodiazepine alternatives such as buspirone can be used. Sedative-hypnotics useful for patients with VaD and sleep disturbances include trazodone, a short-acting benzodiazepine such as temazepam, or non-benzodiazepine alternatives such as zaleplon or zolpidem.

Cholinesterase inhibitors

Cholinesterase inhibitors are indicated for patients with evidence of Alzheimer's disease and associated cerebrovascular disease and in VaD. Vascular dementia is uncommon as the sole pathological diagnosis at autopsy and many patients with a clinical diagnosis of VaD have concomitant degenerative changes at autopsy. Some studies have found a cholinergic deficit in patients with VaD.

Galantamine was shown in a double-blind placebo-controlled trial of patients with VaD to significantly improve cognitive, global, behavioral, and functional ratings compared with those in the placebo group.[105] Treatment benefit was evident both in patients with Alzheimer's disease plus cerebrovascular disease and those with probable VaD. Analyses of symptoms assessed by the Neuropsychiatric Inventory revealed that NPI total score, anxiety and apathy improved significantly from baseline in patients receiving galantamine (Figure 6.10). Delusions became more evident in the placebo group and did not change in the galantamine group. Preliminary observations suggest that other cholinesterase inhibitors may also be beneficial in patients with VaD.[106]

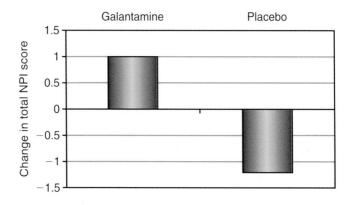

Figure 6.10 In a double-blind placebo-controlled trial galantamine produced an improvement in total NPI score above baseline whereas placebo patients experienced a deterioration below baseline (n = 592 patients).[105]

Management of stroke-related physical disturbances

Incontinence with frequency and urgency is common in VaD, resulting from detrusor muscle hyperactivity following stroke. Many of the agents commonly used to treat this condition such as anticholinergic agents (oxybutynin, dicyclomine) have adverse cognitive consequences in aged and demented individuals. Calcium channel blockers provide an alternative that is effective in some patients.[107]

Spasticity may be managed with tizanidine, baclofen, or dantrolene. Benzodiazepines such as clonezapam may be useful in patients who are unresponsive to other more specific agents.[107] Occasional patients with parkinsonism related to VaD may respond to dopaminergic agents[108] (Chapter 5). Pseudobulbar palsy with emotional incontinence can be stressful to both patients and caregivers. This syndrome has responded to treatment with selective serotonin reuptake inhibitors,[110,111] tricyclic antidepressants,[112] or levodopa.[113]

Treatment of cerebrovascular disease risk factors

Long-term management of cerebrovascular risk factors is critical to prevent further stroke in patients with VaD. Management of hypertension with antihypertensive agents, treatment of hypercholesterolemia with cholesterol-lowering agents, management of diabetes with insulin and other hypoglycemic agents, and treatment of congestive heart failure or arrhythmias with the appropriate cardioactive agents should be pursued to reduce the risk of recurrent stroke and associated cognitive decline.

References

1. Roman GC, Tatemichi TK, Erkinjuntti T *et al*. Vascular dementia: diagnostic criteria for research studies: report of the NINDS-AIREN international workshop. *Neurology* 1993;43:250–60.
2. White KE, Cummings J. Neuropsychiatric aspects of Alzheimer's disease and other dementing illnesses. In: Yudofsky S, Hales RE (eds) *The American Psychiatric Press Textbook of Neuropsychiatry*. Washington, DC: American Psychiatric Press, 1997: 823–54.
3. Gold G, Giannakopoulos P, Montes-Paixao C *et al*. Sensitivity and specificity

of newly proposed clinical criteria for possible vascular dementia. *Neurology* 1997;49:690–4.

4. Gold G, Bouras C, Canuto A *et al.* Clinicopathological validation study of four sets of clinical criteria for vascular dementia. *Am J Psychiatry* 2002;159:82–7.

5. Lopez OL, Larumbe MR, Becker JT *et al.* Reliability of NINDS-AIREN clinical criteria for the diagnosis of vascular dementia. *Neurology* 1994;44:1240–5.

6. Chui H, Mack WJ, Jackson JA *et al.* Clinical criteria for the diagnosis of vascular dementia. *Arch Neurol* 2000;57:191–6.

7. Ross GW, Petrovitch H, White LR *et al.* Characterization of risk factors for vascular dementia: the Honolulu-Asia Aging Study. *Neurology* 1999;53: 337–43.

8. Parnetti L, Mecocci P, Santucci C *et al.* Is multi-infarct dementia representative of vascular dementias? A retrospective study. *Acta Neurol Scand* 1990; 81:484–7.

9. Wallin A, Blennow K, Gottfries C-G. Subcortical symptoms predominate in vascular dementia. *Int J Geriatr Psychiatry* 1991;6:137–45.

10. Cummings JL, Benson DF. *Dementia: A Clinical Approach*, 2nd edn. Boston: Butterworth-Heinemann, 1992.

11. Erkinjuntti T. Types of multi-infarct dementia. *Acta Neurol Scand* 1987; 75:391–9.

12. Loeb C. Vascular dementia: terminology and classification. In: Chopra JS, Jagannathan K, Sawhney IMS *et al.* (eds) *Progress in Cerebrovascular Disease: Current Concepts in Stroke and Vascular Dementia*. New York: Elsevier, 1990: 73–82.

13. Bowler J, Hachinski V. History of the concept of vascular dementia: two opposing views on current definitions and criteria for vascular dementia. In: Prohovnik I, Wade J, Knezevic S *et al.* (eds) *Vascular Dementia: Current Concepts*. New York: John Wiley & Sons, 1996: 1–28.

14. Desmond DW, Tatemichi TK, Paik MC *et al.* Risk factors for cerebrovascular disease as correlates of cognitive function in a stroke-free cohort. *Arch Neurol* 1993;50:162–6.

15. Launer LJ, Masaki KH, Petrovitch H *et al.* The association between midlife blood pressure levels and late-life cognitive function. *JAMA* 1995;274: 1846–51.

16. Moroney JT, Tang M-X, Berglund L *et al.* Low-density lipoprotein cholesterol and the risk of dementia with stroke. *JAMA* 1999;282:254–60.

17. Starr JM, Whalley LJ, Inch S *et al.* Blood pressure and cognitive function in healthy old people. *J Am Geriatr Soc* 1993;41:753–6.

18. You R, McNeil JJ, O'Malley HM *et al.* Risk factors for lacunar infarction syndromes. *Neurology* 1995;45:1483–7.

19. Desmond DW, Moroney JT, Paik MC *et al.* Frequency and clinical determinants of dementia after ischemic stroke. *Neurology* 2000;54:1124–31.

20. Henon H, Durieu I, Guerouaou D *et al.* Poststroke dementia: incidence and relationship to prestroke cognitive decline. *Neurology* 2001;57:1216–22.

21. Liu CK, Miller BL, Cummings JL *et al.* A quantitative MRI study of vascular dementia. *Neurology* 1992;42:138–43.

22. Tatemichi TK, Desmond DW, Mayeux R *et al.* Dementia after stroke: base-

line frequency, risks, and clinical features in a hospitalized cohort. *Neurology* 1992;42:1185–93.

23. Tatemichi TK, Desmond DW, Paik MC *et al.* Clinical determinants of dementia related to stroke. *Ann Neurol* 1993;33:568–75.

24. Hachinski VC, Iliff LD, Zilhka E *et al.* Cerebral blood flow in dementia. *Arch Neurol* 1975;32:632–7.

25. Moroney JT, Bagiella E, Desmond DW *et al.* Meta-analysis of the Hachinski Ischemic Score in pathologically verified dementias. *Neurology* 1997;49: 1096–105.

26. Briley DP, Wasay M, Sergent S *et al.* Cerebral white matter changes (leukoaraiosis), stroke, and gait disturbance. *J Am Geriatr Soc* 1997; 45:1434–8.

27. Thompson PD, Marsden CD. Gait disorder of subcortical arteriosclerotic encephalopathy: Binswanger's disease. *Mov Disord* 1987;2:1–8.

28. Dubinsky RM, Jankovic J. Progressive supranuclear palsy and a multi-infarct state. *Neurology* 1987;37:570–6.

29. Cummings JL, Trimble MR. *Concise Guide to Neuropsychiatry and Behavioral Neurology.* Washington, DC: American Psychiatric Association, 2001.

30. Reichman WR, Cummings JL, McDaniel KD *et al.* Visuoconstructional impairment in dementia syndromes. *Behav Neurol* 1991;4:153–62.

31. Fukuda H, Kobayashi S, Okada K *et al.* Frontal white matter lesions and dementia in lacunar infarction. *Stroke* 1990;21:1143–9.

32. Ishii N, Nishihara Y, Imamura T. Why do frontal lobe symptoms predominate in vascular dementia with lacunes? *Neurology* 1986;36:340–5.

33. McPherson S, Cummings J. Neuropsychological aspects of vascular dementia. *Brain Cogn* 1996;31:269–82.

34. Corbett A, Bennett H, Kos S. Cognitive dysfunction following subcortical infarction. *Arch Neurol* 1994;51:999–1007.

35. Paul R, Cohen R, Moser D *et al.* Performance on the hooper visual organizational test in patients diagnosed with subcortical vascular dementia: relation to naming performance. *Neuropsychiatry Neuropsychol Behav Neurol* 2001;14:93–7.

36. Wolfe N, Linn R, Babikian VL *et al.* Frontal systems impairment following multiple lacunar infarcts. *Arch Neurol* 1990;47:129–32.

37. Moser D, Cohen DA, Paul R *et al.* Executive function and magnetic resonance imaging subcortical hyperintensities in vascular dementia. *Neuropsychiatry Neuropsychol Behav Neurol* 2001;14:89–92.

38. Powell AL, Cummings JL, Hill MA *et al.* Speech and language alterations in multi-infarct dementia. *Neurology* 1988;38:717–19.

39. Doody RS, Massman PJ, Mawad M *et al.* Cognitive consequences of subcortical magnetic resonance imaging changes in Alzheimer's disease: comparison to small vessel ischemic vascular dementia. *Neuropsychiatry Neuropsychol Behav Neurol* 1998;11:191–9.

40. Kertesz A, Clydesdale S. Neuropsychological deficits in vascular dementia vs Alzheimer's disease. *Arch Neurol* 1994;51:1226–31.

41. Looi JCL, Sachdev PS. Differentiation of vascular dementia from AD on neuropsychological tests. *Neurology* 1999;53:670–8.

42. Tierney MC, Black SE, Szalai JP *et al.* Recognition memory and verbal

fluency differentiate probable Alzheimer disease from subcortical ischemic vascular dementia. *Arch Neurol* 2001;58:1654–9.

43. Cannata AP, Alberoni M, Franceschi M, Mariani C. Frontal impairment in subcortical ischemic vascular dementia in comparison to Alzheimer's disease. *Dement Geriatr Cogn Disord* 2002;13:101–11.

44. Caplan LR. Binswanger's disease-revisited. *Neurology* 1995;45:626–33.

45. Roman GC. Senile dementia of the Binswanger type. *JAMA* 1987;258: 1782–8.

46. Ylikoski R, Ylikoski A, Erkinjuntti T *et al*. White matter changes in healthy elderly persons correlate with attention and speed of mental processing. *Arch Neurol* 1993;50:818–24.

47. Bennett DA, Wilson RS, Gilley DW *et al*. Clinical diagnosis of Binswanger's disease. *J Neurol Neurosurg Psychiatry* 1990;53:961–5.

48. Cummings JL, Mega M, Gray K *et al*. The Neuropsychiatric Inventory: comprehensive assessment of psychopathology in dementia. *Neurology* 1994; 44:2308–14.

49. Aharon-Peretz J, Kliot D, Tomer R. Behavioral differences between white matter lacunar dementia and Alzheimer's disease: a comparison on the Neuropsychiatric Inventory. *Dement Geriatr Cogn Disord* 2000;11:294–8.

50. Cummings JL, Miller B, Hill MA *et al*. Neuropsychiatric aspects of multi-infarct dementia and dementia of the Alzheimer type. *Arch Neurol* 1987; 44:389–93.

51. Lyketsos CG, Steinberg M, Tschanz JT *et al*. Mental and behavioral disturbances in dementia: findings from the Cache County Study on Memory in Aging. *Am J Psychiatry* 2000;157:708–14.

52. Sultzer DL, Levin HS, Mahler ME *et al*. A comparison of psychiatric symptoms in vascular dementia and Alzheimer's disease. *Am J Psychiatry* 1993; 150:1806–12.

53. Flynn FG, Cummings J, Scheibel J *et al*. Monosymptomatic delusions of parasitosis associated with ischemic cerebrovascular disease. *J Geriatr Psychiatry Neurol* 1989;2:134–9.

54. Lawrence RM, Hillam JC. Psychiatric symptomatology in early-onset Binswanger's disease: two case reports. *Behav Neurol* 1995;8:43–6.

55. Flynn FG, Cummings JL, Gornbein J. Delusions in dementia syndromes: investigation of behavioral and neuropsychological correlates. *J Neuropsychiatry Clin Neurosci* 1991;3:364–70.

56. Binetti G, Bianchetti A, Padovani A *et al*. Delusions in Alzheimer's disease and multi-infarct dementia. *Acta Neurol Scand* 1993;88:5–9.

57. Ghika-Schmid F, Bogousslavsky J. The acute behavioral syndrome of anterior thalamic infarction: a prospective study of 12 cases. *Ann Neurol* 2000;48:220–7.

58. Dian L, Cummings JL, Petry S *et al*. Personality alterations in multi-infarct dementia. *Psychosomatics* 1990;31:415–19.

59. Cummings JL, Petry S, Dian L *et al*. Organic personality disorder in dementia syndromes: an inventory approach. *J Neuropsychiatry Clin Neurosci* 1990;2:261–7.

60. Richfield EK, Twyman R, Berent S. Neurological syndrome following bilateral damage to the head of the caudate nuclei. *Ann Neurol* 1987;22:768–71.

61. Mendez MF. Pathological stealing in dementia. *J Am Geriatr Soc* 1988;36:825–6.
62. Cummings J, Mega M. *Neuropsychiatry and Clinical Neuroscience*. New York: Oxford University Press (in press).
63. Shimoda K, Robinson RG. The relationship between poststroke depression and lesion location in long-term follow-up. *Biol Psychiatry* 1999;45:187–92.
64. Starkstein SE, Pearlson GD, Boston J *et al*. Mania after brain injury: a controlled study of causative factors. *Arch Neurol* 1987;44:1069–73.
65. Chacko RC, Corbin MA, Harper RG. Acquired obsessive-compulsive disorder associated with basal ganglia lesions. *J Neuropsychiatry Clin Neurosci* 2000;12:269–72.
66. Laplane D, Levasseur M, Pillon B *et al*. Obsessive-compulsive and other behavioural changes with bilateral basal ganglia lesions. *Brain* 1989;112: 699–725.
67. Pullicino P, Benedict RHB, Capruso DX *et al*. Neuroimaging criteria for vascular dementia. *Arch Neurol* 1996;53:723–8.
68. Choi SH, Na DL, Chung CS *et al*. Diffusion-weighted MRI in vascular dementia. *Neurology* 2000;54:83–9.
69. Boone K, Miller BL, Lesser IM *et al*. Neuropsychological correlates of white-matter lesions in healthy elderly subjects. *Arch Neurol* 1992;49:549–54.
70. Cahn DA, Malloy PF, Salloway S *et al*. Subcortical hyperintensities on MRI and activities of daily living in geriatric depression. *J Neuropsychiatry Clin Neurosci* 1996;8:404–11.
71. de Groot JC, de Leeuw F-E, Oudkerk M *et al*. Cerebral white matter lesions and cognitive function: the Rotterdam Scan study. *Ann Neurol* 2000;47:145–51.
72. Matsubayashi K, Shimada K, Kawamoto A *et al*. Incidental brain lesions on magnetic resonance imaging and neurobehavioral functions in the apparently healthy elderly. *Stroke* 1992;23:175–80.
73. Kwan LT, Reed B, Eberling JL *et al*. Effects of subcortical cerebral infarction on cortical glucose metabolism and cognitive function. *Arch Neurol* 1999; 56:809–14.
74. Mielke R, Herholz K, Grond M *et al*. Severity of vascular dementia is related to volume of metabolically impaired tissue. *Arch Neurol* 1992;49:909–13.
75. Reed B, Eberling JL, Mungas D *et al*. Frontal lobe hypometabolism predicts cognitive decline in patients with lacunar infarcts. *Arch Neurol* 2001; 58:493–7.
76. Sultzer DL, Mahler ME, Cummings J *et al*. Cortical abnormalities associated with subcortical lesions in vascular dementia. *Arch Neurol* 1995;52:773–80.
77. Leys D, Bogousslavsky J. Mechanisms of vascular dementia. In: Leys D, Scheltens P (eds) *Vascular Dementia*. Dordrecht, The Netherlands: ICG Publications, 1994: 121–32.
78. Filley CM. *The Behavioral Neurology of White Matter*. New York: University Press, 2001.
79. Nolan KA, Lino MM, Seligmann AW *et al*. Absence of vascular dementia in an autopsy series from a dementia clinic. *J Am Geriatr Soc* 1998;46:597–604.
80. Hulette C, Nochlin D, McKeel D *et al*. Clinical-neuropathologic findings in multi-infarct dementia: a report of six autopsied cases. *Neurology* 1997;48: 668–72.

81. Gearing M, Mirra SS, Hedreen JC *et al.* The consortium to establish a registry for Alzheimer's disease (CERAD). Part X. *Neurology* 1995;45:461–6.

82. Erkinjuntti T, Haltia M, Palo J *et al.* Accuracy of the clinical diagnosis of vascular dementia: a prospective clinical and post-mortem neuropathological study. *J Neurol Neurosurg Psychiatry* 1988;51:1037–44.

83. del Ser T, Bermejo F, Portera A *et al.* Vascular dementia: a clinicopathological study. *J Neurol Sci* 1990;96:1–17.

84. Markesbery WR. Vascular dementia. In: Markesbery WR (ed) *Neuropathology of Dementing Disorders.* New York: Arnold, 1998: 293–311.

85. De Reuck J. Neuropathology of vascular dementia. In: Leys D, Scheltens P (eds) *Vascular Dementia.* Dordrecht, The Netherlands: ICG Publications, 1994: 9–17.

86. Munoz DG, Hastak SM, Harper B *et al.* Pathologic correlates of increased signals of the centrum ovale on magnetic resonance imaging. *Arch Neurol* 1993;50:492–7.

87. Pantoni L, Garcia JH. Pathogenesis of leukoaraiosis. *Stroke* 1997;28:652–9.

88. Erkinjuntti T, Benavente O, Eliasziw M *et al.* Diffuse vacuolization (spongiosis) and arteriolosclerosis in the frontal white matter occurs in vascular dementia. *Arch Neurol* 1996;53:325–32.

89. Arvanitakis Z, Hachinksi V. Vascular cognitive impairment: what else do we need to learn? In: Terry RD, Katzman R, Bick KL, Sisodia SS (eds) *Alzheimer Disease,* 2nd edn. Philadelphia: Lippincott Williams and Wilkins, 1999:147–60.

90. Snowdon DA, Greiner LH, Mortimer JA *et al.* Brain infarction and the clinical expression of Alzheimer disease; the Nun Study. *JAMA* 1997;277:813–17.

91. Moroney JT, Bagiella E, Tatemichi TK *et al.* Dementia after stroke increases the risk of long-term stroke recurrence. *Neurology* 1997;48:1317–25.

92. Adams HP Jr, del Zoppo GJ, von Kummer R. *Management of Stroke: A Practical Guide for the Prevention, Evaluation and Treatment of Acute Stroke.* Caddo, OK: Professional Communications, 1998.

93. Meyer JS, Obara K, Muramatsu K *et al.* Cognitive performance after small strokes correlates with ischemia, not atrophy of the brain. *Dementia* 1995; 6:312–22.

94. Starkstein SE, Manes F. Apathy and depression following stroke. *CNS Spectrums* 2000;5:43–50.

95. Wiart L, Petit H, Joseph PA *et al.* Fluoxetine in early poststroke depression: a double-blind placebo-controlled study. *Stroke* 2000;31:1829–32.

96. Andersen G, Vestergaard K, Lauritzen L. Effective treatment of poststroke depression with the selective serotonin reuptake inhibitor citalopram. *Stroke* 1994;25:1099–104.

97. Robinson RG, Schultz SK, Castillo C *et al.* Nortriptyline versus fluoxetine in the treatment of depression and in short-term recovery after stroke: a placebo-controlled, double-blind study. *Am J Psychiatry* 2000;157:351–9.

98. Lipsey JR, Robinson RG, Pearlson GD *et al.* Nortriptyline treatment of post-stroke depression: a double-bind study. *Lancet* 1984;1:297–300.

99. Martensson B, Murray V, von Arbin M *et al.* Alternative treatment for post-stroke depression. *Am J Psychiatry* 1997;154:583–4.

100. Masand P, Murray GB, Pickett P. Psychostimulants in post-stroke depression. *J Neuropsychiatry Clin Neurosci* 1991;3:23–7.

101. Simpson S, Baldwin RC, Jackson A *et al.* Is subcortical disease associated with a poor response to antidepressants? Neurological, neuropsychological and neuroradiological findings in late-life depression. *Psychol Med* 1998; 28:1015–26.
102. Currier MB, Murray GB, Welch C. Electroconvulsive therapy for post-stroke depressed geriatric patients. *J Neuropsychiatry Clin Neurosci* 1992;4:140–4.
103. De Deyn PP, Rabheru K, Rasmussen A *et al.* A randomized trial of risperidone, placebo, and haloperidol for behavioral symptoms of dementia. *Neurology* 1999;53:946–55.
104. Katz IR, Jeste DV, Mintzer JE *et al.* Comparison of risperidone and placebo for psychosis and behavioral disturbances associated with dementia: a randomized, double-blind trial: Risperidone Study Group. *J Clin Psychiatry* 1999;60:107–15.
105. Erkinjuntti T, Kurz A, Gauthier S *et al.* Efficacy of galantamine in probable vascular dementia and Alzheimer's disease combined with cerebrovascular disease: a randomised trial. *Lancet* 2002;359:1283–90.
106. Mendez MF, Younesi FL, Perryman KM. Use of donepezil for vascular dementia: preliminary clinical experience. *J Neuropsychiatry Clin Neurosci* 1999;11:268–70.
107. Brandeis GH, Resnick NM. Urinary incontinence. In: Duthie EHJ, Katz PR (eds) *Practice of Geriatrics*. Philadelphia: WB Saunders, 1998: 189–98.
108. Standaert DG, Young AB. Treatment of central nervous system degenerative disorders. In: Hardman JG, Limbird L (eds) *Goodman & Gilman's The Pharmacological Basis of Therapeutics*. New York: McGraw-Hill Medical Publishing Division, 2001: 549–68.
109. Mark MH, Sage J, Walters AS *et al.* Binswanger's disease presenting as levodopa-responsive parkinsonism: clinicopathologic study of three cases. *Mov Disord* 1995;10:450–4.
110. Andersen G, Vestergaard K, Riis JO. Citalopram for post-stroke pathological crying. *Lancet* 1993;342:837–9.
111. Nahas Z, Arlinghaus KA, Kotrla KJ *et al.* Rapid response of emotional incontinence to selective serotonin reuptake inhibitors. *J Neuropsychiatry Clin Neurosci* 1998;10:453–5.
112. Robinson RG, Parikh RM, Lipsey JR *et al.* Pathological laughing and crying following stroke: validation of a measurement scale and a double-blind treatment study. *Am J Psychiatry* 1993;150:286–93.
113. Udaka F, Yamao S, Nagata H *et al.* Pathologic laughing and crying treated with levodopa. *Arch Neurol* 1984;42:1095–6.

chapter 7

Frontotemporal lobar degeneration

Frontotemporal lobar degeneration (FTLD) is a progressive neurological disorder producing a dementia syndrome with prominent aphasia, neuropsychiatric features, or both. The disease typically has an onset in the mid- or early fifties and leads to death in approximately a decade. Many cases are familial and some have an identified mutation on chromosome 17. Abnormal tau metabolism is the underlying neuropathological feature that links the disparate clinical phenotypes of FTLD. Three clinical syndromes[1] are recognized manifestations of FTLD: frontotemporal dementia (FTD) is characterized by behavioral disinhibition, coarsened interpersonal interactions, impulsivity and executive dysfunction progressing to dementia; progressive nonfluent aphasia (PNA) features a progressive nonfluent aphasia; semantic dementia (SD) is characterized by a progressive semantic aphasia and associative agnosia. There can be substantial overlap between the three syndromes, as well as with other clinical disorders such as corticobasal degeneration and progressive supranuclear palsy. All eventually worsen and develop a dementia syndrome. FTLD is superior to 'dementia' as a generic term for this group of disorders, since patients may have progressive neurological dysfunction for substantial periods of time before meeting criteria for a dementia syndrome.

Frontotemporal lobar degeneration tends to be markedly asymmetric in a substantial number of patients, giving rise to left- and right-sided syndromes, with the left-sided disorders manifesting primarily language abnormalities, whereas the right-sided disorders tend to exhibit more marked neuropsychiatric disturbances. Left frontal (PNA) and left temporal (SD) syndromes can be distinguished, as well as right frontal and right temporal syndromes.

Clinical features

All of the FTLD syndromes share certain demographic and clinical characteristics. Onset of the disorder is usually between the ages of 45 and 70, and nearly all cases begin before the age of 65, although occasional late-onset cases have been observed.[2] Likewise, cases may occasionally have their onset as early as the 20s. The length of illness is highly variable, ranging from 2 to 20 years, with an average duration of approximately 8 years. It is often difficult to determine exactly when the disease began since onset may be with subtle behavioral changes such as apathy, and some degree of frontal dysfunction may be present throughout life in cases carrying mutations.[3]

A family history of dementia is present in approximately half of the first-degree relatives.[4,5] Hereditary FTLD has an autosomal dominant inheritance pattern and 30% of such families have known mutations.[6,7] Mutations are very rare among sporadic FTLD cases.

Three types of elementary neurological signs have been identified in patients with FTLD. One subgroup develops motor neuron disease with fasciculations, wasting, and weakness. Motor neuron disease has been seen in combination with all of the major subtypes of FTLD (FTD, PNA, SD), but is most common in those with FTD or PNA.[1] Parkinsonism also occurs in patients with FTLD. Akinesia, rigidity, and tremor have been seen in the late phases of all the FTLD syndromes. Primitive reflexes consistent with a loss of supranuclear control of primitive survival motor behaviors occur earlier in the course of FTLD than in other dementia syndromes such as Alzheimer's disease. Grasping, pouting, and sucking responses may all be seen.[2]

Frontotemporal dementia

Frontotemporal dementia is the most dramatic of the FTLD syndromes in terms of its neuropsychiatric manifestations (Box 7.1). Patients display an early loss of personal awareness with neglect of personal hygiene, poor grooming, and a disheveled appearance. Disinhibition is a characteristic feature; patients may make unrestrained lewd or sexual remarks, engage in inappropriate behaviors, make jokes at others' expense, and be inappropriately jocular. They lack empathy and have difficulty taking the feelings of others into account. Patients are commonly impulsive, acting on or saying the first idea that comes to mind without reflection on potential consequences. Distractibility and impersistence are evident in the behavior of many patients. There is early loss of insight with no appreciation of the changes in behavior that have occurred. Emotional unconcern, with indifference, apathy, and remoteness, is common. Lack of emotions and social avoidance are more common in FTD than in other types of FTLD.[8] Patients may have a bizarre, disconnected affect. Depression, anxiety, and hypochondriasis are evident in some patients. Not uncommonly, patients may be misdiagnosed as suffering from a primary psychiatric illness.[9] They tend to be rigid and inflexible in terms of behavior and may have changes in diet such as overeating, indiscriminate eating, or indulging themselves in high carbohydrate diets.[10] Stereotyped and perseverative behavior, including rituals and compulsions are not uncommon in FTD. In later stages of the disease, utilization behaviors with inappropriate use of objects, and imitation behaviors manifested by imitating the acts of others may appear.

Box 7.1 The clinical diagnostic features of frontotemporal dementia (FTD)[1]

Character change and disordered social conduct are the dominant features initially and throughout the disease course. Instrumental functions of perception, spatial skills, praxis and memory are intact or relatively well preserved

Core diagnostic features
- Insidious onset and gradual progression
- Early decline in social interpersonal conduct
- Early impairment in regulation of personal conduct

continued

Box 7.1 *continued*

- Early emotional blunting
- Early loss of insight

Supportive diagnostic features
- Behavioral disorder
  - Decline in personal hygiene and grooming
  - Mental rigidity and inflexibility
  - Distractibility and impersistence
  - Hyperorality and dietary changes
  - Perseverative and stereotyped behavior
  - Utilization behavior
- Speech and language
  - Altered speech output
    Aspontaneity and economy of speech
    Press of speech
  - Stereotypy of speech
  - Echolalia
  - Perseveration
  - Mutism
- Physical signs
  - Primitive reflexes
  - Incontinence
  - Akinesia, rigidity, and tremor
  - Low and labile blood pressure
- Investigations
  - Neuropsychology: significant impairment on frontal lobe tests in the absence of severe amnesia, aphasia, or perceptuospatial disorder
  - Electroencephalography: normal on conventional EEG despite clinically evident dementia
  - Brain imaging (structural and/or functional): predominant frontal and/or anterior temporal abnormality
- Clinical features
  - Onset before 65 years: positive family history of similar disorder in first-degree relative
  - Bulbar palsy, muscular weakness and wasting, fasciculations (associated motor neuron disease present in a minority of patients)

In those without an aphasic disorder (described below) there is commonly a progressive reduction of speech to a mute state. Patients may continue to write, gesture, and display substantial cognitive ability despite the absence of spoken language. While speech is still present, stereotyped output with repetition of words, phrases, or themes is common. Patients may tell the same joke over and over, or retell the same story many times per day. Echolalia may be evident in late-stage patients who are not mute.[11]

Repetitive stereotyped behaviors may include repetitive speech, stereotyped behaviors such as rocking or clapping, compulsive counting, and, occasionally, self-injurious behavior.[12,13] In some cases the impulsive behavior and disregard for civil mores leads to antisocial behavior including assault, indecent exposure, shoplifting, and reckless driving.[14] These socially undesirable traits are more common when the right hemisphere is affected predominantly.[15]

Elements of the Kluver-Bucy syndrome have also been reported in patients with FTD. Oral and dietary changes in combination with hypersexuality, hypermetamorphosis (including utilization behavior), visual agnosia, and auditory agnosia may be seen in various combinations.[16]

Patients with the FTD behavioral syndrome have disproportionate right hemisphere degeneration.[17,18] The disinhibition syndrome appears to require involvement of the right anterior structures and these symptoms emerge in patients with the progressive aphasic disorders as the brain disease progressively involves more brain areas including right frontotemporal regions.[19]

In general, three behavioral subtypes of the FTD syndrome have been described, a disinhibited type characterized by jocularity, unconcern, and breakdown of social and interpersonal behaviors; an apathetic subtype featuring inertia, aspontaneity, loss of volition, unconcern, mental rigidity and perseveration; and a stereotypic type with pronounced behavioral stereotypes, compulsions, and ritualistic behavior.[2] The apathetic subtype corresponds to more involvement of dorsolateral and medial frontal involvement; the disinhibited type corresponds to orbital frontal predominance of degeneration, and the stereotypic type is most strongly related to greater involvement of the striatum along with involvement of frontal and temporal cortex.

The behavioral features that best distinguish FTD and Alzheimer's disease are shown in Table 7.1 and Figure 7.1. A loss of personal

Table 7.1 Behavioral and neuropsychiatric features that distinguish frontotemporal dementia (FTD) from Alzheimer's disease (AD)

Clinical feature	Frontotemporal dementia	Alzheimer's disease
Loss of personal awareness	Common, earlier	Common, later
Alterations in eating	Hyperorality, dietary 'fads', carbohydrate craving	Anorexia and weight loss more common
Stereotyped behavior	Common	Rare
Reduction of speech	Common	Occurs late, if at all
Disinhibition	Common	Occurs but is less severe
Euphoria	Common	Rare
Apathy	Common and severe	Common, less severe
Self-neglect/poor self-care	Common	Rare until late
Memory impairment	Delayed until later in the course	Occurs early, severe
Executive dysfunction	Early, progressive	Late in most cases
Visuospatial skills	Relatively preserved	Involved early
Arithmetic skills	Relatively preserved	Involved early

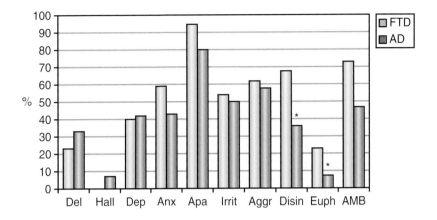

Figure 7.1 *Percentage of patients with frontotemporal lobar degeneration and Alzheimer's disease with symptoms as demonstrated by the Neuropsychiatric Inventory[22] (30 patients with Alzheimer's disease and 17 patients with frontotemporal dementia (FTD) were included in this sample). Mean Mini-Mental State Examination score of the AD patients was 17.5 and of the FTD patients was 14.9; *indicates significant differences (p > 0.05). DEL, delusions; HALL, hallucinations; DEP, depression; ANX, anxiety; APA, apathy; IRRIT, irritability; AGGR, aggression/agitation; DISIN, disinhibition; EUPH, euphoria; AMB, aberrant motor behavior.*

awareness, hyperorality, stereotyped and perseverative behavior, reduction of speech, self-neglect, and euphoria are all more characteristic of FTD than AD.[14,19–22] Psychosis is more common in patients with Alzheimer's disease than in FTD.[22–24] In combination with the earlier age of onset of FTD and the appearance of behavioral changes before cognitive abnormalities, the patients with FTD can usually be distinguished from those with Alzheimer's disease.

Several rating scales have been developed to attempt to capture and quantify the unique features of FTD. The Neuropsychiatric Inventory (NPI)[25] has been used to characterize the profile of neuropsychiatric symptoms in patients with FTD. Compared with patients with Alzheimer's disease, FTD patients had significantly more apathy, aberrant motor behavior, disinhibition, and euphoria. They also tended to be less depressed than patients with Alzheimer's disease[22] (Figure 7.1). A Frontal Behavioral Inventory has been developed specifically to characterize the behavioral features of FTD and has been shown to distinguish FTD from patients with Alzheimer's disease or major depression.[26] Similarly, the Frontal Temporal Behavioral Scale found that loss of self-monitoring, self-neglect, increase in self-centered behavior, and mood and affect disturbances are more common in FTD than in Alzheimer's disease.[21]

Progressive nonfluent aphasia

Progressive aphasia is the FTLD syndrome corresponding to degeneration of the left frontal cortex (Box 7.2). Patients exhibit a progressively worsening nonfluent spontaneous output with agrammatism (omission or incorrect use of grammatical terms including articles, prepositions, etc.), phonemic paraphasias with sound-based errors, and anomia. Stuttering and oral apraxia commonly accompany the dementia syndrome. Repetition of words or phrases is interrupted by paraphasic intrusions and both reading and writing are nonfluent, effortful, and agrammatic. In the early stages of the illness, comprehension is preserved for word meaning but impaired for syntactic relationships. Nonlanguage cognitive skills and demeanor are largely normal, although evolution to dementia with features of FTD is common after several years of progressive linguistic changes.[1,27–31]

Alzheimer's disease can present primarily as an aphasic syndrome if the pathologic changes involve the left hemisphere disproportionately. In most cases the aphasia of Alzheimer's disease begins with an anomic type of output and progresses to a transcortical sensory aphasia. The language syndrome associated with Alzheimer's disease can usually be distinguished from PNA but is more difficult to differentiate from SD with progressive fluent aphasia (described below).

Semantic dementia

Patients with FTLD can exhibit a progressive fluent aphasia as well as the PNA syndrome described above[32] (Box 7.3). When progressive fluent

Box 7.2 The clinical diagnostic features of progressive nonfluent aphasia (PNA)[1]

Disorder of expressive language is the dominant feature initially and throughout the disease course. Other aspects of cognition are intact or relatively well preserved

Core diagnostic features
- Insidious onset and gradual progression
- Nonfluent spontaneous speech with at least one of the following: agrammatism, phonemic paraphasias, anomia

Supportive diagnostic features
- Speech and language
  - Stuttering or oral apraxia
  - Impaired repetition
  - Alexia, agraphia
  - Early preservation of word meaning
  - Late mutism
- Behavior
  - Early preservation of social skills
  - Late behavioral changes similar to FTD
- Physical signs: late contralateral primitive reflexes, akinesia, rigidity, and tremor
- Investigations
  - Neuropsychology: nonfluent aphasia in the absence of severe amnesia or perceptuospatial disorder
  - Electroencephalography: normal or minor asymmetric abnormality predominantly affecting dominant (usually left) hemisphere
- Clinical features
  - Onset before 65 years: positive family history of similar disorder in first-degree relative
  - Bulbar palsy, muscular weakness and wasting, fasciculations (associated motor neuron disease present in a minority of patients)

Box 7.3 The clinical diagnostic features of progressive semantic dementia (SD)[1]

Semantic disorder (impaired understanding of word meaning and/or object identity) is the dominant feature initially and throughout the disease course. Other aspects of cognition, including autobiographic memory, are intact or relatively well preserved

Core diagnostic features
- Insidious onset and gradual progression
- Language disorder characterized by
  - Progressive, fluent, empty spontaneous speech
  - Loss of word meaning, manifest by impaired naming *and* comprehension
  - Semantic paraphasias *and/or*
- Perceptual disorder characterized by
  - Prosopagnosia: impaired recognition of identity of familiar faces *and/or*
  - Associative agnosia: impaired recognition of object identity
- Preserved perceptual matching and drawing reproduction
- Preserved single-word repetition
- Preserved ability to read aloud and write to dictation orthographically regular words

Supportive diagnostic features
- Speech and language
  - Press of speech
  - Idiosyncratic word usage
  - Absence of phonemic paraphasias
  - Surface dyslexia and dysgraphia
  - Preserved calculation
- Behavior
  - Loss of sympathy and empathy
  - Narrowed preoccupations
  - Parsimony
- Physical signs
  - Absent or late primitive reflexes
  - Akinesia, rigidity, and tremor

Box 7.3 *continued*

- Investigations
  - Neuropsychology
    Profound semantic loss, manifest in failure of word comprehension
    and naming and/or face and object recognition
    Preserved phonology and syntax, and elementary perceptual
    processing, spatial skills, and day-to-day memorizing
  - Electroencephalography: normal
  - Brain imaging (structural and/or functional): predominant anterior
    temporal abnormality (symmetric or asymmetric)
  - Clinical features
    Onset before 65 years: positive family history of similar disorder in
    first-degree relative
    Bulbar palsy, muscular weakness and wasting, fasciculations
    (associated motor neuron disease present in a minority of patients)

aphasia is combined with associative visual agnosia the term semantic dementia (SD) is applied.[1,31] Patients with this syndrome have fluent, well-articulated and syntactically correct spontaneous speech. They are anomic, however, and the content of the speech is empty. Patients have a marked deficit in single-word comprehension with a breakdown of the semantic meaning of words. Autobiographical and day-to-day episodic memory is well preserved.[28,33–36] Compared with patients with FTD, patients with SD are more likely to manifest depression.[19]

Semantic dementia can be difficult to distinguish from Alzheimer's disease. Both manifest a progressive fluent aphasic disorder. In nearly all cases, patients with Alzheimer's disease will exhibit an amnestic type of memory impairment and concomitant visuospatial changes in addition to their fluent aphasic output. Attention to these details of the neuro-behavioral assessment (Chapter 2) will help in distinguishing these two similar syndromes.

Studies with the NPI show that compared with patients with FTD, SD patients exhibit less apathy and less aberrant motor behavior, but more anxiety.[37]

An unusual number of patients with primary progressive aphasia of the fluent type or SD have had the emergence of artistic talent in their dementia syndrome[38–40] (Figures 7.2 and 7.3). This may reflect the

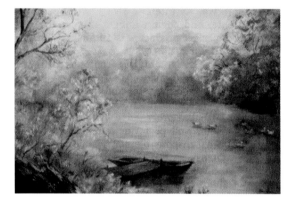

Figure 7.2 *Painting by a patient with frontotemporal lobar degeneration with progressive nonfluent aphasia who developed an interest in painting after the onset of this disease (Miller et al. 1998[39] with permission).*

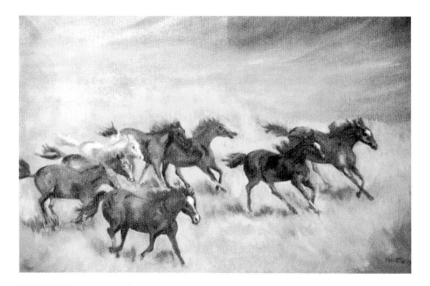

Figure 7.3 *Painting by a patient with frontotemporal lobar degeneration with progressive nonfluent aphasia whose artistic talent emerged after the onset of this disease (not the same patient as Figure 7.2) (Miller et al. 1998[39] with permission).*

preservation of visuospatial skills associated with the integrity of the right hemisphere, progressive aphasia with disinhibition of right hemisphere activity, and preoccupation and compulsive repetition common to FTLD syndromes.

Dementia syndrome

The dementia syndrome that evolves in the early to middle phases of FTD and may appear in the later phases of PNA and SD has characteristic neuropsychological features. Executive abilities are disproportionately compromised. Verbal fluency (number of animals or members of specific categories named in 1 minute) and performance on the Wisconsin Card Sort Test are particularly sensitive to the deficits exhibited by patients with FTD. Visuospatial abilities tend to be disproportionately preserved, although segmentation and planning difficulties may be evident in copying complex figures. Patients may exhibit a retrieval deficit syndrome on memory testing, with better recognition of previously learned material than spontaneous recall.[41-44]

Executive abilities are mediated primarily by the dorsolateral prefrontal cortex and when the degeneration is confined to the orbitofrontal cortex patients may exhibit marked behavioral and comportment abnormalities while performing relatively normally on tests of executive function.[45] Patients with primarily left-sided FTLD (PNA or SD) exhibit a syndrome that differs from that of patients with right FTLD. Patients with predominantly right-sided involvement have more difficulty with performance items of the Weschler Adult Intelligence Scale, are more impaired on design fluency than verbal fluency, and have more difficulty with picture arrangement than word sequencing. Patients with left FTLD exhibit the opposite pattern, with greater difficulty with verbal intelligence, word generation, and word sequencing. Left FTLD patients are more anomic, while those with right FTLD make more errors and have more perseverate responses on the Wisconsin Card Sort Test.[17,46] Memory tests, psychomotor speed, and visual, perceptual, and constructional tasks do not distinguish between the two groups.

Neuropsychological testing can aid in distinguishing FTLD from Alzheimer's disease (Table 7.2). Executive functions tend to be more severely compromised in FTLD than in AD, particularly in tasks such as the Wisconsin Card Sort Test. This is particularly evident in distinguishing FTLD from Alzheimer's disease.[47] Patients with FTLD have reduced verbal fluency that may be disproportionately severe and they may exhibit more perseverations than patients with Alzheimer's disease. Tests such as the 'social dilemma' test where patients must recognize that one of two potential solutions to a problem is more ethically correct, may be particularly sensitive to early changes of FTD.[48] Patients with FTD tend to perform better than patients with Alzheimer's disease on tasks of word list recall, constructions, and calculations.[49-52] None of these features individually distinguish Alzheimer's disease from FTLD. In most cases, the pattern of greater memory than executive deficits characteristic of Alzheimer's disease can be distinguished from the reverse pattern of greater executive than memory deficits in FTD.[53] Even patients with the frontal variant of Alzheimer's disease (discussed in Chapter 2) have an amnestic type of memory defect and visuospatial disturbances in addition to their executive abnormalities. Onset of disease earlier in life and the appearance of behavioral deficits antedating cognitive changes further aid in distinguishing FTLD syndromes from Alzheimer's disease.[54]

Neuroimaging

Structural and functional imaging can both be useful in the diagnosis of FTLD and in aiding in the identification of specific FTLD subtypes. Studies with computerized tomography (CT) demonstrate that patients with frontotemporal dementia may evidence marked frontal and temporal atrophy (symmetric or asymmetric).[55] Magnetic resonance imaging (MRI) reveals atrophy with greater involvement of left temporal lobe structures in patients with semantic dementia. The left anterior temporal lobe atrophy is more severe in SD than in Alzheimer's disease and there is a quantitative relationship between the degree of semantic memory impairment in SD and the degree of left temporal atrophy.[56,57] Patients

Table 7.2 Neuropsychological features distinguishing frontotemporal lobar dementia (FTLD) from Alzheimer's disease (AD)

Clinical feature	FTLD	AD
Attention	More distractable, impersistent	Less distractable
Memory	Retrieval deficit syndrome (poor recall, preserved recognition)	Amnestic-type memory disturbance (poor recall and recognition)
	SD: Autobiographical memory better preserved than remote memory	Remote memory better preserved than recent memory
Language	FTD: reduced spontaneous speech progressing to mutism	Fluent anomic aphasia progressing to transcortical sensory aphasia
	PPA: nonfluent aphasia	
	SD: fluent aphasia with loss of semantic comprehension	
Visuospatial skills	Relatively preserved	Impaired early in clinical course
	Route-finding normal	Route-finding impaired
Executive function	FTD: compromised early	Compromised later in clinical course
	PNA/SD: impaired later in clinical course	
	Verbal fluency reduced	Verbal fluency reduced (fewer perseverations)
Calculation	Relatively spared	Affected early in course
Order of cognition/behavioral change	Behavior > executive > memory	Memory > executive > behavior

with FTD have more atrophy of the right dorsolateral prefrontal cortex while those with SD have greater left anterior temporal atrophy.[58] The rate of atrophy over time is greater in those with FTD than those with primarily temporal atrophy.[59] T2 and proton density-weighted MRI images reveal an increase in white matter signal intensity in the frontal and temporal lobes in patients with FTLD.[60] Sagittal MRI sections reveal that the anterior corpus callosum is more atrophic in patients with FTLD than in those with AD or normal elderly controls.[61] In some cases the atrophy is more widespread than the clinical syndromes suggest and bilateral temporal atrophy is often evident in patients with PNA.

Functional neuroimaging may be abnormal when structural imaging does not reveal significant atrophy. Studies of cerebral perfusion using single photon emission computer tomography (SPECT) reveal fairly widespread anterior temporal and frontal lobe reductions in cerebral blood flow but the intensity of the reduction generally reflects the clinical syndrome. Patients with predominant language abnormalities (PNA and SD) have asymmetrical cerebral perfusion with the greatest reductions in the left frontal or temporal regions[30,62,63] (Figure 7.4). Those with the FTD syndrome have bilateral or right predominant hypoperfusion.[17,18] Within the FTD syndrome those with predominant disinhibition have reduced perfusion primarily involving the ventral

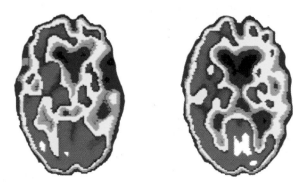

Figure 7.4 *Single photon emission computed tomogram showing reduced left frontotemporal perfusion of a patient with primary progressive aphasia (courtesy of J Felix, Laboratory of Neuroimaging, UCLA School of Medicine).*

orbitofrontal cortex, while those with an apathetic syndrome have reductions in perfusion involving primarily the dorsal medial prefrontal cortex.[64] Positron emission tomography (PET) using fluorodeoxyglucose tends to confirm the observations made with SPECT[65,66] (Figure 7.5).

Genetics

Approximately 40% of FTLD patients have a positive family history of a similar disorder in a first-degree relative;[4,5] 10% of the familial cases and 0–3% of sporadic cases have been linked to specific mutations. Most of these mutations occur in the tau gene on chromosome 17,[67,68] although rare cases of familial motor neuron disease with FTLD have been linked to chromosome 9 and rare cases of familial FTLD have been linked to chromosome 3.[69,70] There is substantial phenotypic heterogeneity among

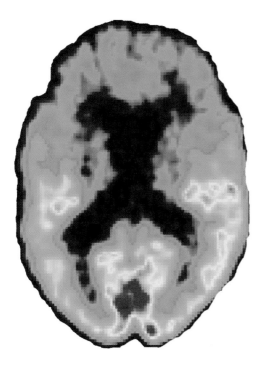

Figure 7.5
Fluorodeoxyglucose (FDG) positron emission tomogram (PET) showing reduced frontotemporal metabolism in a patient with FTD (courtesy of J Felix, Laboratory of Neuroimaging, UCLA School of Medicine).

patients with chromosome 17 mutations. All of the identified mutations result in some form of tau protein abnormality and interruption of microtubule-associated protein function in assembly and stabilization of microtubules. There is also pathologic heterogeneity associated with chromosome 17 mutations; some patients have had Pick bodies indicative of the Pick's disease form of FTLD while others have not.[71,72] Pick's bodies are present in approximately 25% of patients with FTLD.[73] Box 7.4 lists clinical syndromes that have been linked to chromosome 17.

Other disorders with abnormal tau metabolism include corticobasal degeneration, progressive supranuclear palsy, neurofibrillary tangle dementia, and frontotemporal dementia with motor neuron disease.[74]

Neuropathology

At autopsy, the brains of patients with FTLD show marked frontal and temporal atrophy with relative preservation of the posterior gyri (Figure 7.6). Three basic types of neuropathological changes have been identified in FTLD.[11,74] Tau positive inclusions (Figure 7.7) have been described

---

Box 7.4 Clinical disorders linked to chromosome 17

Pick's disease
FTD (without Pick bodies)
FTD with parkinsonism
Pallido-nigral-luysian degeneration
Pallido-ponto-nigral degeneration
FTD with parkinsonism and seizures
Disinhibition-dementia-parkinsonism-amyotrophy complex
Hereditary dysphoric disinhibition dementia
Familial atypical progressive supranuclear palsy
Multiple system tauopathy with presenile dementia
Dementia lacking distinctive histopathology (tauless tauopathy)
Progressive subcortical gliosis
Progressive nonfluent aphasia

in Pick's disease and in FTLD with parkinsonism linked to chromosome 17. There is associated neuronal loss and gliosis in the frontal and temporal regions. The changes may be asymmetric. Frontotemporal lobar degeneration lacking distinct histopathologic features has neither tau nor ubiquitin positive inclusions. There is microvacuolation and mild to moderate astrocytic gliosis affecting chiefly the upper lamina of the cortex. In the substantia nigra there may be mild to moderate loss of pigmented neurons. In this disorder there is a loss of tau protein function ('tauless tauopathy'), which may be functionally related to abnormal tau aggregation in other forms of FTLD.[75] In the third neuropathologic syndrome, FTLD is characterized by neuronal loss and gliosis with ubiquitin positive, tau negative inclusions. Frontotemporal degeneration with motor neuron disease and some cases of SD and patients with FTLD with marked striatal degeneration have had this pathology.[35,74,76] Tau positive inclusions also are evident in corticobasal degeneration, progressive supranuclear palsy, and neurofibrillary tangle dementia.[74]

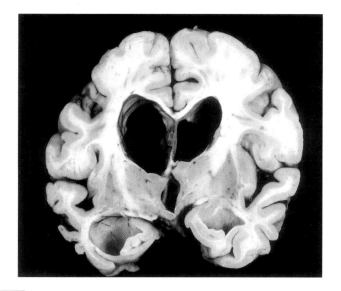

Figure 7.6 *Brain of FTD patient. Note asymmetric atrophy especially prominent in the left temporal lobe with dramatic shrinkage of the left, middle, and inferior temporal gyri. The left, frontal, and cingulated gyri are atrophic (courtesy of H Vinters, MD, Division of Neuropathology, UCLA School of Medicine).*

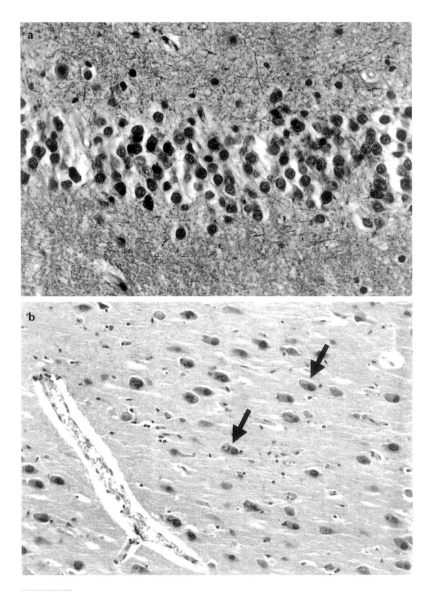

Figure 7.7 *Pick bodies. (a) Bielschowsky-stained section, granule cell layer of hippocampus. (b) Tau-immunostained section (magnification 435 × 220) (courtesy of H Vinters, MD, Division of Neuropathology, UCLA School of Medicine).*

Neurochemical studies reveal preserved neocortical cholinergic function and decreased serotonergic function in patients with FTLD.[77,78]

Treatment

The serotonergic deficit of FTLD suggests that at least some of the symptoms may be mediated via serotonergic mechanisms. An open-label study of selective serotonin reuptake inhibitors revealed decreased disinhibition, depression, carbohydrate craving, and compulsions in over half of patients receiving treatment.[24] Side effects were modest. Adrenergic agonists, specifically idazoxan, have been reported to improve performance on tests of planning, attention, fluency, and episodic memory.[79,80]

References

1. Neary D, Snowden JS, Gustafson L *et al.* Frontotemporal lobar degeneration: a consensus on clinical diagnostic criteria. *Neurology* 1998;51:1546–54.
2. Snowden JS, Neary D, Mann DMA. *Fronto-Temporal Lobar Degeneration. Fronto-Temporal Dementia, Progressive Aphasia, Semantic Dementia.* New York: Churchill Livingstone, 1996.
3. Geschwind DH, Robidoux J, Alarcon M *et al.* Dementia and neurodevelopmental predisposition: cognitive dysfunction in presymptomatic subjects precedes dementia by decades in frontotemporal dementia. *Ann Neurol* 2001; 50:741–6.
4. Chow TW, Miller BL, Hayashi VN *et al.* Inheritance of frontotemporal dementia. *Arch Neurol* 1999;56:817–22.
5. Stevens M, van Duijn CM, Kamphorst W *et al.* Familial aggregation in frontotemporal dementia. *Neurology* 1998;50:1541–5.
6. Houlden H, Baker M, Adamson J *et al.* Frequency of tau mutations in three series of non-Alzheimer's degenerative dementia. *Ann Neurol* 1999;46:243–8.
7. Poorkaj P, Grossman M, Steinbart E *et al.* Frequency of tau gene mutations in familial and sporadic cases of non-Alzheimer dementia. *Arch Neurol* 2001; 58:383–7.
8. Snowden J, Bathgate D, Varma A *et al.* Distinct behavioural profiles in frontotemporal dementia and semantic dementia. *J Neurol Neurosurg Psychiatry* 2001;70:323–32.
9. Gregory CA, Hodges JR. Frontotemporal dementia: use of consensus criteria and prevalence of psychiatric features. *Neuropsychiatry Neuropsychol Behav Neurol* 1996;9:145–53.

10. Bathgate D, Snowden JS, Varma A *et al.* Behaviour in frontotemporal dementia, Alzheimer's disease and vascular dementia. *Acta Neurol Scand* 2001; 103:367–78.
11. Lund and Manchester Groups. Consensus statement: clinical and neuropathological criteria for frontotemporal dementia. *J Neurol Neurosurg Psychiatry* 1994;57:416–18.
12. Ames A, Cummings J, Wirshing WC *et al.* Repetitive and compulsive behavior in frontal lobe degenerations. *J Neuropsychiatry Clin Neurosci* 1994;6: 100–13.
13. Mendez MF, Bagert BA, Edwards-Lee T. Self-injurious behavior in frontotemporal dementia. *Neurocase* 1997;3:231–6.
14. Miller BL, Darby A, Benson DF *et al.* Aggressive, socially disruptive and antisocial behaviour associated with fronto-temporal dementia. *Br J Psychiatry* 1997;170:150–5.
15. Mychack P, Kramer JH, Boone K *et al.* The influence of right frontotemporal dysfunction on social behavior in frontotemporal dementia. *Neurology* 2001;56:S11–S15.
16. Cummings JL, Duchen LW. Klüver-Bucy syndrome in Pick disease: clinical and pathologic correlations. *Neurology* 1981;31:1415–22.
17. Edwards-Lee T, Miller BL, Benson DF *et al.* The temporal variant of frontotemporal dementia. *Brain* 1997;120:1027–40.
18. Miller BL, Chang L, Mena I *et al.* Progressive right frontotemporal degeneration: clinical, neuropsychological, and SPECT characteristics. *Dementia* 1993;4:204–13.
19. Bozeat S, Gregory CA, Ralph MAL *et al.* Which neuropsychiatric and behavioural features distinguish frontal and temporal variants of frontotemporal dementia from Alzheimer's disease? *J Neurol Neurosurg Psychiatry* 2000; 69:178–86.
20. Barber R, Snowden JS, Craufurd D. Frontotemporal dementia and Alzheimer's disease: retrospective differentiation using information from informants. *J Neurol Neurosurg Psychiatry* 1995;59:61–70.
21. Lebert F, Pasquier F, Souliez L *et al.* Frontotemporal behavioral scale. *Alzheimer Dis Assoc Disord* 1998;12:335–9.
22. Levy ML, Miller BL, Cummings J *et al.* Alzheimer disease and frontotemporal dementias: behavioral distinctions. *Arch Neurol* 1996;53:687–90.
23. Mendez MF, Perryman KM, Miller BL *et al.* Behavioral differences between frontotemporal dementia and Alzheimer's disease: A comparison on the BEHAVE-AD rating scale. *Int Psychogeriatr* 1998;10:155–62.
24. Swartz JR, Miller BL, Lesser IM *et al.* Behavioral phenomenology in Alzheimer's disease, frontotemporal dementia, and late-life depression: a retrospective analysis. *J Geriatr Psychiatry Neurol* 1997;10:67–74.
25. Cummings JL, Mega M, Gray K *et al.* The Neuropsychiatric Inventory: comprehensive assessment of psychopathology in dementia. *Neurology* 1994; 44:2308–14.
26. Kertesz A, Davidson W, Fox H. Frontal behavioral inventory: diagnostic criteria for frontal lobe dementia. *Can J Neurol Sci* 1997;24:29–36.
27. Weintraub S, Rubin N, Mesulam MM. Primary progressive aphasia, longitudinal course, neuropsychological profile, and language features. *Ann Neurol* 1990;31:174–83.

28. Hodges JR, Patterson K. Nonfluent progressive aphasia and semantic dementia: a comparative neuropsychological study. *J Int Neuropsychol Soc* 1996;2: 511–24.
29. Karbe H, Kertesz A, Polk M. Profiles of language impairment in primary progressive aphasia. *Arch Neurol* 1993;50:193–201.
30. Snowden J, Neary D, Mann D *et al.* Progressive language disorder due to lobar atrophy. *Ann Neurol* 1992;31:74–83.
31. Mesulam MM. Primary progressive aphasia. *Ann Neurol* 2001;49:425–32.
32. Neary D, Snowden JS. Clinical features of frontotemporal dementia. In: Pasquier F, Lebert F, Scheltens P (eds) *Frontotemporal Dementia*. Dordrecht, The Netherlands: ICG Publications, 1996: 31–47.
33. Hodges JR, Patterson K, Oxbury S *et al.* Semantic dementia. Progressive fluent aphasia with temporal lobe atrophy. *Brain* 1992;115:1783–806.
34. Kertesz A, Davidson W, McCabe P. Primary progressive semantic aphasia: a case study. *J Int Neuropsychol Soc* 1998;4:388–98.
35. Rossor MN, Revesz T, Lantos PL *et al.* Semantic dementia with ubiquitin-positive tau-negative inclusion bodies. *Brain* 2000;123:267–76.
36. Snowden JS, Goulding PJ, Neary D. Semantic dementia: a form of circumscribed cerebral atrophy. *Behav Neurol* 1989;2:167–82.
37. Hokoishi K, Ikeda M, Maki N *et al.* Frontotemporal lobar degeneration: a study in Japan. *Dement Geriatr Cogn Disord* 2001;12:393–9.
38. Miller BL, Ponton M, Benson DF *et al.* Enhanced artistic creativity with temporal lobe degeneration. *Lancet* 1996;348:1744.
39. Miller BL, Cummings J, Mishkin F *et al.* Emergence of artistic talent in frontotemporal dementia. *Neurology* 1998;51:978–82.
40. Miller BL, Boone K, Cummings J *et al.* Functional correlates of musical and visual ability in frontotemporal dementia. *Br J Psychiatry* 2000;176:458–63.
41. Elfgren C, Passant U, Risberg J. Neuropsychological findings in frontal lobe dementia. *Dement Geriatr Cogn Disord* 1993;4:214–19.
42. Miller BL, Cummings JL, Villaneuva-Meyer J *et al.* Frontal lobe degeneration: clinical, neuropsychological and SPECT characteristics. *Neurology* 1991;41: 1374–82.
43. Pasquier F, Lebert F, Grymonprez L *et al.* Verbal fluency in dementia of frontal lobe type and dementia of Alzheimer type. *J Neurol Neurosurg Psychiatry* 1995;58:81–4.
44. Zakzanis KK. Neurocognitive deficit in fronto-temporal dementia. *Neuropsychiatry Neuropsychol Behav Neurol* 1998;11:127–35.
45. Gregory CA, Serra-Mestres J, Hodges JR. Early diagnosis of the frontal variant of frontotemporal dementia: how sensitive are standard neuroimaging and neuropsychologic tests? *Neuropsychiatry Neuropsychol Behav Neurol* 1999; 12:128–35.
46. Boone K, Miller BL, Lee A *et al.* Neuropsychological patterns in right versus left frontotemporal dementia. *J Int Neuropsychol Soc* 1999;5:616–22.
47. Perry RJ. Differentiating frontal and temporal variant frontotemporal dementia from Alzheimer's disease. *Neurology* 2000;54:2277–84.
48. Gregory CA, Orrell M, Sahakian B *et al.* Can frontotemporal dementia and Alzheimer's disease be differentiated using a brief battery of tests? *Int J Geriatr Psychiatry* 1997;12:375–83.

49. Lindau M, Almkvist O, Johansson S-E et al. Cognitive and behavioral differentiation of dementia of the non-Alzheimer type and Alzheimer's disease. Dement Geriatr Cogn Disord 1998;9:205–13.

50. Mendez MF, Cherrier M, Perryman KM et al. Frontotemporal dementia versus Alzheimer's disease: differential cognitive features. Neurology 1996; 47:1189–94.

51. Binetti G, Locascio JJ, Corkin S et al. Differences between Pick disease and Alzheimer disease in clinical appearance and rate of cognitive decline. Arch Neurol 2000;57:225–32.

52. Elfgren C, Brun A, Gustafson L et al. Neuropsychological tests as discriminators between dementia of Alzheimer type and frontotemporal dementia. Int J Geriatr Psychiatry 1994;9:635–42.

53. Pachana N, Boone K, Miller BL et al. Comparison of neuropsychological functioning in Alzheimer's disease and frontotemporal dementia. J Int Neuropsychol Soc 1996;2:505–10.

54. Mendez MF, Selwood A, Mastri AR et al. Pick's disease versus Alzheimer's disease: a comparison of clinical characteristics. Neurology 1993;43:289–92.

55. Knopman DS, Christensen KJ, Schut LJ et al. The spectrum of imaging and neuropsychological findings in Pick's disease. Neurology 1989;39:362–8.

56. Chan D, Fox NC, Scahill RI et al. Patterns of temporal lobe atrophy in semantic dementia and Alzheimer's disease. Ann Neurol 2001;49:433–42.

57. Mummery CJ, Patterson K, Price CJ et al. A voxel-based morphometry study of semantic dementia: relationship between temporal lobe atrophy and semantic memory. Ann Neurol 2000;47:36–45.

58. Rosen HJ, Gorno-Tempini ML, Goldman WP et al. Patterns of brain atrophy in frontotemporal dementia and semantic dementia. Neurology 2002; 58:198–208.

59. Chan D, Fox NC, Jenkins R et al. Rates of global and regional cerebral atrophy in AD and frontotemporal dementia. Neurology 2001;57:1756–63.

60. Kitagaki H, Mori E, Hirono N et al. Alteration of white matter MR signal intensity in frontotemporal dementia. Am J Neuroradiol 1997;18:367–78.

61. Kaufer DI, Miller BL, Itti L et al. Midline cerebral morphometry distinguishes frontotemporal dementia and Alzheimer's disease. Neurology 1997;48:978–85.

62. Grossman M, Payer F, Onishi K et al. Language comprehension and regional cerebral defects in frontotemporal degeneration and Alzheimer's disease. Neurology 1998;50:157–63.

63. Turner RS, Kenyon LC, Trojanowski JQ et al. Clinical, neuroimaging, and pathologic features of progressive nonfluent aphasia. Ann Neurol 1996;39: 166–73.

64. Didic M, Giusiano B, de Laforte C et al. Identification of clinical subtypes of fronto-temporal dementia and cerebral blood flow on SPECT: preliminary results. Alzheimer's Reports 1998;1:179–85.

65. Chawluk JB, Mesulam MM, Hurtig H et al. Slowly progressive aphasia without generalized dementia: studies with positron emission tomography. Ann Neurol 1986;19:68–74.

66. Kamo H, McGeer PL, Harrop R et al. Positron emission tomography and histopathology in Pick's disease. Neurology 1987;37:439–45.

67. Foster NL, Wilhemsen K, Sima AFS et al. Frontotemporal dementia and

parkinsonism linked to chromosome 17: a consensus conference. *Ann Neurol* 1997;41:706–15.

68. Reed LA, Wszolek ZK. Phenotypic correlations in FTDP-17. *Neurobiol Aging* 2001;22:89–107.

69. Hosler BA, Siddique T, Sapp PC *et al*. Linkage of familial amyotrophic lateral sclerosis with frontotemporal dementia to chromosome 9q21-q22. *JAMA* 2000;284:1664–9.

70. Clark LN, Wilhelmsen KC. The genetics of Pick complex and adult-onset dementia. In: Kertesz A, Munoz DG (eds) *Pick's Disease and Pick Complex*. New York: Wiley-Liss, 1998: 269–80.

71. Pickering-Brown S, Baker M, Yen S-H *et al*. Pick's disease is associated with mutations in the tau gene. *Ann Neurol* 2000;48:859–67.

72. Rosso SM, van Herpen E, Deelen W *et al*. A novel tau mutation, S320F, causes a tauopathy with inclusions similar to those in Pick's disease. *Ann Neurol* 2002;51:373–6.

73. Brun A. Frontal lobe degeneration of non-Alzheimer type. 1-Neuropathology. *Arch Gerontol Geriatr* 1987;6:193–208.

74. McKhann GM, Albert MS, Grossman M *et al*. Clinical and pathological diagnosis of frontotemporal dementia. Report of the Work Group on Frontotemporal Dementia and Pick's Disease. *Arch Neurol* 2001;58:1803–9.

75. Zhukareva V, Vogelsberg-Ragaglia V, Van Deerlin VMD *et al*. Loss of brain tau defines novel sporadic and familial tauopathies with frontotemporal dementia. *Ann Neurol* 2001;49:165–75.

76. Mann DMA, South PW, Snowden JS *et al*. Dementia of frontal lobe type: neuropathology and immunohistochemistry. *J Neurol Neurosurg Psychiatry* 1993;56:605–14.

77. Francis PT, Holmes C, Webster M-T *et al*. Preliminary neurochemical findings in non-Alzheimer dementia due to lobar atrophy. *Dement Geriatr Cogn Disord* 1993;4:172–7.

78. Sparks DL, Markesbery WR. Altered serotonergic and cholinergic synaptic markers in Pick's disease. *Arch Neurol* 1991;48:796–9.

79. Sjogren M, Blennow K, Minthon L *et al*. Neurochemical and treatment studies on frontotemporal dementia. In: Pasquier F, Lebert F, Scheltens P (eds) *Frontotemporal Dementia*. Dordrecht, The Netherlands: ICG Publications, 1996: 91–8.

80. Sahakian BJ, Coull JJ, Hodges JR. Selective enhancement of executive function by idazoxan in a patient with dementia of the frontal lobe type. *J Neurol Neurosurg Psychiatry* 1994;57:120–1.

chapter 8

Creutzfeldt-Jakob disease and other prion disorders

Prion diseases are a unique group of disorders that may be transmitted under rare circumstances and may be inherited in others. Prion (imaginatively derived from the words 'proteinaceous infectious particle') disorders are the only known condition with this unique dual pathogenesis. Prion protein is encoded by a gene on the short arm of chromosome 20. Mutations in the gene are responsible for the inherited form of the illness, whereas the transmissible forms of the disorder are caused by recruiting normal cellular prion protein and commandeering its conversion to the disease-causing form of the protein (Figures 8.1 and 8.2).[1] Four human illnesses are recognized as prion disorders: Creutzfeldt-Jakob disease (CJD), Kuru, Gerstmann-Straussler-Scheinker disease, and fatal familial insomnia. Several variants of CJD are known. Neuropsychiatric presentations of CJD are common and have been particularly striking in the new variant CJD (nvCJD) transmitted from cows with bovine spongiform encephalopathy (BSE, 'mad cow disease').

Creutzfeldt-Jakob disease

Demography and clinical features

The incidence of sporadic CJD is approximately one case per million in the population (among persons aged 60–74 the incidence changes to approximately 5 per million). Cases have been described in individuals

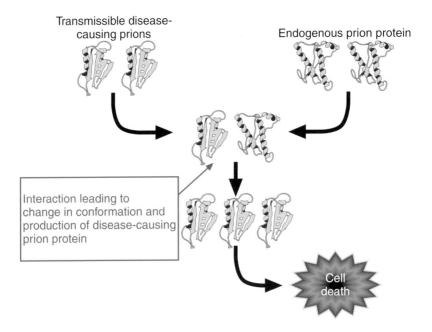

Figure 8.1 *Sporadic Creutzfeldt-Jakob disease. Transmissible disease-causing proteins recruit the normal endogenous prion protein and interact to produce a conformational change into the disease-causing form and production of the lethal prion protein.[2]*

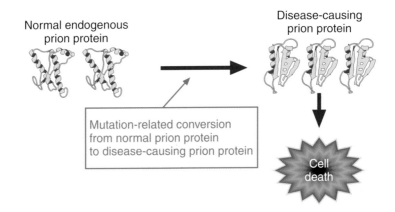

Figure 8.2 *Familial Creutzfeldt-Jakob disease. Normal endogenous prion proteins spontaneously convert to disease-causing prion protein.[2]*

as young as 17 and as old as 83. Sporadic CJD accounts for 85% of all cases of prion diseases in humans.[2] Box 8.1 presents diagnostic criteria for sporadic CJD. Probable CJD is based on a combination of myoclonus, pyramidal signs, characteristic EEG findings, cerebellar abnormalities, and extrapyramidal signs.[3] The average age of onset is 60 years and the average duration of disease is 8 months. Approximately 10% of patients have a long duration form of the illness, surviving for 2–10 years.[4]

Creutzfeldt-Jakob disease proceeds through three phases: a prodromal phase, a period of rapid clinical deterioration, and a phase of advanced disability with mutism and immobility. Neuropsychiatric symptoms are especially common in the prodromal phase.

In the course of the illness, 100% of the patients exhibit memory deterioration and memory loss, approximately 60% have behavioral disturbances, and 70% have abnormalities of higher cortical functions. Cerebellar signs are seen in 71%, oculomotor abnormalities in 42%,

---

Box 8.1 Criteria for diagnosis of Creutzfeldt-Jakob disease (CJD)[3]

Definite
- Neuropathologically confirmed spongiform encephalopathy in a case of progressive dementia with at least one of the clinical features listed

Probable
- Myoclonus
- Pyramidal signs
- Characteristic EEG
- Cerebellar signs
- Extrapyramidal signs
- Neuropathologically unconfirmed

Possible
- History, without medical records, allowing confirmation of progressive dementia, with: 1) myoclonus and a course of <3 years; or 2) a member of the family having transmissible definite or probable CJD; or 3) at least two of the clinical features listed together with the appearance of prominent and early signs of lower motor neuron involvement (the amyotrophic form of CJD)

myoclonus in 78%, pyramidal tract signs in 62%, extrapyramidal signs in 56%, and evidence of lower motor neuron disease in 12% of patients. Seizures occur in 70% of patients and classical periodic EEG with triphasic waves or a burst-suppression pattern are present in 60%.[5] Aphasia is a common manifestation of CJD and mixed transcortical aphasia with echolalia[6] is often observed. Neuropsychiatric features may include apathy, depression, anxiety, irritability, delusions and bizarre or uncharacteristic behavior.

Laboratory studies are helpful in the diagnosis of CJD. Periodic sharp wave complexes are the characteristic EEG findings in patients with CJD but are not present in all cases. They have a sensitivity of approximately 70% and a specificity of approximately 85%.[7] Magnetic resonance imaging in CJD reveals bilateral symmetric high signal intensities on T2-weighted images in the basal ganglia of approximately 70% of patients. Similar abnormalities are rare in other dementias.[8,9] Perfusion-weighted imaging reveals increased signal intensity in affected cortical and subcortical regions.[10,11] Studies with fluorodeoxyglucose (FDG) positron emission tomography (PET) reveal irregular areas of diminished cortical metabolism.[11,12] Several studies indicate that detection of the 14-3-3 protein in the cerebrospinal fluid is both sensitive and specific for diagnosis of CJD.[13,14] Others, however, have found that the test may be positive in non-CJD causes of dementia.[15] Clinical and EEG criteria (Box 8.1) are the current gold standard for the diagnosis of CJD.

Classic neuropathologic features of CJD include spongiform degeneration with vacuolation of the neuropil and an exuberant fibrous astrogliosis with marked proliferation of the fibrous astrocytes. Prion protein positive plaques are present in approximately 10% of CJD[2,16] (Figure 8.3).

Familial Creutzfeldt-Jakob disease

Familial CJD, Gerstmann-Straussler-Scheinker, and fatal familial insomnia are all dominantly inherited prion diseases caused by mutations of the prion protein.[2] The prion protein gene is located on the short arm of

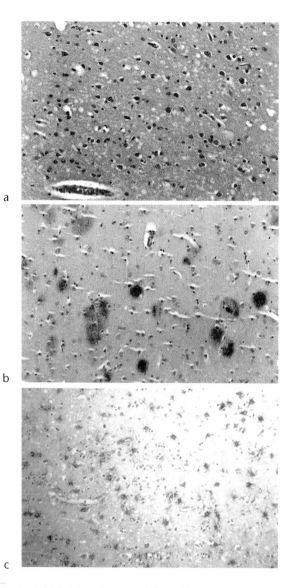

a

b

c

Figure 8.3 Creutzfeldt-Jakob disease. (a) Spongiform change evident as microvacuolation of the neocortex. (b) Section immunostained with antibody to prion protein showing prion protein plaques. (c) Astrocytic gliosis shown by immunostaining (brown) with anti-GFAP antibody in a region of spongy change (courtesy of H Vinters, MD, Division of Neuropathology, UCLA School of Medicine).

chromosome 20. Two types of pathogenic changes have been reported to cause familial CJD: 1) point mutations within the coding sequence resulting in amino acid substitutions in the prion protein; 2) insertions coding additional integral copies of an octapeptide repeat in the normal protein.[17] Patients with CJD produced by point mutations have a clinical phenotype similar to classic sporadic CJD. Patients whose disease is a result of insertional mutations have highly variable phenotypes. For example, the age of onset varies between 21 and 82 years of age and disease duration varies between 2 months and 18 years among reported cases.[18] The type of insertion determines the phenotype of the disease.

Genetic factors predispose to sporadic CJD. Individuals who are homozygous for valine or methionine at codon 129 are at increased risk for the disease.[17]

New variant Creutzfeldt-Jakob disease

A new variant of CJD was observed in the United Kingdom in concert with the epidemic of bovine spongiform encephalopathy. The variant form has demographic, clinical, and pathological features that differ from those of classic CJD.[19,20] Typically the disease has an earlier age of onset, more prolonged duration of illness, prominent early psychiatric symptoms, and an earlier age at death. The median age at onset is 29 years with a range of 18–53. The median duration of the illness is 14 months with a range of 8–38 months among reported cases.[20] The presenting psychiatric symptoms are heterogeneous and have included social withdrawal, anxiety, depression, delusions, emotional lability, aggression, apathy, and agitation.[21] Many patients received an initial psychiatric diagnosis such as major depression, anxiety, schizophrenia, or hysteria. Sensory abnormalities such as dysesthesias or hyperesthesias also may occur. The appearance of neurological signs is often delayed (average 6 months) after the onset of the illness. Early neurological signs include ataxia, rapidly progressive cognitive impairments, and involuntary movements. Progression is rapid, with patients progressing from unsteadiness to being bed bound in approximately 6 months.[21]

Myoclonus occurs in nearly all cases, but is a late feature in some. The characteristic pattern of periodic sharp waves on EEGs is rare in patients with nvCJD. Slow waves are common. Neuropathologically nvCJD is unusual; histological features include numerous prion protein positive amyloid plaques surrounded by intense spongiform degeneration.[19] Box 8.2 provides diagnostic criteria for nvCJD.[20]

Box 8.2 Diagnostic criteria for new variant Creutzfeldt-Jakob disease (nvCJD)[20]

Definite: IA (progressive neuropsychiatric disorder) and neuropathological confirmation of nvCJD§
Probable: I; 4/5 of II; IIIA and B
Possible: I; 4/5 of II; IIIA

I. Necessary criteria
  A. Progressive neuropsychiatric disorder
  B. Duration of illness >6 months
  C. Routine investigations do not suggest an alternative diagnosis
  D. No history of potential iatrogenic exposure
II. Supportive clinical features
  A. Early psychiatric symptoms*
  B. Persistent painful sensory symptoms†
  C. Ataxia
  D. Myoclonus or chorea or dystonia
  E. Dementia
III. Supportive laboratory feature
  A. EEG does not show the typical appearance of sporadic CJD‡ (or no EEG performed)
  B. Bilateral pulvinar high signal on MRI scan

*Depression, anxiety, apathy, withdrawal, delusions.[14]
†These include frank pain and unpleasant dysesthesia.
‡Generalized triphasic periodic complexes at approximately one per second.
§Spongiform changes and extensive prion protein deposition with florid plaques throughout the cerebrum and cerebellum.[12]
EEG, electroencephalogram; MRI, magnetic resonance imaging.

Other forms of CJD

In addition to familial, sporadic, and nvCJD, iatrogenic cases are also recognized.[19] Prions have been transmitted in human growth hormone extracts, improperly sterilized depth electrodes, transplanted corneas, transplanted dura mater, and gonadotropins derived from cadaveric pituitaries.[19,22]

There are several recognized clinical variants of CJD, including a panencephalic type with extensive white matter involvement;[23] a disorder featuring a progressive spastic gait disturbance and dementia without cerebellar signs or myoclonus;[24] the Heidenhain variant featuring prominent disorders of perception progressing to cortical blindness;[25] an amyotropic variant with lower motor neuron signs that occur late in the clinical course following the occurrence of a prominent dementia and cerebellar signs;[26] and a Kuru-like ataxic variant presenting with cerebellar abnormalities (Box 8.3).

Box 8.3 Human prion diseases

Creutzfeldt-Jakob disease
- Etiologic variants
  - Sporadic
  - Familial
  - New variant (associated with bovine spongiform encephalopathy)
  - Iatrogenic
- Clinical variants
  - Classical type
  - Heidenhain (visual disturbances)
  - Panencephalitic type
  - Familial spastic paraparesis with dementia
  - Amyotrophic type
  - Ataxic type

Other prion diseases
- Kuru (Fore people of New Guinea)
- Gerstmann-Straussler-Scheinker disease
- Fatal familial insomnia

Other prion diseases

Other recognized prion disorders include Kuru, Gerstmann-Straussler-Scheinker disease, and fatal familial insomnia. *Kuru* is a disorder of the Fore people of New Guinea transmitted through cannibalistic practices and manifesting initially as a cerebellar ataxia progressing to dementia and death. The condition is rapidly decreasing in frequency as cannibalistic practices are relinquished.

Gerstmann-Straussler Scheinker disease is a rare familial variety of transmissible spongiform encephalopathy that is distinguished from CJD by an earlier age at onset, more prominent cerebellar signs, and a longer duration of illness. Patients usually experience the onset of the illness in their mid-30s to mid-60s and survive for 2–2.5 years.[27,28] At autopsy amyloid plaques with prion protein are widespread throughout the cerebrum and cerebellum. Neurofibrillary tangles can be seen in the cerebral cortex and hippocampus.[28,29] Most families have a mutation at codon 102 of the prion protein gene, but a variety of other point mutations have been described.[28]

Fatal familial insomnia is a rapidly progressive familial disease characterized clinically by untreatable insomnia, dysautonomia, and motor signs.[30] Pathological changes are most marked in the anterior ventral and medial dorsal thalamic nuclei, where there is neuronal loss and marked astrogliosis.[30,31] The disease is linked to a mutation at codon 178 of the prion protein gene.[32] There is substantial phenotypic heterogeneity in families with this mutation; patients may present with fatal familial insomnia, autosomal dominant cerebellar ataxia, or characteristic features of CJD.[33] Fluorodeoxyglucose PET in patients with fatal familial insomnia reveals hypometabolism in the thalamus with variable degrees of cortical involvement.[34,35]

Treatment of prion disorders

There is no available proven treatment for any prion disease. Two agents approved for use in other settings – quinacrine, an antimalarial, and thorazine, an antipsychotic agent – are active against prion proteins in laboratory settings. Quinacrine was more effective than chlorpromazine.[36] Development of derivatives of these compounds may lead to effective pharmacotherapy.

References

1. Prusiner SB, Hsiao KK. Human prion diseases. *Ann Neurol* 1994;35:385–95.
2. Prusiner SB. Shattuck lecture – neurodegenerative diseases and prions. *N Engl J Med* 2001;344:1516–26.
3. Brandel JP, Delasnerie-Laupretre N, Laplanche JL *et al.* Diagnosis of Creutzfeldt-Jakob disease: effect of clinical criteria on incidence estimates. *Neurology* 2000;54:1095–9.
4. Brown P, Rodgers-Johnson P, Cathala F *et al.* Creutzfeldt-Jakob disease of long duration: clinicopathological characteristics, transmissibility, and differential diagnosis. *Ann Neurol* 1984;16:295–304.
5. Brown P, Gibbs CJ, Rodgers-Johnson P *et al.* Human spongiform encephalopathy: the National Institutes of Health series of 300 cases of experimentally transmitted disease. *Ann Neurol* 1994;35:513–29.
6. McPherson SE, Kuratani JD, Cummings JL *et al.* Creutzfeldt-Jakob disease with mixed transcortical aphasia: insights into echolalia. *Behav Neurol* 1994; 7:197–203.
7. Steinhoff B, Racker S, Herrendorf G *et al.* Accuracy and reliability of periodic sharp wave complexes in Creutzfeldt-Jakob disease. *Arch Neurol* 1996;53:162–6.
8. Schroter A, Zerr I, Henkel K *et al.* Magnetic resonance imaging in the clinical diagnosis of Creutzfeldt-Jakob disease. *Arch Neurol* 2000;57:1751–7.
9. Mittal S, Farmer P, Kalina P *et al.* Correlation of diffusion-weighted magnetic resonance imaging with neuropathology in Creutzfeldt-Jakob disease. *Arch Neurol* 2002;59:128–34.
10. Demaerel P, Heiner L, Robberecht W *et al.* Diffusion-weighted MRI in sporadic Creutzfeldt-Jakob disease. *Neurology* 1999;52:205–8.
11. Na DL, Suh CK, Choi SH *et al.* Diffusion-weighted magnetic resonance imaging in probable Creutzfeldt-Jakob disease. *Arch Neurol* 1999;56:951–7.
12. Goldman S, Laird A, Flament-Durand J *et al.* Positron emission tomography and histopathology in Creutzfeldt-Jakob disease. *Neurology* 1993;43:1828–30.
13. Lemstra A, Meegen MT, Vreyling JP *et al.* 14-3-3 testing diagnosing Creutzfeldt-Jakob disease: a prospective study in 112 patients. *Neurology* 2000;55:514–16.
14. Zerr I, Pocchiari M, Collins S *et al.* Analysis of EEG and CSF 14-3-3 proteins as aids to the diagnosis of Creutzfeldt-Jakob disease. *Neurology* 2000;55:811–15.
15. Burkhard PR, Sanchez J-C, Landis T *et al.* CSF detection of the 14-3-3 protein in unselected patients with dementia. *Neurology* 2001;56:1528–33.
16. Kretzschmar HA, Ironside JW, DeArmond SJ *et al.* Diagnostic criteria for sporadic Creutzfeldt-Jakob disease. *Arch Neurol* 1996;53:913–20.

17. Collinge J, Palmer MS. Human prion diseases. In: Collinge J, Palmer MS (eds) *Prion Diseases*. New York: Oxford University Press, 1997: 18–56.
18. Gambetti P, Petersen RB, Parchi P *et al*. Inherited prion diseases. In: Prusiner SB (ed) *Prion Biology and Diseases*. Cold Spring Harbor, NY: Cold Spring Harbor Laboratory Press, 1999: 509–83.
19. Prusiner SB. Prion diseases and the BSE crisis. *Science* 1997;389:389–423.
20. Will RG, Zeidler M, Stewart GE *et al*. Diagnosis of new variant Creutzfeldt-Jakob disease. *Ann Neurol* 2000;47:575–82.
21. Zeidler M, Johnstone EC, Bamber RWK *et al*. New variant Creutzfeldt-Jakob disease: psychiatric features. *Lancet* 1997;350:908–10.
22. Billete de Villemeur T, Deslys J-P, Pradel A *et al*. Creutzfeldt-Jakob disease from contaminated growth hormone extracts in France. *Neurology* 1996;47:690–5.
23. Shyu W-C, Lee C-C, Hsu Y-D *et al*. Panencephalitic Creutzfeldt-Jakob disease unusual presentation of magnetic resonance imaging and proton magnetic resonance spectroscopy. *J Neurol Sci* 1996;138:157–60.
24. Kitamoto T, Amano N, Terao Y *et al*. A new inherited prion disease (PrP-P105L mutation) showing spastic paraparesis. *Ann Neurol* 1993;34:808–13.
25. Kropp S, Schulz-Schaeffer WJ, Finkenstaedt M *et al*. The Heidenhain variant of Creutzfeldt-Jakob disease. *Arch Neurol* 1999;56:55–61.
26. Salazar AM, Masters CL, Gajdusek DC *et al*. Syndromes of amyotrophic lateral sclerosis and dementia: relation to transmissible Creutzfeldt-Jakob disease. *Ann Neurol* 1983;14:17–26.
27. Farlow MR, Yee RD, Dlouhy SR *et al*. Gerstmann-Straussler-Scheinker disease. I. Extending the clinical spectrum. *Neurology* 1989;39:1446–52.
28. Majtenyi C, Brown P, Cervenakova L *et al*. A three-sister sibship of Gerstmann-Straussler-Scheinker disease with a CJD phenotype. *Neurology* 2000;54:2133–7.
29. Ghetti B, Tagliavini F, Masters CL *et al*. Gerstmann-Straussler-Scheinker disease. II. Neurofibrillary tangles and plaques with PrP-amyloid coexist in an affected family. *Neurology* 1989;39:1453–61.
30. Medori R, Tritschler H-J, LeBlanc A *et al*. Fatal familial insomnia, a prion disease with mutation at codon 178 of the prion protein gene. *N Engl J Med* 1992;326:444–9.
31. Parchi P, Castellani R, Cortelli P *et al*. Regional distribution of protease-resistant prion protein in fatal familial insomnia. *Ann Neurol* 1995;38:21–9.
32. Rossi G, Macchi G, Porro M *et al*. Fatal familial insomnia: genetic, neuropathologic, and biochemical study of a patient from a new Italian kindred. *Neurology* 1998;50:688–92.
33. McLean CA, Storey E, Gardner RJM *et al*. The D178N (cis-129M) 'fatal familial insomnia' mutation associated with diverse clinicopathologic phenotypes in an Australian kindred. *Neurology* 1997;49:552–8.
34. Cortelli P, Perani D, Parchi P *et al*. Cerebral metabolism in fatal familial insomnia: relation to duration, neuropathology, and distribution of protease-resistant prion protein. *Neurology* 1997;49:126–33.
35. Perani D, Cortelli P, Lucignani G *et al*. [18F] FDG PET in fatal familial insomnia: the functional effects of thalamic lesions. *Neurology* 1993;43:2565–9.
36. Korth C, May BCH, Cohen FE *et al*. Acridine and phenothiazine derivatives as pharmacotherapeutics for prion disease. *Proc Natl Acad Sci USA* 2001;98: 9836–41.

Neurobiology of neuropsychiatric symptoms in dementias

Evolving understanding of the neurobiology of the dementing disorders, the relationship of neuropathologic and neurochemical changes to clinical abnormalities, and the correlation between histologic and neurotransmitter changes and behavioral abnormalities provide insight into the neurobiological mediation of neuropsychiatric symptoms in dementing disorders. This chapter links observations concerning molecular biologic, neuropathologic and neurochemical changes in dementia syndromes to neuropsychiatric and behavioral manifestations of these disorders.

A hierarchical model of brain–behavior relationships

Figure 9.1 provides a hierarchical model integrating observations from several levels of observation relevant to understanding brain–behavior relationships. Molecular events (e.g. abnormalities of amyloid peptide protein processing in Alzheimer's disease) lead to cellular changes (dysfunction and death). Cell death is not a global occurrence in the central nervous system but has regional preferences and this regional distribution of neuronal dysfunction and death underlies many of the specific clinical manifestations of each dementing disorder.

Cell death in specific brain nuclei responsible for transmitter synthesis leads to deficits in a variety of transmitter systems including the cholinergic system following involvement of the nucleus basilis of Mynert, the noradrenergic system reflecting involvement of the locus ceruleus, serotonergic deficits secondary to effects on the raphe nuclei of the brain stem, and dopaminergic deficits due to involvement of the substantia nigra and ventral tegmental area of the midbrain. Transmitter deficits also have preferential regional involvement and contribute to the clinical phenotype.

The pattern of distribution of neuronal and transmitter changes leads to dysfunction of neural systems. Two neural networks have been recognized as particularly important to the mediation of neuropsychiatric disturbances: the limbic system and the system comprised of frontal-subcortical circuits. The limbic system mediates normal human emotional experience.[1] This system is responsible for assigning the valence of emotional value to human experiences. Frontal-subcortical circuits mediate executive function (dorsolateral prefrontal-subcortical circuits), motivation (medial prefrontal/anterior cingulate-subcortical circuit), and control of behavior in social contexts (orbitofrontal-subcortical circuit), as well as motor (premotor-subcortical circuit) and eye movement

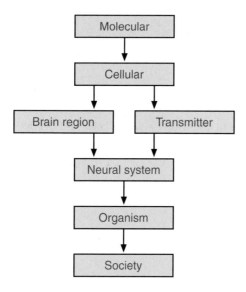

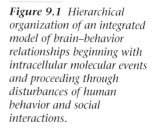

Figure 9.1 Hierarchical organization of an integrated model of brain–behavior relationships beginning with intracellular molecular events and proceeding through disturbances of human behavior and social interactions.

(oculomotor-subcortical circuit) functions.[2] Transmitters involved in dementia syndromes also exert their influence through these neural systems. The dopaminergic system projects to basal ganglia and medial frontal regions; cholinergic, noradrenergic, and serotonergic projections disperse widely from subcortical sites to cortical targets.

Neural system dysfunction is evident in the behavior of the organism in the form of cognitive abnormalities and neuropsychiatric symptoms. Motor and sensory disturbances are present when these systems are involved by the neurobiological changes of the dementing disorder.

Humans interact in social systems and some central nervous system disorders become particularly evident in the context of this social milieu. Orbitofrontal-subcortical circuit disorders render the usual socially relevant constraints on behavior dysfunctional, resulting in socially inappropriate behavior. Interpersonal disinhibition, tactless comments, lewd behavior and verbalizations, and psychopathological behavior are evident in conditions such as the frontotemporal lobar degenerations.

Thus, inherited frontotemporal lobar degeneration, a mutation in chromosome 17, leads to abnormal tau processing, regionally predominant dysfunction in anterior temporal and frontal lobe regions, disturbance of frontal-subcortical systems, and abnormalities of human behavior particularly in interpersonal settings. In Alzheimer's disease, abnormalities in processing of the amyloid precursor protein yielding increased production or aggregation of the beta-amyloid peptide leads to regional dysfunction in medial temporal and posterior hemispheric structures evident as disabilities in memory, language, and visuospatial skills and disrupting the success of the individual in social and occupational function. Figure 9.2 illustrates how the hierarchical model of behavior (Figure 9.1) applies to dementia syndromes leading from changes in protein metabolism to social and occupational disability.

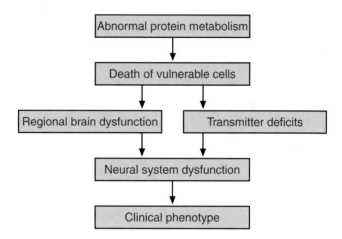

Figure 9.2 *Hierarchical model of behavior applied to dementia disorders. Changes in protein metabolism lead to cell death and transmitter deficits in neural systems that produce clinical phenotypes and lead to social and occupational disability.*

Protein metabolism abnormalities in degenerative dementias

Protein metabolism abnormalities are present in most degenerative dementias and are associated with characteristic histopathological changes (Box 9.1).[3] Each proteinopathy is associated with a distinct anatomic pattern of degeneration. Alzheimer's disease is associated primarily with the abnormal production and accumulation of beta-amyloid with more limited abnormalities of tau and synuclein protein. This is true of both sporadic and familial forms of the disorder. Abnormalities of tau protein metabolism occur in the frontotemporal lobar degenerations, pallido-ponto-nigral degeneration, progressive supranuclear palsy, Guamanian amyotrophic lateral sclerosis-parkinsonism dementia complex and corticobasal degeneration.[4–7] Secondary tauopathies where tau protein abnormalities appear to be secondary to other identifiable cellular changes include Alzheimer's disease, dementia with Lewy bodies, dementia pugilistica, Creutzfeldt-Jakob disease, Gerstmann-

Box 9.1 Classification of degenerative dementias and related disorders based on protein abnormalities

Amyloidopathy (with limited tauopathy and alpha-synucleinopathy)
- Alzheimer's disease
  - Sporadic
  - Familial with amyloid precursor protein mutation
  - Familial with presenilin 1 mutation
  - Familial with presenilin 2 mutation
  - Down's syndrome with Alzheimer's disease (trisomy 21)

Tauopathies
- Frontotemporal lobar degeneration
  - Pick's disease
  - Frontotemporal lobar degeneration with parkinsonism linked to chromosome 17
  - Frontotemporal lobar degeneration lacking distinct histopathologic features
  - Frontotemporal lobar degeneration with motor neuron disease
  - Hereditary disinhibition dysphasic dementia
- Pallidopontonigral degeneration
- Progressive supranuclear palsy
- Guamanian amyotrophic lateral sclerosis-parkinsonism dementia complex
- Corticobasal degeneration
- Secondary tauopathies
  - Alzheimer's disease
  - Dementia with Lewy bodies
  - Dementia pugilistica
  - Hallervorden-Spatz disease
  - Creutzfeldt-Jakob disease
  - Gerstmann-Straussler-Scheinker disease
  - Neimann-Pick disease (type C)
  - Subacute sclerosing panencephalitis

Synucleinopathies
- Parkinson's disease
  - Sporadic
  - Familial with alpha-synuclein mutations

continued

Box 9.1 *continued*

- – MPTP-induced
- • Dementia with Lewy bodies (with amyloidopathy and limited tauopathy)
- • Cortical Lewy body disease
- • Multiple system atrophy
  - – Shy-Drager syndrome
  - – Olivopontocerebellar atrophy
  - – Striatonigral degeneration
- • Neurodegeneration with brain iron accumulation
  - – Hallervorden-Spatz disease
  - – Neuroaxonal dystrophy
- • Secondary synucleinopathies
  - – Alzheimer's disease
  - – Traumatic brain injury
  - – Amyotrophic lateral sclerosis

Prion protein disorders
- • Creutzfeldt-Jakob disease
  - – Sporadic
  - – Familial
  - – New variant
  - – Iatrogenic
- • Kuru
- • Fatal familial insomnia
- • Sporadic fatal insomnia
- • Gerstmann-Straussler-Scheinker disease
- • Familial progressive subcortical gliosis

MPTP, 1-methyl-1-phenyl-1,2,3,6-tetrahydropyridine.

Straussler-Scheinker disease, Neimann-Pick disease, and subacute sclerosing panencephalitis. Synucleinopathies involving primarily alpha-synuclein protein disorders include Parkinson's disease (sporadic, those associated with synuclein mutations, and MTPT-induced parkinsonism), dementia with Lewy bodies, cortical Lewy body disease, multiple system atrophies, and degeneration associated with brain iron accumulation

(Hallervorden-Spatz disease and neuroaxonal dystrophy).[8] Disorders of prion protein metabolism include Creutzfeldt-Jakob disease (sporadic, familial, new variant, and iatrogenic), Kuru, fatal familial insomnia, sporadic familial insomnia, Gerstmann-Straussler-Scheinker disease, and familial progressive subcortical gliosis.[3]

Alzheimer's disease and dementias with Lewy bodies (amyloidopathies) affect posterior hemispheric structures preferentially (Figure 9.3). Primary tauopathies such as frontotemporal lobar degenerations may result in tau aggregation in the form of neurofibrillary tangles or other tau-protein aggregates. Some tauopathies ('tauless') disrupt the function without producing the aggregation. The tauopathies affect primarily the frontal lobes or related structures and produce frontal-subcortical clinical syndromes. Other tau-modifying conditions and tau abnormalities in Alzheimer's disease also have a predilection to affect frontal and limbic cortical neurons. When tau abnormalities are disproportionately prominent in Alzheimer's disease, they involve the frontal cortex and result in unusually severe frontal disturbances including executive functional abnormalities, psychosis and agitation (Figure 9.4).[9–11]

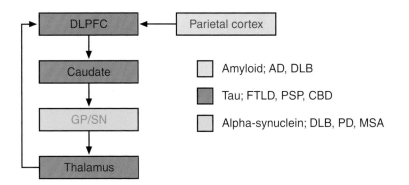

Figure 9.3 *Differential anatomic vulnerability to major types of protein metabolic abnormalities involved in dementing disorders. DLPFC, dorsolateral prefrontal cortex; GP/SN, globus pallidus/substantia nigra; FTLD, frontotemporal lobar degeneration; PSP, progressive supranuclear palsy; CBD, corticobasal degeneration; DLB, dementia with Lewy bodies; PD, Parkinson's disease; MSA, multiple system atrophies; AD, Alzheimer's disease.*

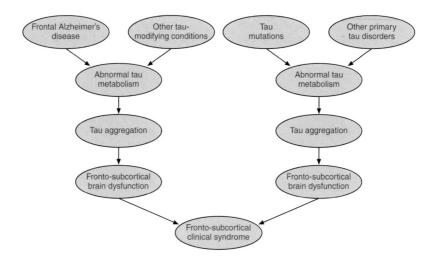

Figure 9.4 *Primary and secondary tauopathies have their primary impact on frontal-subcortical circuits and produce frontal-subcortical clinical syndromes.*

Thus, a unifying principle of degenerative dementias is that they reflect abnormalities of protein metabolism. Specific cellular populations are vulnerable to different types of protein metabolic abnormalities. The hippocampal, medial temporal, and posterior hemispheric neurons are most susceptible to abnormalities of A-beta metabolism. Frontal and basal ganglionic neurons are predominantly affected in tau metabolism disturbances resulting in frontal and subcortical abnormalities manifested as frontal and subcortical dementia syndromes. Alpha-synuclein disturbances involve brain stem, basal ganglia, and limbic system neurons. Prion protein abnormalities affect the central nervous system more diffusely, but individual mutational events in the familial prion disorders result in differential topography of brain involvement; fatal familial insomnias, for example, involve the thalamus preferentially; Gerstmann-Straussler-Scheinker disease often presents with ataxia and a cerebellar syndrome; new variant Creutzfeldt-Jakob disease preferentially involves the basal ganglia; and Kuru presents with a tremor and cerebellar syndrome. Thus, genotype–phenotype and molecular–clinical/behavioral correlations are linked. Specific protein disturbances lead to abnormalities of vulnerable neural systems and manifest as specific clinical and behavioral syndromes. Preliminary linkages can be made between specific proteinopathies and clinical phenotypes. Disinhibition is most frequent in patients with primary (frontotemporal dementia, progressive supranuclear palsy) or secondary (Alzheimer's disease) tauopathies (Figure 9.5). Visual hallucinations are most common among patients with alpha-synucleinopathies (dementia with Lewy bodies, Parkinson's disease with dementia) (Figure 9.6).

The limbic system and emotional function in the dementias

Disorders of emotional function in dementia syndromes include both dysfunction of normal emotions and the appearance of psychopathology. Relationships of drive, emotion, motivation, and mood are complex and linkages between normal emotion and psychopathology or neuropsychiatric symptoms are ill understood. Drives involve the basic

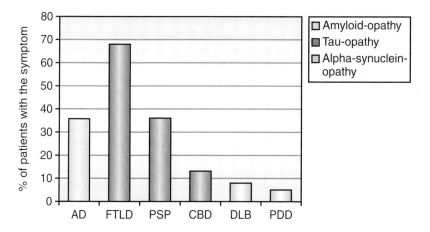

Figure 9.5 Disinhibition is most common in disorders with abnormalities of the metabolism. FTLD and PSP are primary tauopathies; AD is a secondary tauopathy. AD, Alzheimer's disease; FTLD, frontotemporal dementia; PSP, progressive supranuclear palsy; CBD, corticobasal degeneration; DLB, dementia with Lewy bodies; PDD, Parkinson's disease with dementia.

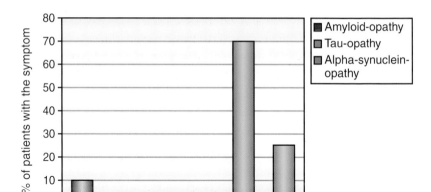

Figure 9.6 *Visual hallucinations are most common in disorders involving alpha-synuclein dysmetatabolism. AD, Alzheimer's disease; FTLD, frontotemporal dementia; PSP, progressive supranuclear palsy; CBD, corticobasal degeneration; DLB, dementia with Lewy bodies; PDD, Parkinson's disease with dementia.*

survival functions including satiation of hunger, thirst, and reproduction as well as the need for safety. Emotions on which some degree of consensus has been achieved include amusement, anger, awe, contempt, contentment, disgust, embarrassment, excitement, fear, guilt, interest, pride in achievement, relief, sadness, satisfaction, sensory pleasure, and shame.[12] These words are labels summarizing complex experiences that have subjective, somatic, autonomic, and affective dimensions. The subjective experience of emotions is mediated primarily by limbic system structures (Figure 9.7), whereas perception and interpretation of emotional signals are mediated primarily by right posterior hemispheric cortical structures and emotional expression is mediated primarily through right anterior cortical structures and the basal ganglia. Mood refers to happiness, sadness, irritability, lability (rapid shifts in mood), and possibly anxiety.

While substantial studies have been devoted to neuropsychiatric and behavioral abnormalities in patients with dementia syndromes (Chapters 3–8) relatively little attention has been given to the assessment of normal emotions. Patients with Alzheimer's disease evidence a reduction of emotional intensity of many normal emotions and have diminished inflection in their spontaneous speech. Patients with clinical syndromes of frontotemporal lobar degeneration (Chapter 7) often have dramatic changes in goals and values, reflecting fundamental alterations in their emotional processing and assignment of emotional valence to specific life objectives and behaviors.[13] Patients with Parkinson's disease and other parkinsonian syndromes have diminished facial expression and vocal inflection giving rise to a subdued repertoire of overt emotional responses.

The linkages between psychopathology and abnormalities of normal emotional function remain to be worked out in detail. Models of potential relationships between normal CNS function and psychopathology are provided below for apathy, depression, psychosis, and agitation.

The limbic system includes both cortical and subcortical structures integrated into a functionally related circuitry involved in emotional processing of sensory stimuli. Cortical regions included in the limbic

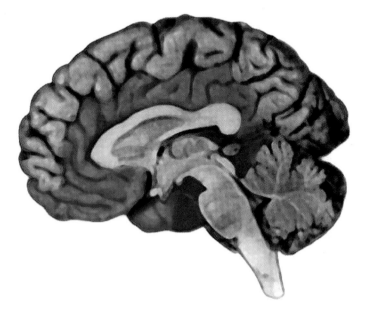

Figure 9.7 *Key elements of the limbic system (blue).*

system include the hippocampal formation and dentate gyrus, anterior hippocampal gyrus, cingulate gyrus, subcallosal (genu) cortical regions, temporal pole, insula, and posterior orbitofrontal cortex[14,15] (Figure 9.7). Subcortical structures involved in the limbic system include the amygdala, septal area, and substantia innominata.[15]

The nucleus basilis of Mynert is included in the septal nuclei and is involved in all dementia syndromes with a cholinergic disturbance (reflecting involvement of cholinergic neurons). Alzheimer's disease, dementia with Lewy bodies, and Parkinson's disease with dementia all involve the nucleus basilis and have a disconnection between the limbic system and the neocortex. Thus, neocortical structures are deprived of critical input from limbic system regions when the nucleus basilis and cholinergic system is affected. A limbic/cortical disconnection syndrome is created by the atrophy of nucleus basilis.

Frontal-subcortical circuits

Five frontal-subcortical circuits linking frontal lobe regions to subcortical structures and back to frontal lobe areas have been described[16–18] (Figure 9.8). Five frontal-subcortical circuits are recognized: one mediating volitional control of eye movements, one involved with volitional action

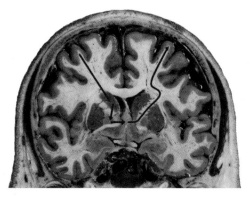

Figure 9.8 *Anatomy of frontal-subcortical circuits (afferents to thalamus are shown on the left, efferents from thalamus are shown on the right).*

and motor system control, a dorsolateral prefrontal circuit mediating executive function, an anterior cingulate-subcortical circuit mediating motivation, and an orbitofrontal-subcortical circuit mediating social–interpersonal behaviors. Each of the circuits begins in a separate defined area of the frontal cortex, which project to defined areas within the striatum (caudate nucleus, putamen, or nucleus accumbens); these in turn project to defined areas of substantia nigra or globus pallidus; these structures project to discrete thalamic nuclei; and thalamic neurons project back to frontal cortical regions. In each case a direct pathway connects striatum to globus pallidus interna, while an indirect pathway projects from striatum to globus pallidus externa thence to subthalamic nucleus and to globus pallidus interna. The direct and indirect pathways create a dynamic balance between inhibitory and excitatory input to globus pallidus interna which in turn either stimulates or inhibits thalamic nuclei.[17] This dynamic balance determines the appropriate output from thalamus to cortex and creates the circumstance for disease-related abnormalities of thalamo-cortical connections. Abnormalities of frontal-subcortical circuits have been identified or inferred in a variety of behavioral disturbances including apathy, disinhibition, depression, obsessive-compulsive disorder, addictions, attention deficit hyperactivity disorder, and schizophrenia.[2,18,19] Figure 9.9 demonstrates the anatomical relationships of the three behaviorally relevant frontal-subcortical circuits mediating executive function, motivation, and civil behavior.

Frontal-subcortical circuitry is vulnerable to a variety of types of pathology (Figure 9.10). Abnormalities of tau metabolism disproportionately affect frontal-subcortical circuits and produce frontal-subcortical circuit disorders. Tau abnormalities involve the frontal lobe and to a lesser extent the basal ganglia in the frontotemporal lobar degenerations. Tau abnormalities involve the basal ganglia in corticobasal degeneration and the Guamanian amyotrophic lateral sclerosis-parkinsonism dementia complex. Tau disturbances are evident in the diencephalic nuclei in progressive supranuclear palsy and in the globus pallidus and brain stem structures in pallido-pontonigral degeneration. Alpha-synuclein disorders also affect frontal-subcortical circuits, particularly brain stem and basal ganglia structures in Parkinson's disease, dementia with Lewy

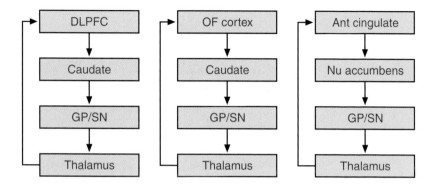

Figure 9.9 *Three behaviorally relevant frontal-subcortical circuits. The dorsolateral prefrontal-subcortical circuit mediates executive function. The orbitofrontal-subcortical circuit mediates socially appropriate behavior and the anterior cingulate-subcortical circuit mediates motivation. DLPFC, dorsolateral prefrontal cortex; GP, globus pallidus; SN, substantia nigra; Nu accumbens, nucleus accumbens; Ant cingulate, anterior cingulate; OF, orbitofrontal.*

bodies, neurodegenerations with iron accumulation, and the multiple system atrophies (Box 9.1). Patients with vascular dementia have prominent frontal-subcortical system dysfunction. Binswanger's disease produces ischemic demyelination of projections from frontal lobe to caudate nuclei and from the thalamus to the frontal lobe. In addition, lacunar infarctions in vascular dementia may involve the caudate, putamen, or thalamus. Creutzfeldt-Jakob disease and related prion disorders may involve frontal-subcortical structures at cortical, basal ganglia, or thalamic levels. White matter disorders such as multiple sclerosis and leukoencephalopathies produce demyelination of white matter tracks and may disconnect dorso-lateral prefrontal regions from subcortical nuclei, producing frontal-subcortical disorders (Figure 9.10).

Executive disturbances are the cognitive markers of involvement of frontal-subcortical circuits. Executive abnormalities are evident in difficulties with set shifting, abstraction, planning, judgment, behavioral inhibition, and motor programming (Chapter 2). The typical memory disturbance evident in patients with frontal-subcortical circuit abnormalities is a retrieval deficit syndrome with poor recall and relatively preserved recognition. If the thalamus is involved, typical executive

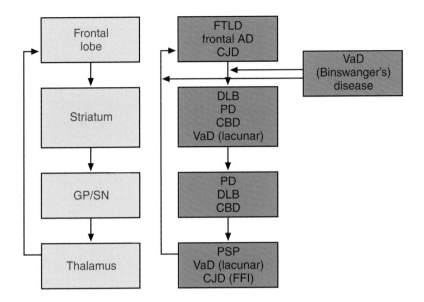

Figure 9.10 *Regional involvement of frontal-subcortical circuits by dementia syndromes. FTLD, frontotemporal lobar degeneration; AD, Alzheimer's disease; CJD, Creutzfeldt-Jakob disease; VaD, vascular dementia; DLB, dementia with Lewy bodies; PD, Parkinson's disease; CBD, corticobasal degeneration; PSP, progressive supranuclear palsy; FFI, fatal familial insomnia; GP/SN, globus pallidus/substantia.*

abnormalities co-exist with a true amnestic disorder with poor recall and poor recognition.[18] Executive disturbances are the hallmark of subcortical dementia.[20] Alzheimer's disease is the typical cortical dementia and involves primarily posterior cortical structures producing amnesia, aphasia, and visuospatial disturbances.[20] Dementia with Lewy bodies shares features of both posterior cortical and frontal-subcortical dysfunction.

Pathophysiology of major neuropsychiatric syndromes in dementia

The precise pathophysiology of neuropsychiatric symptoms occurring in dementing disorders remains to be delineated in detail. However, converging observations suggest preliminary models that can guide hypothesis-driven research directed at revealing the pathophysiology of these syndromes. Models of the potential pathophysiological underpinnings of apathy, depression, psychosis, and agitation are described here.

Apathy

Apathy is a common neuropsychiatric syndrome in patients with dementia. Studies with the Neuropsychiatric Inventory (NPI)[21] show that apathy is present in up to 70% of patients with Alzheimer's disease; 90% of those with frontotemporal dementia, dementia with Lewy bodies, and progressive supranuclear palsy; 40% of those with corticobasal degeneration; and 20% of those with Parkinson's disease[22-27] (Figure 9.11). There are many factors potentially contributing to apathetic behavior (Figure 9.12). Parietal disorders present in Alzheimer's disease, corticobasal degeneration, and dementia with Lewy bodies may contribute to lack of concern and denial of abnormalities. Neocortical involvement present in Alzheimer's disease, dementia with Lewy bodies, and frontotemporal lobar degeneration produces impaired cognition that may affect engagement with intellectual challenges. Placidity is a common behavior observed in patients with bilateral medial temporal lobe disorders exhibiting the Kluver-Bucy syndrome. Dysfunction of the dorsolateral prefrontal cortex may lead to loss of engagement with the environment and apathetic behavior. Impaired emotional memory associated with medial temporal lobe involvement may cause lack of recognition of the emotional importance of environmental events and lead to apathetic behavior. Limbic system dysfunction may cause decreased emotional engagement with environmental stimuli and subsequent apathy. Right hemisphere dysfunction may cause an inability to process emotional stimuli and loss of motivated behavior. The most neurobiologically

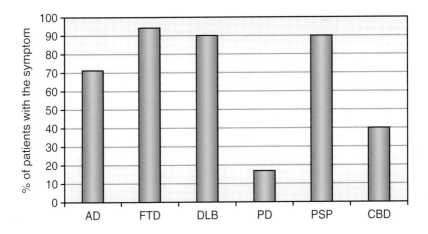

Figure 9.11 *Percent of patients exhibiting apathy. AD, Alzheimer's disease; FTD, frontotemporal dementia; DLB, dementia with Lewy bodies; PD, Parkinson's disease; CBD, corticobasal degeneration; PSP, progressive supranuclear palsy. (Figure derived from the Neuropsychiatric Inventory; references in text.)*

salient abnormalities related to apathy appear to be diminished motivation secondary to involvement of anterior cingulate and related subcortical structures. Studies with single photon emission tomography and positron emission tomography reveal diminished cerebral blood flow in the anterior cingulate regions in patients with Alzheimer's disease and prominent apathy.[28,29] Other syndromes with prominent apathy have histological involvement of frontal lobes and related subcortical structures (frontotemporal lobar degeneration, dementia with Lewy bodies, progressive supranuclear palsy). Focal lesions of this anterior cingulate region also reduce motivational behavior.

Apathy is a multi-dimensional construct that involves lack of motivation, diminished engagement with intellectual material, reduced interest in activities that provided pleasure and stimulation in the past, reduced affective expression of emotion, and reduced motor activity. Involvement of different cortical and subcortical structures may lead to apathetic syndromes comprised of differing elements. Figure 9.12 presents a summary of components contributing to apathy in dementing disorders.

Apathy has an ameliorating influence on some other behaviors that may

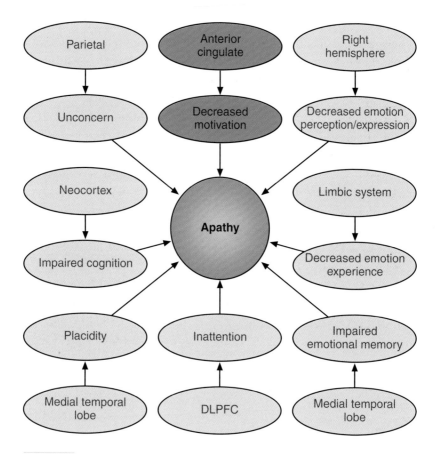

Figure 9.12 *A model of central nervous system dysfunction contributing to the clinical syndrome of apathy. DLPFC, dorsolateral prefrontal cortex.*

co-occur in patients with dementia syndromes. Patients with prominent apathy tend to exhibit less severe forms of disinhibition and agitation.[24]

Depression

Depression is common in patients with dementia syndromes. In many cases patients do not meet criteria for a major depressive episode but have symptoms similar to those for the criteria presented for depression in Alzheimer's disease discussed in Chapter 3. Depression has been identified in 35–50% of patients with Alzheimer's disease, frontotemporal lobar degeneration, dementia with Lewy bodies, and Parkinson's disease.[22–24,27] Depression is less common in progressive supranuclear palsy and more common in patients with corticobasal degeneration[25,26] (Figure 9.13).

Like apathy, depression is a multi-dimensional syndrome with emotional, cognitive, neurovegetative, endocrine, motivational, and psychomotor aspects (Figure 9.14). A model of central nervous system mediation of depression needs to account for these diverse aspects of the depression syndrome. Limbic system dysfunction contributes to disturbances of pleasure, happiness, and sense of achievement. Involvement of the dorsolateral prefrontal cortex and an inability to generate new ideas may contribute to the sense of helplessness and worthlessness. Neurovegetative disturbances result from dysfunction of the hypothalamus (abnormalities of sleep, appetite, and sexual desire) and psychomotor retardation reflects involvement of basal ganglia. Hypothalamic abnormalities may also contribute to endocrine disturbances such as changes in the dexamethasone suppression test. Anterior cingulate involvement results in decreased motivation, which may be prominent

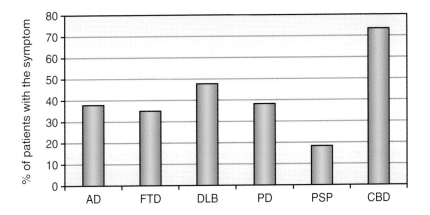

Figure 9.13 *Percent of patients with degenerative dementias exhibiting depressive symptoms. AD, Alzheimer's disease; FTD, frontotemporal dementia; DLB, dementia with Lewy bodies; PD, Parkinson's disease; CBD, corticobasal degeneration; PSP, progressive supranuclear palsy. (Percentages derived from the Neuropsychiatric Inventory; references in text.)*

in some patients with depression.[30] Dysfunction of the nucleus accumbens may contribute to a diminished sense of reward from usually pleasurable activities. Right hemisphere involvement and an inability to correctly interpret facial and vocal expressions may contribute importantly to a sense of loneliness and isolation.

Transmitter disturbances have been implicated in the mediation of depression, particularly given the effectiveness of antidepressant agents

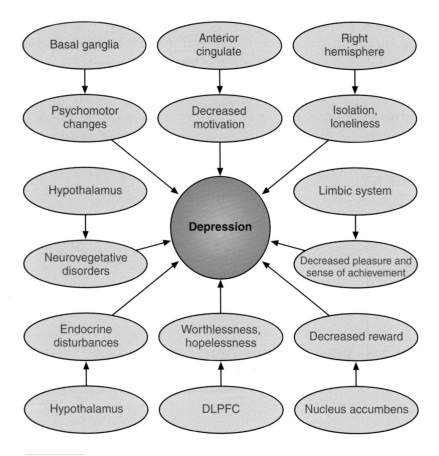

Figure 9.14 *Model of pathophysiology of depression with regional central nervous system dysfunction contributing component symptoms. DLPFC, dorsolateral prefrontal cortex.*

in relieving depressive symptoms. Serotonergic and noradrenergic projections from brain stem nuclei have diffuse cortical and subcortical targets and may mediate features of the depression syndrome. In addition, depression is prominent in disorders with dopaminergic abnormalities and dopamine disturbances may contribute importantly to the depression syndrome.

Psychosis

Psychosis is a more uncommon phenomenon in dementing disorders than apathy, depression, or agitation. In studies with the NPI it has been identified in approximately 20% of patients with Alzheimer's disease and 30% of those with Parkinson's disease and dementia. It is less common in corticobasal degeneration, progressive supranuclear palsy or frontotemporal dementia. It is particularly frequent as a manifestation of dementia with Lewy bodies.[22–27] Figure 9.15 shows the prevalence of delusions in patients with these degenerative dementing disorders. Psychosis in patients with dementia is commonly manifested by a combination of delusions and hallucinations. Delusions are more common than

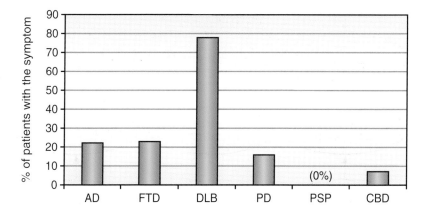

Figure 9.15 *Percent of patients with degenerative disorders exhibiting psychosis. AD, Alzheimer's disease; FTD, frontotemporal dementia; DLB, dementia with Lewy bodies; PD, Parkinson's disease; CBD, corticobasal degeneration; PSP, progressive supranuclear palsy. (Percentages derived from the Neuropsychiatric Inventory; references in text.)*

hallucinations in all syndromes except dementia with Lewy bodies. In most cases hallucinations are endorsed as veridical externally originating phenomena and thus entail a delusional component. Although delusions are relatively uncommon in Alzheimer's disease, the high frequency of this disorder in the elderly (approximately 4 million cases within the United States) places this disorder as the second most common cause of psychosis in the population following schizophrenia. Thus, degenerative dementias must be seen as common causes of major mental illnesses in addition to being common etiologies for progressive late-life cognitive disorders.

There are many competing theories regarding the pathophysiology of delusions. Some authors favor cognitive constructs, whereas others favor noncognitive explanations involving dysfunction of the limbic system. A limbic system-based model for delusions is presented in Figure 9.16. In this model, limbic dysfunction is posited to contribute to an abnormal perception of threat in the environment. The limbic system is normally responsible for the experience of fear and discovery of threat in the environment, a function critical for organismic survival. When limbic

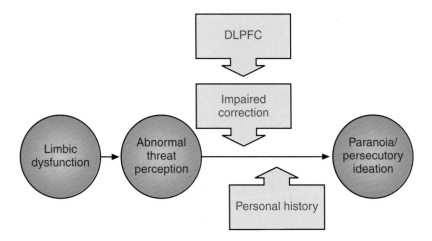

Figure 9.16 *Model for the production of delusions with paranoid and persecutory ideation reflecting limbic system dysfunction, abnormal threat perception, and failure to correct the accuracy of perceptions because of cognitive dysfunction. DLPFC, dorsolateral prefrontal cortex.*

system dysfunction (common in the dementias) occurs, threat may be perceived where none exists. This abnormal perception of threat would not be challenged or corrected because of the associated cognitive and judgment deficits. The social, cultural, and individual history of the individual would contribute to the specific delusional content assigned to the abnormal threat perception. Thus, delusions of infidelity, theft, persecution, identity change, or abandonment would all reflect the experience of the specific individual exhibiting the delusional disorder. Clinically, this interaction of personal history, abnormal limbic system function, and impaired cognition would manifest as a delusional disorder.

Agitation

Agitation is a common disorder in patients with dementia syndromes (Figure 9.17). It is particularly common in Alzheimer's disease where it becomes more frequent and more severe with advancing cognitive decline.[27] It is not uncommon in patients with frontotemporal lobar degeneration, dementia with Lewy bodies, Parkinson's disease (particularly those with dementia), and corticobasal degeneration.[22–24,26] The co-occurrence of apathy does not eliminate the occurrence of agitation and

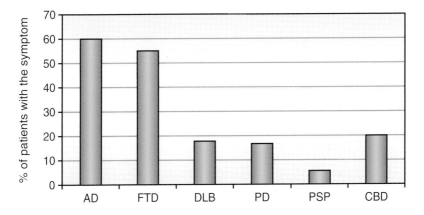

Figure 9.17 *Percent of patients with degenerative disorders exhibiting agitation. AD, Alzheimer's disease; FTD, frontotemporal dementia; DLB, dementia with Lewy bodies; PD, Parkinson's disease; CBD, corticobasal degeneration; PSP, progressive supranuclear palsy. (Percentages derived from the Neuropsychiatric Inventory; references in text.)*

both syndromes may occur in the same patient. However, severe apathy tends to ameliorate the frequency or severity of agitation.

Agitation is most common in patients with the frontal variant of Alzheimer's disease or in patients with frontotemporal lobar degeneration.[11,24] Figure 9.18 provides a model of the pathophysiology of agitation that includes both intrinsic central nervous system factors and environmental provocations. Agitation is not a syndrome that occurs on its own; it is accompanied by other comorbid psychopathology such as psychosis, depression, anxiety, irritability, or disinhibition. In addition, agitation in patients with dementia may be provoked by environmental circumstances such as an overstimulating environment, an aggressive room-mate, adverse interactions with a caregiver, pain, or physical distress. We hypothesize that when psychopathology is present or an environmental provocation occurs, patients with frontal dysfunction have an inappropriate unmodulated behavioral response recognized clinically as agitation. Agitation is manifested as physical aggression, verbal aggression, and active resistance to care. This model provides the basis for understanding the diverse pharmacologic and environmental interventions that may impact agitation (Chapter 10).

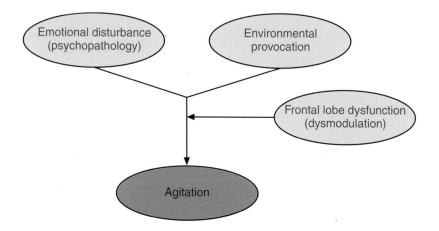

Figure 9.18 *Model of agitation with emotional disturbances or environmental provocations leading to agitation reflecting abnormal modulation of emotional responses secondary to frontal lobe dysfunction.*

References

1. Heilman K. The neurobiology of emotional experience. In: Salloway S, Malloy P, Cummings J (eds) *The Neuropsychiatry of Limbic and Subcortical Disorders*. Washington, DC: American Psychiatric Press, 1997: 133–42.
2. Mega MS, Cummings JL. Frontal subcortical circuits. anatomy and function. In: Salloway SP, Malloy PF, Duffy JD (eds) *The Frontal Lobes and Neuropsychiatric Illness*. Washington, DC/London: American Psychiatric, 2001.
3. Prusiner SB. Shattuck lecture – neurodegenerative diseases and prions. *N Engl J Med* 2001;344:1516–26.
4. Giasson BI, Wilson CA, Trojanowski JQ et al. Tau and α-synuclein in neurodegenerative diseases. In: Chesselet M-F (ed) *Contemporary Clinical Neuroscience: Molecular Mechanisms of Neurodegenerative Diseases*. Totowa, NJ: Humana Press, 2001: 151–76.
5. Hong M, Trojanowski JQ, Lee VM-Y. Tau-based neurofibrillary lesions. In: Clark CM, Trojanowski JQ (eds) *Neurodegenerative Dementias: Clinical Features and Pathological Mechanisms*. New York: McGraw-Hill, 2000: 161–75.
6. McKhann G, Albert M, Grossman M et al. Clinical and pathological diagnosis of frontotemporal dementia. *Arch Neurol* 2001;58:1803–9.
7. Perl DP. Amyotrophic lateral sclerosis-parkinsonism-dementia complex of Guam. In: Markesbery WR (ed) *Neuropathology of Dementing Disorders*. New York: Arnold, 1998: 268–92.
8. Galvin J, Lee VM-Y, Trojanowski JQ. Synucleinopathies: clinical and pathological implications. *Arch Neurol* 2001;58:186–90.
9. Farber NB, Rubin EH, Newcomer JW et al. Increased neocortical neurofibrillary tangle density in subjects with Alzheimer disease and psychosis. *Arch Gen Psychiatry* 2000;57:1165–73.
10. Johnson JK, Head E, Kim R et al. Clinical and pathological evidence for a frontal variant of Alzheimer's disease. *Arch Neurol* 1999;56:1233–9.
11. Tekin S, Mega MS, Masterman DL et al. Orbitofrontal and anterior cingulate cortex: neurofibrillary tangle burden is associated with agitation in Alzheimer's disease. *Ann Neurol* 2001;49:355–61.
12. Ekman P. All emotions are basic. In: Ekman P, Davidson RJ (eds) *The Nature of Emotion*. New York: Oxford University Press, 1994: 15–19.
13. Miller BL, Seeley WW, Mychack P et al. Neuroanatomy of the self: evidence from patients with frontotemporal dementia. *Neurology* 2001;57:817–21.
14. Carpenter MB. *Core Text of Neuroanatomy*, 4th edn. Baltimore: Williams and Wilkins, 1991.
15. Mesulam M-M. Behavioral neuroanatomy: large-scale networks, association cortex, frontal syndromes, the limbic system, and hemispheric specializations. In: Mesulam M-M (ed) *Principles of Behavioral and Cognitive Neurology*. New York: Oxford University Press, 2000: 1–120.
16. Alexander GE, DeLong MR, Strick PL. Parallel organization of functionally segregated circuits linking basal ganglia and cortex. *Annu Rev Neurosci* 1986;9:357–81.
17. Alexander GE, Crutcher MD. Functional architecture of basal ganglia circuits: neural substrates of parallel processing. *Trends Neurosci* 1990;13:260–76.

18. Lichter DG, Cummings JL. Introduction and Overview. In: Lichter DG, Cummings JL (eds) *Frontal-Subcortial Circuits in Psychiatric and Neurological Disorders*. New York: The Guilford Press, 2001: 1–43.

19. Cummings JL. Frontal-subcortical circuits and human behavior. *Arch Neurol* 1993;50:873–80.

20. Cummings JL, Benson DF. *Dementia: A Clinical Approach*, 2nd edn. Boston: Butterworth-Heinemann; 1992.

21. Cummings JL, Mega M, Gray K *et al.* The Neuropsychiatric Inventory: comprehensive assessment of psychopathology in dementia. *Neurology* 1994; 44:2308–14.

22. Aarsland D, Larsen JP, Lim NG *et al.* Range of neuropsychiatric disturbances in patients with Parkinson's disease. *J Neurol Neurosurg Psychiatry* 1999;67:492–6.

23. Hirono N, Mori E, Tanimukai S *et al.* Distinctive neurobehavioral features among neurodegenerative dementias. *J Neuropsychiatry Clin Neurosci* 1999;11:498–503.

24. Levy ML, Miller BL, Cummings JL *et al.* Alzheimer disease and frontotemporal dementias: behavioral distinctions. *Arch Neurol* 1996;53:687–90.

25. Litvan I, Mega MS, Cummings JL *et al.* Neuropsychiatric aspects of progressive supranuclear palsy. *Neurology* 1996;47:1184–9.

26. Litvan I, Cummings JL, Mega M. Neuropsychiatric features of corticobasal degeneration. *J Neurol Neurosurg Psychiatry* 1998;65:717–21.

27. Mega MS, Cummings JL, Fiorello T *et al.* The spectrum of behavioral changes in Alzheimer's disease. *Neurology* 1996;46:130–5.

28. Craig AH, Cummings JL, Fairbanks L *et al.* Cerebral blood flow correlates of apathy in Alzheimer's disease. *Arch Neurol* 1996;53:1116–20.

29. Migneco O, Benoit M, Koulibaly PM *et al.* Perfusion brain SPECT and statistical parametric mapping analysis indicate that apathy is a cingulate syndrome: a study of Alzheimer's disease and non-demented patients. *Neuroimage* 2001;13:896–902.

30. Cummings JL. The neuroanatomy of depression. *J Clin Psychiatry* 1993;54: 14–20.

chapter 10

Management of neuropsychiatric aspects of dementia

Treatment of neuropsychiatric symptoms in Alzheimer's disease (AD) and other dementias provides an opportunity to reduce the distress experienced by the patient in association with these symptoms, reduce the distress experienced by caregivers as a result of behavioral disturbances in the family member for whom they are caring, improve the quality of life of the patient and caregiver, and reduce the risk of institutionalization. Treatment of behavioral disturbances also may improve functional ability, decrease dependency, and facilitate the use of cognitive resources by the dementia patient. In previous chapters, the specific treatments of each disease have been considered. In this chapter, working with caregivers, nonpharmacologic interventions for behavioral disorders, and general principles of pharmacologic management of individuals with dementia-associated neuropsychiatric symptoms are presented. Developing an alliance with caregivers is described first since caregivers are the ones most likely to employ nonpharmacologic management strategies and to supervise pharmacologic interventions.

Caregivers

More than 70% of all dementia patients are cared for at home by family caregivers, usually spouses.[1] Family caregivers often provide supervised care to dementia patients, 24 hours per day. They are responsible for ensuring that the patient eats, bathes, sleeps, does not wander, and is not exposed to harmful circumstances. Caregiving is often associated with a sense of being captive, burdened, and distressed. Burden refers to the physical, psychological or emotional, social, and financial problems that affect family members caring for impaired older adults.[2] Caregivers manifest psychological symptoms, particularly depression and anxiety, and may have more physical illness than non-caregiving older adults.[1,3,4]

Neuropsychiatric symptoms contribute importantly to the distress experienced by caregivers and the ensuing decrease in the quality of life (Figure 10.1). Agitated behaviors have been linked to caregiver depression[5,6] and caregivers rank behavioral disturbances among the most distressing issues that arise while caring for persons with dementia.[7,8] Troublesome behaviors contribute to the decision to institutionalize individuals with dementia[9] and agitated patients who are aggressive towards caregivers are also more likely to be abused by caregivers.[9] The absence of the usual affection and emotional engagement from patients towards caregivers is also a source of distress.[5,6]

The Neuropsychiatric Inventory (NPI)[10] measures the distress experienced by the caregiver associated with each of the behavioral domains

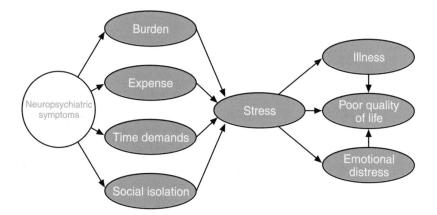

Figure 10.1 Model showing how neuropsychiatric symptoms lead to burden, expense, time demands, and social isolation for caregivers; these produce stress and its consequences including physical illness, emotional distress, and reduced quality of life.

assessed by the instrument. Figure 10.2 shows that many behaviors are associated with at least moderate levels of distress as reported by caregivers.[11]

A variety of interventions have been shown to be helpful in decreasing the burden experienced by family caregivers. Educational programs decrease depression and delay nursing home placement.[12,13] Family counseling to increase family support of the caregiver and decrease family disagreements also reduces the burden experienced by family caregivers.[14] Comprehensive home-based case management focusing on support of caregivers diminishes anxiety and depression.[15] Some caregivers may experience depression, anxiety, or substance use disorders of sufficient severity to warrant individual therapy or psychopharmacologic intervention. Assessing the physical and mental health of the caregiver is an essential aspect of providing care to dementia patients. Referral to community resources such as the local chapter of the Alzheimer's Association or Alzheimer's Disease International allies the caregiver with those

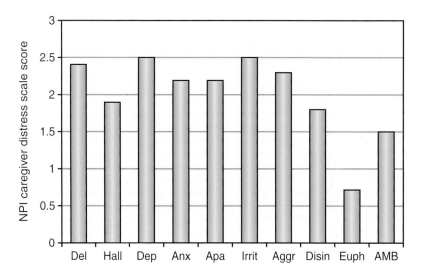

Figure 10.2 *Caregiver distress scores from the Neuropsychiatric Inventory (NPI). The highest possible distress score for each domain is 5.[11] Del, delusions; Hall, hallucinations; Dep, depression; Anx, anxiety; Apa, apathy; Irrit, irritability; Aggr, aggression/agitation; Disin, disinhibition; Euph, euphoria; AMB, aberrant motor behavior.*

providing caregiver support and knowledge about community resources. Caregivers must be reassessed periodically as burden and distress change in concert with advancing dementia in the patient.

Nonpharmacologic interventions

Pharmacologic interventions should be used for treatment of behavioral disturbances in dementia patients only when nonpharmacologic treatments are not feasible or have failed. In many cases, nonpharmacologic management can be used in conjunction with pharmacotherapy to amplify the results and minimize the required doses. Nonpharmacologic management strategies are based largely on changing caregiver behavior or restructuring the environment in a variety of ways to decrease problematic behaviors. Psychotherapeutic interventions for the patient are often limited by memory and cognitive disturbances. Changing caregiver behavior is itself a challenging proposition and may at least temporarily add to the burden experienced by caregiving family members. The clinician must be aware of the increased stress for the caregiver that may accompany nonpharmacologic treatment strategies.

A useful approach to helping caregivers reduce problem behaviors in patients is to teach them the four 'Rs': Reassure, Reorient, Remind, and Redirect. Reassurance is helpful in diffusing confrontation and helping the patient know that he/she is in a supportive, affectionate environment. Reorienting allows the patient to know where he/she is and in what task he/she is engaged. Reminding the patient reacquaints them with what will happen in the immediate future and what they are to do in each circumstance. Redirecting diminishes problematic behaviors by distracting the patient's attention from a frustrating and anger-producing circumstance to one with a more benign emotional content. Thus, the patient who is aggressively resisting bathing or other daily tasks may be redirected to working in the yard, looking at family pictures, or taking a ride. The desired activity can be returned to later in the day when it may more acceptable.

A variety of potential nonpharmacologic interventions have been recommended for use with patients with dementia and behavioral disturbances.[16,17] These include changes in the physical environment, patient-related activities, family caregiver activities, and professional caregiver educational programs. Music, simulated sounds of nature, bright lights, and creation of a homelike setting in institutions have all been recommended as means of diminishing behavioral disturbances in patients with more advanced dementia. Walking, cognitive remediation activities, simulated presence with videos or audio tapes of a family member, massage, pet therapy, and participation in adult day-care activities are all designed to involve patients in activities and redirect them from problematic behaviors.

Support groups, educational programs, family counseling, respite care, telephone helplines, and computer chat rooms may all be of benefit to family caregivers. Professional caregivers require education about AD, dementias, and behavioral disturbances associated with these brain disorders. They also require assistance in recognizing neuropsychiatric symptoms in patients with dementia. Depression is particularly likely to go undetected. Professional caregivers (e.g. nurses, nursing assistants, aides, and social workers) require education about recognition of neuropsychiatric symptoms, the use of medications, and how best to survey patients for the appearance of side effects. Box 10.1 summarizes common nonpharmacologic interventions that are useful in diminishing behavioral changes in patients with dementia.

Many caregivers (both family and professional) regard neuropsychiatric symptoms as reactive or intentional and under the patient's voluntary control. Caregivers require education concerning the brain-based nature of neuropsychiatric symptoms in dementia syndromes and the concomitant decrease in coping and adapting skills caused by the brain disorder (Figure 10.3). These educational strategies assist the caregivers in avoiding blaming the patients for the presence of behavioral disturbances.

Pharmacologic management

Pharmacologic strategies that are useful in dementias address the underlying disease process, any comorbid medical conditions that require

Box 10.1 Nonpharmacologic interventions used to diminish behavioral disturbances in patients with dementia

Physical environment
• Music
• Simulated sounds of nature
• Bright lights
• Homelike setting in institution
• White noise
• Wandering areas

Patient activities
• Walking
• Cognitive remediation activities
• Adult day-care
• Simulated presence
• Massage
• Pet therapy
• Reminiscence
• Exercise
• Touch
• Sensory stimulation

Patient treatment
• One-on-one interaction
• Behavior therapy
• Cognitive therapy
• Structured activities
• Pain management
• Hearing aids
• Classes

Caregiver activities
• Support groups
• Educational programs
• Family counseling
• Respite care
• Telephone helpline
• Computer chat room

Professional caregivers' activities
• Education about behavior management
• Education about neuropsychiatric symptom recognition
• Education about drugs and side effects

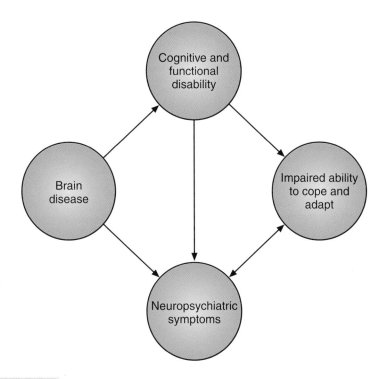

Figure 10.3 *Brain diseases produce neuropsychiatric symptoms, cognition deficits, and loss of functional ability. Cognition and functional loss exacerbate behavioral disturbances. Brain dysfunction also reduces the patient's ability to cope and adjust.*

therapy (e.g. hypertension, cardiac disease, gastrointestinal illnesses), and treatment of behavioral disturbances that fail to respond or respond inadequately to nonpharmacologic interventions. Medications may also be used in the management of associated consequences of dementing disorders including parkinsonism, incontinence, and spasticity. The latter is particularly common in patients with upper motor neuron involvement such as those with vascular dementia (Chapter 6) or frontotemporal lobar degeneration with an accompanying amyotrophic lateral sclerosis-like disorder (Chapter 7). Treatment of parkinsonism is summarized in Chapter 5.

Treatment of the underlying dementing disorder may have behavioral ramifications. Treatment of AD with vitamin E and selegiline simultaneously decreases the emergence of behavioral disturbances (Chapter 3). Likewise, cholinesterase inhibitors have been shown to decrease existing behaviors and to ameliorate the emergence of new behaviors in patients with AD (Chapter 3). Cholinesterase inhibitors also reduce behavioral disturbances in patients with dementia with Lewy bodies (Chapter 4), patients with Parkinson's disease (Chapter 5) and patients with vascular dementia (Chapter 6). Management of vascular risk factors in patients with vascular dementia may diminish the risk of additional ischemic injury and any associated behavioral changes.

Comorbid medical conditions are common in elderly patients with AD and other dementias. A majority of aged patients with dementia have conditions requiring medical management in addition to treatment of their dementia syndrome. Medical illness is not correlated with behavioral disturbances as measured by the Neuropsychiatric Inventory,[18] but optimal management of medical illnesses and avoiding drug interactions will lessen the chance of delirium and delirium-associated behavioral changes.

Use of psychopharmacologic agents in elderly and demented individuals requires expertise. These agents have powerful effects in reducing behavioral disturbances and may have marked side effects. Box 10.2 introduces guidelines to be considered when administering medications to patients with dementia. An accurate diagnosis should be made for both the dementing disorder and any concurrent neuropsychiatric symptoms. A careful medication history should be taken including review of over-the-counter medications, nutraceuticals, and responses to previously administered agents. A specific behavioral target symptom is chosen and the response of this symptom to therapy is carefully monitored. Instructions (both verbal and written) should be provided to the patient and caregiver. Starting doses should be one-third to one-half those recommended for use in younger adults (Table 10.1). Dosage increments should be small, but dosage escalation should continue until an optimal response has been obtained or intolerable side effects emerge. Partial responses may be acceptable if complete amelioration of the neuropsychiatric symptom

Box 10.2 Guidelines for pharmacotherapy in dementia

- Establish an accurate diagnosis of the dementing disorder as well as any concurrent illnesses
- Minimize the use of medication and seek nonpharmacologic alternatives where possible
- Take a careful medication history including over-the-counter drugs and nutraceuticals
- Review the response to previous drug treatment
- Choose specific behavioral target symptoms for treatment, and carefully monitor the response to therapy
- Provide easily read and easily understood written, as well as verbal, instructions to both the patient and the caregiver
- Introduce pharmacotherapy at one-third to one-half the dose recommended for younger adults
- Optimize the total dose administered
- Accept partial responses if more complete target responses are associated with unacceptable side effects
- Know the pharmacology, side effect profile, and potential drug interactions of each agent administered to the patient
- Avoid multiple drug regimens whenever possible and monitor potential additive toxicity
- Use rational polypharmacy employing drugs with complementary actions when more than one agent is needed
- Review drug regimens frequently, discontinuing unnecessary medications and simplifying dosage schedules in concert with changes in the patient's condition
- Evaluate adherence to treatment instructions
- Obtain serum drug levels when they may help guide dosage decisions
- Monitor side effects regularly
- Do not avoid pharmacotherapy because of the age of the patient or the presence of a dementing disorder

cannot be achieved without unacceptable side effects. Partial responses may allow effective use of nonpharmacologic interventions. Avoid multiple drug regimens whenever possible and beware of potential additive toxicity or drug interactions. Know the side effect profile and drug

Table 10.1 Psychotropic agents used to treat neuropsychiatric symptoms in patients with dementia

Symptom	Agent (commercial name)	Usual dose	Range
Agitation/aggression	Risperidone (Risperdal)	1 mg	0.5–2 mg
	Olanzapine (Zyprexa)	5 mg	5–10 mg
	Quetiapine (Seroquel)	300 mg	50–400 mg
	Haloperidol (Haldol)	2 mg	0.5–3 mg
	Carbamazepine (Tegretol)	400 mg	200–1200 mg
	Divalproex (Depakote)	500 mg	250–3000 mg
	Trazodone (Desyrel)	100 mg	100–400 mg
	Buspirone (Buspar)	30 mg	15–45 mg
	Propranolol (Inderal)	120 mg	80–240 mg
	Lorazepam (Ativan)	1 mg	0.5–6 mg
Delusions	Risperidone (Risperdal)	1 mg	0.5–2 mg
	Olanzapine (Zyprexa)	5 mg	5–10 mg
	Quetiapine (Seroquel)	300 mg	50–400 mg
	Clozapine (Clozaril)	50 mg	12.5–100 mg
	Haloperidol (Haldol)	2 mg	0.5–3 mg
Depression	Fluoxetine (Prozac)	20 mg	20–40 mg
	Sertraline (Zoloft)	50 mg	50–200 mg
	Paroxetine (Paxil)	20 mg	10–50 mg
	Citalopram (Celexa)	20 mg	10–30 mg
	Venlafaxin (Effexor)	100 mg	50–300 mg

Table 10.1 *continued*

Symptom	Agent (commercial name)	Usual dose	Range
Anxiety	Nefazodone (Serzone)	400 mg	200–600 mg
	Mirtazepine (Remeron)	15 mg	7.5–30 mg
	Nortriptyline (Pamelor)	50 mg	50–100 mg
	Oxazepam (Serax)	30 mg	20–60 mg
	Lorazepam (Ativan)	1 mg	0.5–6 mg
	Buspirone (Buspar)	30 mg	15–45 mg
Apathy	Methylphenidate (Ritalin)	10 mg	10–30 mg
	Dextramphetamine (Dexedrine)	5 mg	5–20 mg
	Modafanil (Provigil)	200 mg	100–200 mg
Insomnia	Trazodone (Desyrel)	100 mg	50–200 mg
	Zolpidem (Ambien)	10 mg	5–10 mg
	Temazepam (Restoril)	15 mg	15–30 mg
	Zaloplon (Sonata)	10 mg	10 mg
Sexual aggression (males)	Leuprolide (Lupron)		
	subcutaneous	1 mg	—
	depot i.m.	7.5 mg/month	—
	Medroxyprogesterone		
	i.m.	150/3 month	(150 mg/1–3 months)
	p.o.	5 mg/day	(2.5–10 mg/day)

interaction potential of each agent administered to the patient. When polypharmacy is required, employ a rational strategy using drugs with complementary actions. When following the patient longitudinally, drug regimens should be reviewed frequently and unnecessary medications discontinued. Adherence to the medication regimen should also be evaluated, asking the caregiver about success in having the patient take their medication regularly and inspecting the amount of medication remaining in pill bottles as an indication of regularity of use. In some cases serum levels may be useful in monitoring treatment adherence and guiding doses. Side effects should be assessed regularly, particularly parkinsonism, tardive dyskinesia, and other disorders of the motor system. Pharmacotherapy should not be avoided simply because the patient is elderly or has a dementing disorder. Pharmacologic management should be combined with nonpharmacologic management strategies when possible.

The model of agitation presented in Chapter 9 (Figure 9.18) provides a basis for using a variety of types of interventions to modify agitation (Figure 10.4).

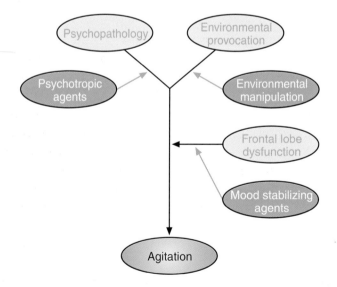

Figure 10.4 *Model showing the factors contributing to agitation (light orange) and their modification (dark orange).*

Treatment of specific neuropsychiatric symptoms

The usual doses as well as the dosage range of psychotropic agents used in dementia patients are presented in Table 10.1. No pharmacologic agent has been approved specifically for the management of behavioral disturbances in dementia, and treatment is guided by limited clinical trials and experience with non-demented individuals.

Agitation is the dementia symptom most often requiring treatment with pharmacologic agents. Data are available regarding treatment of agitation in AD with atypical antipsychotic agents (Chapter 3). It is currently assumed, although unproven, that these agents will be useful in other dementing illnesses as well. Conventional neuroleptics are efficacious but produce more side effects than atypical antipsychotic agents. Neuroleptic agents should be avoided in patients with dementia with Lewy bodies; these patients may experience a marked extrapyramidal syndrome when treated with conventional dopamine-blocking drugs. Anticonvulsant compounds have mood-stabilizing properties and have been used to ameliorate agitation in patients with AD and other dementias. They may be used as monotherapy or in conjunction with atypical antipsychotic agents. Carbamazepine and divalproex have been used most widely in this clinical setting. Newer anticonvulsants such as gabapentin, lamotrigine, and topiramate have been used in bipolar illness and have promising mood-stabilizing properties.[19] These agents may be found to have a role in treatment of agitation in patients with dementing disorders. Trazodone is useful in the treatment of agitation in some patients. It is a sedating agent and may be particularly helpful for treatment of night-time agitation. Buspirone is a nonbenzodiazepine anxiolytic agent that may be especially beneficial in the management of anxiety-related agitation. Propranolol, a beta-blocking agent, is helpful in some patients with aggressive behavior. Benzodiazepines, when used chronically, may produce disinhibition or confusion and exacerbate agitation. They may be useful in the management of acute and infrequent periods of agitation. Benzodiazepines that are well metabolized in the elderly, such as lorazepam or oxazepam, are the agents of choice in this setting. Figure 10.5 presents an algorithm for treatment of agitation in dementia.

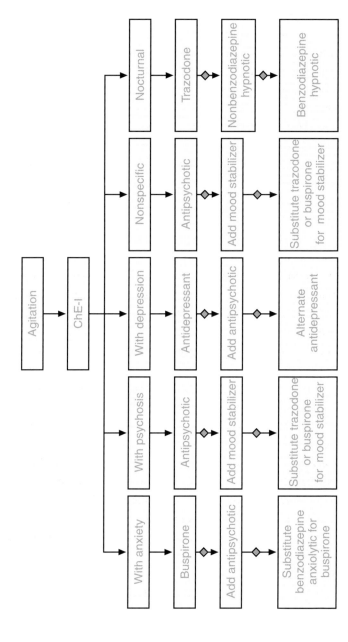

Figure 10.5 *Algorithm for treatment of agitation (cholinesterase inhibitors (ChE-I) would be used only in patients with dementias with cholinergic deficits). (♦ indicates next step if previous intervention is inadequate.)*

Delusions are treated with atypical antipsychotics or occasionally with conventional neuroleptic drugs. Psychosis occasionally responds to selective serotonin reuptake inhibitors.

Depression may be treated with selective serotonin reuptake inhibitors or with agents that have combined transmitter reuptake effects (venlafaxin, nefazodone, mirtazepine). If a tricyclic antidepressant is used, an agent with few anticholinergic side effects such as nortriptyline should be chosen. The presence of subcortical hyperintensities or lacunes reduces the responsiveness of patients to treatment of antidepressant agents and may increase the likelihood of drug-induced confusion (Chapter 6). Figure 10.6 presents an algorithm for treatment of depression in dementia.

Anxiety can be managed with benzodiazepines that are well metabolized in the elderly (oxazepam or lorazepam) or with a nonbenzodiazepine anxiolytic such as buspirone.

Apathy is occasionally sufficiently problematic to be treated with psychostimulants. Methylphenidate, dextroamphetamine, or modafinil may be used in this setting. Some antidepressants (desipramine, fluorxetine) have activating qualities and cholinesterase inhibitors also may reduce apathetic behaviors (Chapter 3).

Insomnia may be treated with sedating antidepressants such as trazodone, with nonbenzodiazepine sedative hypnotics such as zolpidem and zaloplon or with a medium duration benzodiazepine such as temazepam. Sedative hypnotics should be used in conjunction with sleep hygiene measures (Box 10.3) to minimize the dose and duration of use of these agents. Recommendations include maintaining regular bed times and rise times, using the bedroom only for sleep, establishing a quiet and comfortable sleep environment, avoiding the bed while awake, establishing regular meal times, avoiding stimulants and excessive fluid before retiring for bed, avoiding daytime naps, treating any pain symptoms, voiding before going to bed, seeking morning sunlight exposure, and engaging in regular daily exercise. Figure 10.7 provides an algorithm for pharmacologic management of insomnia.

Most sexual aggression in males may be diminished by the use of estrogenic agents (medroxyprogesterone) or antitestosterone agents (leuprolide).

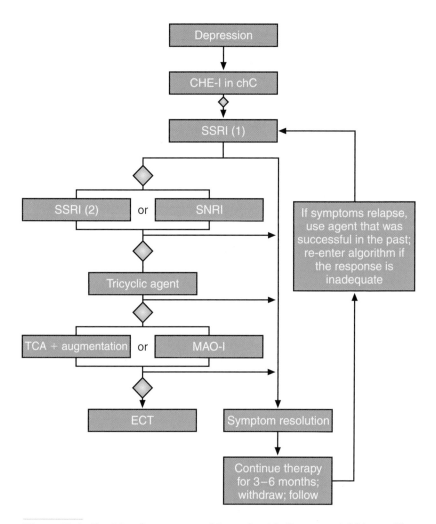

Figure 10.6 *Algorithm for treatment of depression (cholinesterase inhibitors will be used only in patients with dementia with cholinergic deficits). SSRI (1), 1st selective serotonin reuptake inhibitor; SSRI (2), alternate selective serotonin reuptake inhibitor; SNRI, serotonin and norepinephrine reuptake inhibitor; TCA, tricyclic agent; MAO-I, monoamine oxidase inhibitor; ECT, electroconvulsive therapy; AChE-I, acetyle/cholinesterase inhibitor. (↓ indicates next step if response to previous intervention is inadequate.)*

Box 10.3 Sleep hygiene measures to optimize night-time sleep, regularize diurnal behavior patterns, and minimize requirements for sedative-hypnotics

- Maintain regular bed times and rise times
- Use bedroom only for sleep
- Do not stay in bed while awake
- Establish regular meal times
- Avoid alcohol, caffeine, and nicotine
- Avoid excessive evening fluid intake
- Void before retiring to bed
- Avoid daytime naps
- Treat any pain symptoms
- If awakened, do not watch television
- Seek morning sunlight exposure
- Engage in regular daily exercise
- Establish a quiet, comfortable sleep environment
- If donepezil (cholinesterase inhibitor) is being administered, avoid night-time dosing
- Administer psychostimulants and selegiline no later than 6–8 hours before bed time
- Attempt to terminate use of sedative-hypnotics after a regular sleep pattern has been established

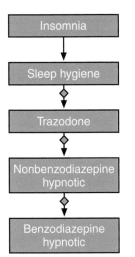

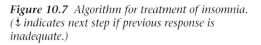

Figure 10.7 *Algorithm for treatment of insomnia. (⇃ indicates next step if previous response is inadequate.)*

Cholinesterase inhibitors are used in AD as well as other dementia syndromes with cholinergic deficits including dementia with Lewy bodies, Parkinson's disease with dementia, mixed AD and cerebrovascular disease, and vascular dementia (Chapters 3, 4, 5 and 6). The use of cholinesterase inhibitors is described in Chapter 3. These agents often have behavioral effects and should be instituted first in dementia patients with neuropsychiatric symptoms to determine the cognitive and behavioral benefits. In some cases, use of additional psychotherapeutic agents will be unnecessary. When behavioral changes are severe and urgent treatment is needed, a psychotropic drug should be administered prior to use of the cholinesterase inhibitor.

Pharmacoeconomic aspects of treatment

Effective management of neuropsychiatric symptoms may reduce caregiver burden and distress and improve quality of life of both patient and caregiver. Neuropsychiatric symptoms result in additional expense in patient care beyond that required for other dementia patients as a result of exaggerated caregiver stress, patient hospitalization, the expense of psychotropic medication, and the increased likelihood of residential placement. Some of the economic consequences of neuropsychiatric symptoms may be reduced through effective pharmacotherapy leading to reduced hospitalization, deferral of residential placement, and reduced caregiver stress (Figure 10.8).

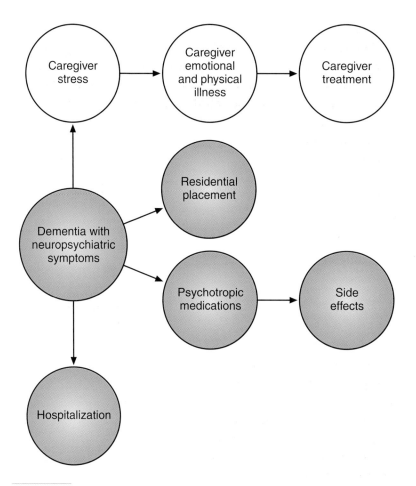

Figure 10.8 *Neuropsychiatric symptoms have many economic consequences including costs associated with caregiver stress, placement of patient in residential care, hospitalization, and psychotropic medications and their side effects.*

References

1. Buckwalter KC. Overview of psychological factors contributing to stress of family caregivers. In: Khachaturian ZS, Radebaugh TS (eds) *Alzheimer's Disease: Causes, Diagnosis, Treatment, and Care.* New York: CRC Press, 1996: 305–12.
2. George LK, Gwyther L. Caregiver well-being: a multidimensional examination of family caregivers of demented adults. *Gerontologist* 1986;26:253–9.

3. Connell CM, Janevic MR, Gallant MP. The costs of caring: impact of dementia on family caregivers. *J Geriatr Psychiatry Neurol* 2001:179–87.

4. Schulz R, O'Brien AT, Bookwala J *et al.* Psychiatric and physical morbidity effects of dementia caregiving: prevalence, correlates, and causes. *Gerontologist* 1995;35:771–91.

5. Pruchno RA, Resch NL. Aberrant behaviors and Alzheimer's disease: mental health effects on spouse caregivers. *J Gerontol* 1989;44:S177–S182.

6. Pruchno RA, Resch NL. Husbands and wives as caregivers: antecedents of depression and burden. *Gerontologist* 1989;29:159–65.

7. Greene JG, Smith R, Gardiner M *et al.* Measuring behavioural disturbance of elderly demented patients in the community and its effects on relatives: a factor analytic study. *Age Ageing* 1982;11:121–6.

8. Rabins PV, Mace NL, Lucas MJ. The impact of dementia on the family. *JAMA* 1982;248:333–5.

9. Coyne A, Reichman W, Berbig L. The relationship between dementia and elder abuse. *Am J Psychiatry* 1993;150:643–6.

10. Cummings JL, Mega M, Gray K *et al.* The Neuropsychiatric Inventory: comprehensive assessment of psychopathology in dementia. *Neurology* 1994; 44:2308–14.

11. Kaufer DI, Cummings JL, Christine D *et al.* Assessing the impact of neuropsychiatric symptoms in Alzheimer's disease: the Neuropsychiatric Inventory Caregiver Distress Scale. *J Am Geriatr Soc* 1998;46:210–15.

12. Kahan J, Kemp B, Staples FR *et al.* Decreasing the burden in families caring for a relative with a dementing illness. *J Am Geriatr Soc* 1985;33:664–70.

13. Mittelman M, Ferris S, Shulman E *et al.* A family intervention to delay nursing home placement of patients with Alzheimer's disease. *JAMA* 1996;276:1725–31.

14. Scott JP, Roberto KA, Hutton JT. Families of Alzheimer's victims: family support to the caregivers. *J Am Geriatr Soc* 1986;34:348–54.

15. Mohide EA, Pringle DM, Streiner DL *et al.* A randomized trial of family caregiver support in the home management of dementia. *J Am Geriatr Soc* 1990;38:446–54.

16. Doody RS, Stevens JC, Beck C *et al.* Practice parameter: management of dementia (an evidence-based review). Report of the Quality Standards Subcommittee of the American Academy of Neurology. *Neurology* 2001; 56:1154–66.

17. Cohen-Mansfield J. Nonpharmacological interventions for inappropriate behaviors in dementia: a review, summary, and critique. *Am J Geriatr Psychiatry* 2001;9:361–81.

18. Tekin S, Fairbanks LA, O'Connor S *et al.* Activities of daily living in Alzheimer's disease: neuropsychiatric, cognitive, and medical illness influences. *Am J Geriatr Psychiatry* 2001;9:81–6.

19. Brambilla P, Barale F, Soares JC. Perspectives on the use of anticonvulsants in the treatment of bipolar disorder. *Int J Neuropsychopharmacol* 2001;4:421–46.

Index